Dr. ORBISON

Univ. Tower
Queens Med Centre
Dept of Med.

Hypertension: Mechanisms, Diagnosis, and Treatment

Other Clinics Books Available

Hypertension: Mechanisms, Diagnosis, and Treatment

Gaddo Onesti, M.D., and
Albert N. Brest, M.D. | Editors

CARDIOVASCULAR CLINICS
Albert N. Brest, M.D. | Editor-in-Chief

 F. A. DAVIS COMPANY, PHILADELPHIA

Cardiovascular Clinics 9/1, Hypertension: Mechanisms, Diagnosis, and Treatment

Copyright © 1978 by F. A. Davis Company

Printed in the United States of America

Library of Congress Cataloging in Publication Data

Main entry under title:

Hypertension : mechanisms, diagnosis, and treatment.

(Cardiovascular clinics; 9/1)
Includes bibliographical references and index.
1. Hypertension. I. Onesti, Gaddo. II. Brest, Albert N. III. Series. [DNLM: 1. Hypertension—Drug therapy. 2. Hypertension—Diagnosis. W1 CA77N v. 9 no. 1 / WG340 H9952]
RC681.A1C27   vol. 9, no. 1 [RC685.H8] 616.1′008s
ISBN 0-8036-6630-6   [616.1′32]   77-25888

Editor's Commentary

The first issue of CARDIOVASCULAR CLINICS, published almost a decade ago, dealt with Hypertensive Cardiovascular Disease. Much new information has accumulated since then. From the physiologic standpoint, particular progress has been made in our understanding of the renin-angiotensin system. This has led to new classifications of primary and secondary hypertension and new diagnostic tools, e.g., angiotensin blockade in renal arterial hypertension. Clinically, there is improved understanding of high blood pressure in children and of the importance of systolic hypertension; also the diagnostic workup has been reassessed more critically than ever before. Therapeutically, new drugs have emerged for use in treating ambulatory patients and also in dealing with hypertensive emergencies. In addition, drug compliance has been recognized as an important consideration and is being managed more successfully. These and many other important aspects of hypertension are discussed in this monograph. I am extremely grateful to Gaddo Onesti for his valuable guidance in the formulation of this issue, and both of us are deeply indebted to the individual authors whose contributions we greatly value.

ALBERT N. BREST, M.D.

Contributors

Leslie Baer, M.D.
Associate Professor of Medicine, College of Physicians and Surgeons of Columbia University, New York, New York

Herbert Benson, M.D.
Associate Professor of Medicine, Harvard Medical School, Boston, Massachusetts

Edward G. Biglieri, M.D.
Professor of Medicine, University of California, San Francisco; Chief, Endocrine Section, San Francisco General Hospital, San Francisco, California

Roger Boucher, Ph.D.
Director, Laboratory of Biochemistry on Hypertension, Clinical Research Institute of Montreal, Montreal, Quebec, Canada

Jan Brod, M.D., Dr. Sc., F.R.C.P. (Lond.)
Professor of Medicine, Hannover Medical School, Hannover, West Germany

Jehoiada J. Brown, M.D.
Consultant Physician, Medical Research Council, Blood Pressure Unit, Western Infirmary, Glasgow, Scotland

James Conway, M.D.
Imperial Chemical Industries, Ltd., Pharmaceutical Division, Macclesfield, Cheshire, England

Allen W. Cowley, Jr., Ph.D.
Professor of Physiology, The University of Mississippi Medical Center, Jackson, Mississippi

Karen D. Crassweller, A.B.
Research Assistant, Harvard Medical School, Boston, Massachusetts

Kathryn Hawes Ehlers, M.D.
Professor of Pediatrics, Associate Director of Pediatric Cardiology, Director, Pediatric Cardiographics Laboratory, The New York Hospital —Cornell University Medical School, New York, New York

Mary Allen Engle, M.D.
Professor of Pediatrics, Director, Pediatric Cardiology, The New York Hospital —Cornell University Medical School, New York, New York

Michael Fernandes, M.D.
Assistant Professor of Medicine, Hahnemann Medical College and Hospital, Philadelphia, Pennsylvania

Robert Fraser, Ph.D.
Biochemist, Medical Research Council, Blood Pressure Unit, Western Infirmary, Glasgow, Scotland

Edward D. Frohlich, M.D.
Vice President, Education and Research, Alton Ochsner Medical Foundation; Director, Division of Hypertensive Disease, Ochsner Clinic, New Orleans, Louisiana

Jacques Genest, M.D.
Professor of Medicine, University of Montreal; Scientific Director, Clinical Research Institute of Montreal, Montreal, Quebec, Canada

Ray W. Gifford, Jr., M.D.
Head, Department of Hypertension and Nephrology, Cleveland Clinic, Cleveland, Ohio

Gordon P. Guthrie, Jr., M.D.
Assistant Professor of Medicine, University of Kentucky Medical School, Lexington, Kentucky

Roger B. Hickler, M.D.
Professor and Chairman, Department of Medicine, University of Massachusetts Medical School, Worcester, Massachusetts

Stevo Julius, M.D., Sc.D.
Professor of Medicine, Director, Division of Hypertension, The University of Michigan Medical School, Ann Arbor, Michigan

Kwan Eun Kim, M.D.
Professor of Medicine, Hahnemann Medical College and Hospital, Philadelphia, Pennsylvania

Arthur A. Klein, M.D.
Assistant Professor of Pediatrics, Assistant Director of Pediatric Cardiology Laboratories, The New York Hospital —Cornell University Medical College, New York, New York

Jamie B. Kotch, A.B.
Research Assistant, Harvard Medical School, Boston, Massachusetts

Otto Kuchel, M.D.
Professor of Medicine, University of Montreal; Director of the Autonomic Nervous System Laboratory, Clinical Research Institute of Montreal, Montreal, Quebec, Canada

Herbert G. Langford, M.D.
Professor of Medicine and Physiology, Chief, Endocrine-Hypertension Division, University of Mississippi School of Medicine, Jackson, Mississippi

Brenda Leckie, Ph.D.
Biochemist, Medical Research Council, Blood Pressure Unit, Western Infirmary, Glasgow, Scotland

Anthony F. Lever, M.D.
Consultant Physician, Medical Research Council, Blood Pressure Unit, Western Infirmary, Glasgow, Scotland

Aaron R. Levin, M.D.
Professor of Pediatrics, Associate Director of Pediatric Cardiology, Director, Pediatric Cardiac Catheterization Laboratory, The New York Hospital—Cornell University Medical Center, New York, New York

James J. Morton, Ph.D.
Biochemist, Medical Research Council, Blood Pressure Unit, Western Infirmary, Glasgow, Scotland

Marvin Moser, M.D.
Clinical Professor of Medicine, New York Medical College, Valhalla, New York; Senior Medical Consultant, National High Blood Pressure Education Program, National Heart, Lung, and Blood Institute

Robert C. Northcutt, M.D.
Assistant Professor of Medicine, Mayo Medical School, Consultant, Division of Endocrinology Metabolism and Internal Medicine, Mayo Clinic and Mayo Foundation, Rochester, Minnesota

Wojciech Nowaczynski, D.Sc.
Director, Steroid Research Laboratory, Clinical Research Institute of Montreal, Montreal, Quebec, Canada

Gaddo Onesti, M.D.
Professor of Medicine, Hahnemann Medical College and Hospital, Philadelphia, Pennsylvania

Paul L. Padfield, M.D.
Senior Registrar in Medicine, Medical Research Council, Blood Pressure Unit, Western Infirmary, Glasgow, Scotland

Jose Z. Parra-Carrillo, M.D.
Associate Professor of Clinical Nephrology, State University, Guadalajara, Mexico

Peter G. Pletka, M.D.
Chief, Renal Section, Associate Professor of Medicine, University of Massachusetts Medical School, Worcester, Massachusetts

Ildiko Radichevich, Ph.D.
Research Associate, Department of Medicine, College of Physicians and Surgeons of Columbia University, New York, New York

A. Jarrell Raper, M.D.
Associate Professor of Medicine, Medical College of Virginia, Virginia Commonwealth University, Richmond, Virginia

David W. Richardson, M.D.
Professor of Medicine, Chairman, Division of Cardiology, Medical College of Virginia, Virginia Commonwealth University, Richmond, Virginia

J. Ian S. Robertson, M.D.
Consultant Physician, Medical Research Council, Blood Pressure Unit, Western Infirmary, Glasgow, Scotland

Peter F. Semple, M.D.
Senior Registrar in Medicine, Medical Research Council, Blood Pressure Unit, Western Infirmary, Glasgow, Scotland

Sheldon G. Sheps, M.D.
Associate Professor of Medicine, Mayo Medical School, Consultant, Division of Cardiovascular Diseases and Internal Medicine, Mayo Clinic and Mayo Foundation, Rochester, Minnesota

Cameron G. Strong, M.D.
Associate Professor of Medicine, Mayo Medical School, Chairman, Division of Nephrology and Internal Medicine, Mayo Clinic and Mayo Foundation, Rochester, Minnesota

Charles D. Swartz, M.D.
Professor of Medicine, Vice Chairman, Department of Medicine, Director, Division of Nephrology and Hypertension, Hahnemann Medical College and Hospital, Philadelphia, Pennsylvania

Robert C. Tarazi, M.D.
Vice-Chairman and Head of Clinical Sciences Research Division, Cleveland Clinic, Cleveland, Ohio

Ross M. Tucker, M.D.
Assistant Professor, Mayo Medical School, Consultant, Nephrology Division, Mayo Clinic, Rochester, New York

Donald G. Vidt, M.D.
Head, Clinical Section, Department of Hypertension and Nephrology, Cleveland Clinic Foundation, Cleveland, Ohio

James W. Woods, M.D.
Professor of Medicine, University of North Carolina School of Medicine, Chapel Hill, North Carolina

Contents

Perspectives on the Physiology of Hypertension

Allen W. Cowley, Jr., Ph.D.

Despite the annual publication of nearly 80,000 original research articles and abstracts related to hypertension and the accumulated work of over 100 years of investigation, the etiology in nearly 90 percent of all hypertensive patients is unclear and the associated disorder is termed "essential hypertension." Although the origins of this condition remain undefined, significant progress has been made in understanding the basic physiologic mechanisms that control arterial blood pressure and the manner in which these mechanisms are altered during the development of hypertension. This chapter will review the current state of knowledge of these physiologic mechanisms and illustrate how our understanding of these basic mechanisms has contributed toward the elucidation of the pathogenesis of various forms of hypertension, including the "essential" form.

The following section briefly reviews the principles of arterial pressure regulation. This is followed by appropriate experimental and clinical observations which illustrate how these principles can be applied to the understanding of hypertensive mechanisms.

PHYSIOLOGIC PRESSURE CONTROL MECHANISMS

Rapid Stabilization of Arterial Pressure

Three general types of mechanisms serve to stabilize moment to moment fluctuations in arterial pressure: autonomic reflex mechanisms, hormonal mechanisms, and physical-mechanical properties of the vascular system. Each of these mechanisms differ in their speed and quantitative ability (gain) to return a pressure back toward its normal control level. Each mechanism also differs in the range of pressures over which it can effectively operate and the duration of time over which it is effective.

Autonomic Reflex Mechanisms

STRETCH RECEPTOR REFLEX MECHANISMS. Figure 1 illustrates the numerous rapidly acting reflex feedback pressure control mechanisms.[1,2] The most important of these for arterial pressure stabilization are the baroreceptor reflexes with tension sensitive receptors located in the muscular walls of the carotid sinus and aortic arch areas. Alterations of arterial pressure sensed by these receptors send nervous signals to the vasomotor center in the medulla oblongata, which in turn elicits appropriate changes in cardiac activity, peripheral arterial tone and venous compliance to return arterial pressure

1

NERVOUS CONTROL OF CARDIOVASCULAR SYSTEM

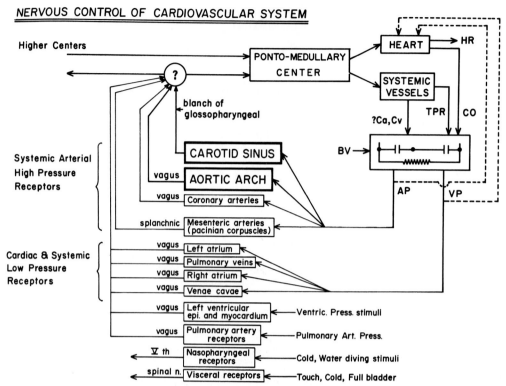

Figure 1. Schematic representation of stretch receptor reflex pathways which participate in rapid arterial pressure regulation by appropriate changes in cardiac function and the systemic vasculature. Reflex pathways involved in release of vasopressin (left atrial vagal afferent pathways), and potential sympathetic-spinal pathways, innervating low pressure receptors, are not shown. Arterial compliance (Ca), venous compliance (Cv), total peripheral resistance (TPR), cardiac output (CO), blood volume (BV), arterial pressure (AP), venous pressure (VP), and heart rate (HR).

back towards its control value.[1] Working together the carotid sinus and aortic arch receptors can return a change in arterial blood pressure nearly two-thirds back to its original control level in less than 20 seconds.[3, 4] The carotid sinus receptors exert their strongest influence at pressures between 40 and 100 mm. Hg, while the aortic arch receptors operate most effectively between arterial pressures of 100 to 180 mm. Hg.[5] In the chronic absence of the baroreceptor reflexes, great liability of arterial pressure is observed as illustrated in Figure 2.

Early investigators reported that a chronic state of "neurogenic hypertension" resulted following afferent denervation of the sinoaortic baroreceptors.[1] Recent evidence indicates, however, that such denervation procedures result only in a transient state of hypertension lasting less than one day. The chronic "neurogenic hypertension" which was observed by earlier investigators appears to have been a laboratory artifact resulting from the fact that even very mild external stimuli or excitement in the absence of these reflex pressure buffering mechanisms result in large arterial pressure elevations. This appears to be a consequence of the laboratory techniques used for measuring arterial pressure which have progressed from painful conscious femoral artery puncture measurements in trained dogs to the use of chronically implanted arterial catheters enabling pressure to be continuously recorded 24 hours per day for many weeks. Computerized analysis and averaging procedures have now been used to quantify over 4400 hours of continuously recorded data and have yielded an average mean arterial pres-

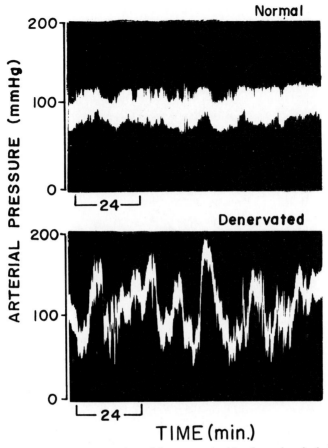

Figure 2. Demonstration of the variability of arterial pressure resulting from chronic denervation of the sinoaortic baroreceptors in contrast to the rather stable pressure pattern normally observed. Both records were obtained in the conscious undisturbed state several weeks following the surgical preparations.

sure value of 106 ± 4 mm. Hg in 42 normal dogs and 107 ± 5 mm. Hg in 50 sinoaortic denervated dogs.[6, 7] Thus, these rapidly responding reflex mechanisms are important in moment to moment *stabilization* but not in the determination of the long-term mean level of arterial pressure. This is illustrated in Figure 3 by the distribution of mean arterial pressure over a 24 hour period in a normal conscious dog compared to the distribution two weeks following sinoaortic baroreceptor denervation.

A very important reason why these reflex mechanisms are only important in short-term stabilization of pressure is that the baroreceptors adapt in one to two days to the pressure to which they are exposed. The consequences of "baroreceptor adaptation,"[8, 9] a general characteristic of all mechanoreceptors yet studied, are illustrated in Figure 4. In these experiments the development of hypertension in normal dogs was compared to sinoaortic baroreceptor denervated dogs.[10] Hypertension in this case was experimentally induced by excess salt and water loading of dogs with reduced renal mass. It is clear from these experiments and others[11, 12] that these reflex mechanisms serve only to slow the rate of pressure rise. The final level of pressure which is obtained does not differ in the two groups, which again demonstrates that these reflexes are not important determinants of the long-term level of arterial pressure.

CHEMORECEPTOR REFLEX MECHANISMS. The chemoreceptors located in the carotid

3

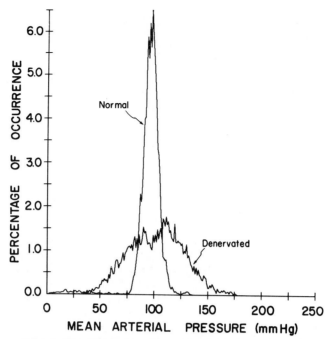

Figure 3. Frequency of distribution of 24 hour, continuously recorded, mean arterial pressure in a conscious normal dog before and after sinoaortic denervation.

and aortic bodies are stimulated as arterial pressure falls below 80 mm. Hg because of decreased oxygen delivery. These receptors in turn signal the autonomic nervous system to return pressure toward normal in a manner similar to that described for the baroreceptor mechanisms.[13] Although this mechanism may contribute to normalization of pressures in hypotensive states, the overall strength of the system, independent of the

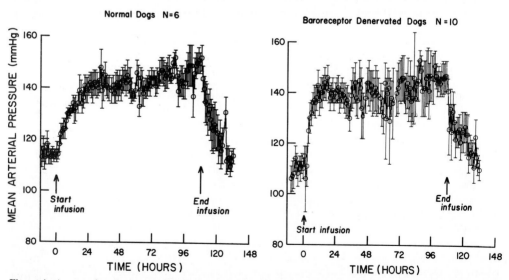

Figure 4. Average hourly mean arterial blood pressure values (±S.D.) obtained during onset of volume loading hypertension in six normal and ten baroreceptor denervated dogs.

baroreceptors, is poorly defined and normally the reflex would not be expected to participate in hypertensive states.

CENTRAL NERVOUS SYSTEM ISCHEMIC REFLEX. At very low levels of arterial pressure, below 40 mm. Hg, the ischemia of the vasomotor center in the lower brain stem elicits a powerful peripheral reflex vasoconstriction and increases cardiac contractility.[14] This reflex appears to be the cause of transient hypertensive states following cerebrovascular accidents which result in increased subdural hydrostatic pressure.

Hormone Stabilization of Arterial Pressure

RENIN-ANGIOTENSIN SYSTEM. Although it has been known for years that the renin-angiotensin system has the potential to be involved in the pathogenesis of some hypertensive states, only in the past five years has the quantitative importance of this hormonal system to arterial pressure homeostasis been established.[15, 16] A decrease of arterial pressure to levels ranging between 50 and 99 mm. Hg will be returned nearly 65 percent of the way back to control levels by the peripheral vasoconstrictor action of angiotensin.[15, 17] The renal mechanisms which sense the fall in pressure and the indirect reflex sympathetic stimulation of renin release have been extensively reviewed.[18] Although renin is immediately released as the arterial pressure is lowered, the time required for maximum pressure response is nearly 15 minutes.[15–18] It is nevertheless a relatively potent system and has pressure compensating ability comparable to the baroreceptor system over its defined operating range. The utility of this system has been demonstrated in conditions of hemorrhage[17] and in the conditions of volume depletion resulting from restricted salt and water intake.[19, 20]

VASOPRESSIN PRESSOR SYSTEM. Evidence recently reviewed suggests a pressor role of vasopressin in various hypotensive states, such as hemorrhage. Although the quantitative importance of this mechanism remains to be determined, the high concentrations of vasopressin seen after hemorrhage have been shown to have considerable pressor effects in baroreceptor-denervated dogs, suggesting that vasopressin may exert such an effect in the normal control of arterial pressure. Until recently, dose-response relationships of vasopressin were obtained in anesthetized animals in which very high circulating control levels of vasopressin obscured most of the pressor activity of vasopressin. In contrast, Figure 5 illustrates that the relative potency of vasopressin favorably compares to that of angiotensin II, the most potent vasoactive peptide known. Since it has been shown that the low pressure, left atrial stretch receptors trigger the release of large amounts of vasopressin in volume depletion, this appears to be a potentially significant factor in the short-term control of pressure.[21, 22]

Physical Mechanisms of Arterial Pressure Control

STRESS RELAXATION MECHANISM. A very rapid physical mechanism which serves to stabilize changes in arterial pressure is the stretch of the blood vessels which occurs when the pressure rises or falls below normal levels.[23] The resistance changes to flow which occur under these circumstances enable the pressure to fall or rise toward its normal level.

CAPILLARY FLUID SHIFT MECHANISM. The shift of plasma water in and out of the vascular system as the arterial pressure rises and falls, resulting in changes of capillary pressure, serves as an escape valve if the arterial pressure is elevated after massive transfusion or reduced during hemorrhage, initiating a sequence of events that slowly, over a period of hours, returns the arterial pressure toward normal levels.[23]

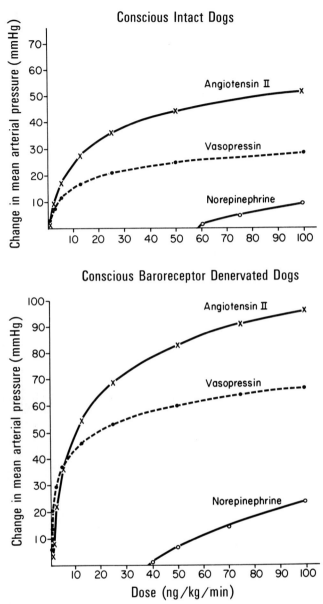

Figure 5. Comparative dose-response effects of angiotensin II, vasopressin and norepinephrine in normal conscious dogs (N = 15) and sinoaortic denervated dogs (N = 15). Absence of baroreceptor reflexes unmasks the potent peripheral pressor activity of the three agents.

Determinants of the Long-Term Average Pressure around Which Daily Fluctuations Occur

The Renal-Body Fluid Mechanism

The long-term arterial pressure level around which moment to moment and daily fluctuations occur is ultimately determined by the steady state relationships of the renal-body fluid volume arterial pressure axis. This is a result of the unique role of the renal circulation which distinguishes it from all others in the body. Other capillary systems

6

filter fluid into an interstitial area from which it is normally returned to the blood volume space by Starling capillary dynamics and through the lymphatic system (Fig. 6). In contrast, a small portion of all water and electrolytes filtered from renal glomerular capillaries is lost irreversibly through continuous urine excretion from the body. Since fluid intake remains rather constant over time, being strongly influenced by habitual patterns, the renal circulation together with tubular transport mechanisms become the major determinants of the rate of body fluids lost over time and thus the major determinants of the interstitial and vascular volumes. Progressive addition of fluid to the extracellular compartment results in elevations of blood volume and pressure within the vascular system. This vascular volume is distributed in the veins and arteries with most of it residing in the venous system (Fig. 6). If the heart is not failing, elevations of venous pressure from volume expansion will elevate venous return and cardiac output.

Figure 7 diagrammatically depicts the interdependence of arterial pressure, renal water loss, and body fluid volume. A circular relationship is apparent whereby arterial pressure determines water loss, which determines body fluid volumes, which determine arterial pressure. This important dependence of daily salt and water loss upon arterial pressure is based on the crucial fact that the renal capillary-tubular fluid dynamics are determined in large measure by hydrostatic pressures in the renal vascular system.

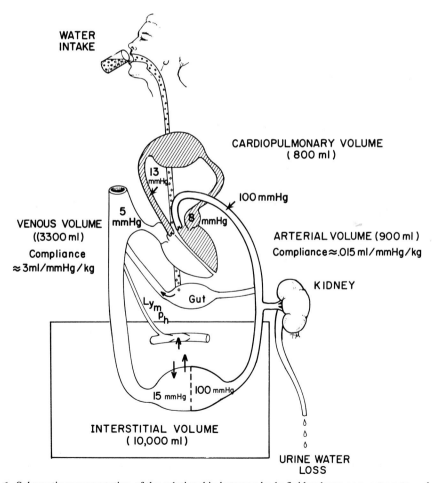

Figure 6. Schematic representation of the relationship between body fluid volume compartments and vascular pressures and fluid volume balance.

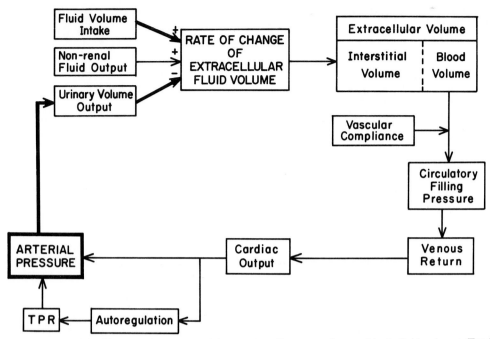

Figure 7. Circular relationship between arterial pressure, urinary excretion, and body fluid volumes. Total peripheral resistance (TPR).

Thus as arterial pressure falls below normal, the renal output of water and salt is reduced, thereby conserving body fluids and maintaining arterial pressure. When arterial pressure rises above normal, urinary output of water and salt increases until the body fluid volume is sufficiently reduced to return arterial pressure toward normal. This relationship has been repeatedly demonstrated in both isolated perfused kidney preparations and in the intact conscious state.

Isolated kidneys, in which extrinsic neurohumoral influences are absent, exhibit about a five- to sevenfold increase in urinary output as renal artery pressure is increased from 100 to 200 mm. Hg. As perfusion is lowered from 100 mm. Hg to 50 mm. Hg, urine excretion falls to zero.[24-26] In the intact chronic state, this relationship is considerably more sensitive, as seen in the ability of the kidney over a period of days to excrete a body salt and water load of nearly 7 times normal intake with only about a 5 mm. Hg rise of arterial pressure, as seen in Figure 8. In this graph each point represents the steady state relationship between arterial pressure and sodium intake obtained after 5 days at different levels of daily sodium intake.[27] The mechanisms which influence this relationship remain to be determined but are believed to be the consequence of multiple interacting neural and hormonal influences superimposed on the underlying physical system and activated under conditions of blood volume changes. An example of just one hormonal influence is seen in the same graph in which a small amount of angiotensin II (5.0 ng./kg./min.) was infused continuously at three levels of sodium and water intake. It is clear that the relationship between salt and water intake is shifted such that equilibrium between sodium intake and loss occurs only at a higher perfusion pressure.

Consequences of Renal-Fluid Balance Pressure Control System

The implications of this circular relationship depicted in Figure 7 have been emphasized by rigorous mathematical system analyses.[28-30] These analyses demonstrated that

8

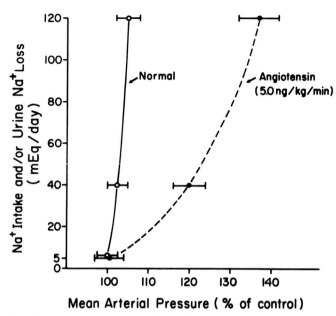

Figure 8. Chronic function curve depicting the relationship between arterial pressure and sodium excretion over a wide range of daily sodium intake. Each point is the steady-state value obtained after five days of the indicated sodium intake which is equal to total sodium loss under steady-state conditions. Angiotensin continuously administered at 5.0 ng./kg./min. alters this relationship so that sodium and water balance occur only at a higher level of arterial pressure.

this system provides the body with the only arterial pressure control system with "infinite" capacity to return a change in arterial blood pressure completely to its normal level. This feature which has been called "the infinite gain" control system is simply the consequence of the fact that the total output of water and salt cannot remain different from the net intake of water and salt for very long. The basic requirement for the body to achieve a balance between salt and water intake and output constitutes the most powerful mechanism for the long-term regulation of arterial pressure. Since the urine output is basically dependent on the arterial pressure, it is this slowly acting volume control system that ultimately overrides all other pressure control systems.

The consequences of this seemingly simple proposition have provided refreshing new insight to our understanding of long-term pressure control and the role of the kidney in hypertension. First, it means that the long-term level of arterial pressure is not determined by total peripheral resistance, but rather by renal resistance to flow or any factors of tubular function which alter the normal relationship of arterial pressure to urinary output. An increase in total peripheral resistance *excluding* renal resistance raises the pressure only as long as is required to cause sufficient volume depletion to return pressure to normal. This is seen in clinical conditions where total peripheral resistance levels are increased abruptly by amputation of limbs or the closing of a large arteriovenous fistula. In time, arterial pressure stabilizes around normal levels at an expanded or contracted state of body fluid volumes. Second, it means that a decrease in venous compliance alone cannot raise the long-term level of arterial blood pressure. Only transient arterial pressure changes are seen until the blood volume is reduced and arterial pressure returns to normal. For example, surgical repairs in patients with extensive long-term venous varicosities do not show long-term alterations in the level of arterial blood pressure.

It is often asked why this slow-acting renal-fluid volume balance control system is really needed since the total action of all the more rapidly acting pressure control systems can to a large extent normalize changes in pressure before the renal-fluid balance control system even has time to act. The answer to this is found in the very nature of these other rapidly acting volume and arterial pressure control systems. Specifically, none of these systems has been found to be capable of returning a change in pressure or volume *completely* to normal levels. The consequences of this slight remaining deviation from normal are readily apparent if we consider what could happen if only 99.9 percent of our daily water intake was removed by the rapid neurohumoral systems. In one year, we would accumulate 430 ml. and over a normal lifetime about 31 liters. It is this unique integral function of the kidney that led Guyton and colleagues to conclude on theoretical grounds that the kidney is the prevailing factor in the long-term control of arterial pressure.[28-30]

By far the most important implication of the renal-fluid volume relationships is that the kidney is the final common pathway for the control of arterial pressure in both normal and hypertensive states. This is not to say that all hypertension originates from renal malfunction. Any number of extrinsic factors influence renal function. The importance of this mechanism to the field of hypertension, however, is broadened when it is considered that there are potentially many extrinsic and intrinsic factors capable of altering renal function and elevating the level of arterial pressure at which body salt and water equilibrium occurs. Various pathologic states affecting the renal vasculature (e.g., nephrosclerosis) and glomerular diseases (e.g., glomerulonephritis) alter the ability of the kidney to excrete salt and water and are generally associated with hypertension. Neurohumoral inputs to the kidney, such as the sympathetic nerves, circulating catecholamines, angiotensin, aldosterone and vasopressin, can strongly influence renal function and can induce hypertension. Thus, there are probably a very large number of initiating factors in hypertension, but if the physiologic concepts of long-term fluid volume and arterial pressure regulation are correct, all must act through the described renal-body fluid volume mechanisms. Similarly, antihypertensive drugs must also act either directly on the kidney as seen with diuretics or indirectly by suppression of extrinsic factors as seen with agents working on the central nervous system. The reason the crucial renal actions are so frequently overlooked in the pharmacology of these drugs is a result of their simultaneous actions on the peripheral vasculature and/or neuroendocrine systems which act to obscure the long-term alterations of renal function which slowly alter the relationship between body fluid volume balance and arterial pressure.

In the following sections, the manner in which these variously described physiologic mechanisms can be applied to some representative categories of hypertension will be discussed.

APPLICATION OF PHYSIOLOGIC CONCEPTS TO HYPERTENSION

Volume-Induced Hypertension

One of the most thoroughly studied experimental models of hypertension is that caused by administration of excess salt and water to animals with a renal mass surgically reduced to about one-third normal.[10, 31-34] This has been a particularly useful model of hypertension because it has provided insight into some fundamental hemodynamic relationships that often participate in the hypertensive process, particularly those between body fluid volumes and arterial pressure.

The role of body fluid volumes in hypertension aroused initial interest during the latter part of the nineteenth century, but the progression of research contraindicated that volumes played an important role in the hypertensive process. The most persuasive indictment against the role of fluid volumes in hypertension resulted from the ability in the early part of the twentieth century to measure blood volume. It was repeatedly found that these volumes were either normal or even below normal in most hypertensive patients. This was followed by development of clinical techniques to measure cardiac output which demonstrated that the elevated levels of pressure in hypertensive patients were being maintained by an increased total peripheral resistance rather than an elevation of cardiac output. These observations were not compatible with those expected if hypertension was a result of body fluid expansion. Pervading interest in the reasons for elevated total peripheral resistance in hypertension led to an explosion of interest in the renin-angiotensin system and the neural control of the circulation from the 1930s to the present time, with the resulting general lack of interest in the role of body fluid volumes.

In the last decade, laboratory and clinical observations of the hemodynamic changes observed in hypertension caused by salt and water expansion have resulted in renewed interest in the role of the body fluid volumes in hypertension. As discussed in the following section these studies have reconciled the seemingly paradoxical observations of earlier investigators and have shown how volume changes are related to arterial pressure and peripheral resistance changes in hypertension.

Hemodynamic Changes in Volume Loading Hypertension

The initiating factor in this type of hypertension, expansion of body fluid volumes, has been carefully documented by numerous investigators.[10, 31-34] Hypertension is a result of the volume changes rather than excess sodium per se. This was shown with the observation that hypertension results from a pure volume expansion when body sodium content is held constant in an experiment performed by hemodialysis of anephric sheep.[35] In contrast, pure sodium expansion at fixed volumes did not result in hypertension. Similarly, hypertension can be produced with continuous administration of vasopressin to dogs with reduced renal mass which results in volume expansion with hyponatremia.[36]

Cardiac output is elevated during the first several days of volume expansion. This in turn is associated with an increased arterial pressure level. Determination of the total peripheral resistance in this period of rising pressure has shown that it is below control levels, a phenomenon resulting from strong baroreceptor reflex activity attempting to counteract the hypertensive process. Interestingly, however, both the increased body fluids and cardiac output reverse direction and return toward normal over a period of 1 to 2 weeks.[10, 34] It is this reversal that has provided important insight for understanding the chronic hemodynamic state observed in volume induced hypertension. The following section discusses the physiology of how expanding fluid volumes are related to cardiac output and total peripheral resistance changes observed in volume induced hypertension.

Peripheral Resistance Changes by "Intrinsic" Regulation of Blood Flow

There are two concepts which are central to the understanding of the changes which are observed in the blood volume, cardiac output and total peripheral resistance changes observed in Figure 9. One is the local "intrinsic" regulation of blood flow and the other is the relationship between vascular size, compliance and volume.

"INTRINSIC" REGULATION OF BLOOD FLOW. The return of cardiac output and blood volume toward normal levels while total peripheral resistance to flow progressively increases (Fig. 9) is best explained on the basis of our present knowledge concerning the intrinsic mechanisms by which tissues regulate their blood flow. Intrinsic mechanisms, although poorly understood, serve the important function of regulating blood flow to the needs of the tissue independently of the autonomic nervous system and hormonal

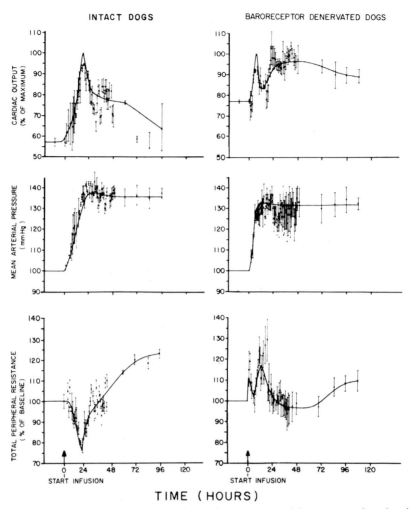

Figure 9. Comparison of average hourly changes in cardiac output, arterial pressure, and total peripheral resistance obtained in normal conscious dogs (left) and sinoaortic baroreceptor denervated dogs (right) during the onset of volume loading hypertension with reduced renal mass.

mechanisms. These local intrinsic mechanisms appear to prevent prolonged overperfusion or underperfusion of tissues despite changes in arterial perfusion pressure. A variety of phenomena participate in this process and have been given various names in the literature. Some of these intrinsic changes occur rapidly, through the mechanism commonly referred to as "autoregulation." It is widely debated whether metabolic or myogenic mechanisms are responsible for this phenomenon, but there is little disagreement that all of the tissues of the body are capable of vasodilating rapidly as arterial pressure is lowered, returning flow toward normal levels.[37, 38] The summated effect of overperfusion of all tissues simultaneously (whole-body autoregulation) has been demonstrated in the absence of the nervous system.[39] Similar findings have been observed in intact, conscious, baroreceptor-denervated dogs.[40] However, this rapid autoregulatory response which occurs in minutes is probably not of much significance in hypertension since opposite changes (rapid increases in resistance to flow) are not observed following a step elevation of arterial pressure above normal.

In contrast, chronic overperfusion of tissues, such as that observed in volume over-

12

loading, triggers other important irtrinsic tissue changes over a period of days and months. One well characterized event is the gradual hypertrophy of vascular walls resulting in a decrease in the basic size of the vessel by increasing wall to lumen ratios.[41] Another mechanism which significantly alters local resistance to blood flow is the degree of vascularization and the opening or closing of collateral flow channels, events clearly observed in retinal blood vessels.[42] It is well known that marked alterations in the arterial vasculature occur in chronic hypertension in which decreased vessel numbers, increased vessel length, and tortuosity are observed in various vascular beds.[43-45]

The intrinsic tissue oriented mechanisms for the local regulation of blood flow clearly provide a logical explanation for the gradual return of cardiac output and the rise in total peripheral resistance observed during hypertension induced by volume overload. Although the precise mechanisms and their long-term potency remain unclear, this intrinsic flow regulating system is capable of normalizing total tissue blood flow in the face of large changes in arterial pressure.

The consequences of these mechanisms in volume induced hypertension are as follows: As the total peripheral resistance gradually increases, an expanded blood volume is no longer necessary to maintain an elevated state of arterial pressure. In the face of a maintained excess volume load, a high arterial pressure level is necessary to maintain normal renal filtration of fluid to keep urine output in balance with fluid intake. The combined effects of total peripheral resistance and cardiac output initially raise the arterial pressure above that level required to maintain fluid balance and the body gradually unloads the excess volume, returning blood volume and cardiac output back toward normal while hypertension is sustained by the increased total peripheral resistance (see Fig. 9). If the arterial pressure should begin to fall from this hypertensive level, fluid volumes would again accumulate and total peripheral resistance would again rise to prevent tissue overperfusion. After months and years of hypertension, cardiac hypertrophy undoubtedly contributes to the sustained level of high arterial pressure, and heart failure finally becomes apparent. Given the ability of the intrinsic tissue mechanism to regulate blood flow, in time only small changes in the volume are capable of initiating large changes in arterial pressure. Thus, when observed in the fully developed chronic state only a slightly elevated blood volume is observed while total peripheral resistance is significantly elevated and appears to be the sustaining factor of the hypertension.

The change of arterial pressure observed with acute expansion of extracellular fluid volume is far less per volume increase than that observed with the chronic expansion of volume. For this reason, the results of acute experiments cannot be extrapolated to the long-term state in which the effects of the local flow regulating mechanisms multiply the resistance changes perhaps as much as tenfold.

RELATIONSHIPS BETWEEN VASCULAR SIZE, VASCULAR VOLUME AND COMPLIANCE. Looking at Figure 6 we can qualitatively deduce what occurs as fluid intake exceeds the renal excretory capacity. When the size of the vascular system remains the same as extracellular volumes increase, the average hydrostatic pressure will rise, unless all the fluid is lost into the interstitial spaces. The resulting average level of vascular hydrostatic pressure is the driving force to move blood through the vascular system and return it to the right heart. As this force increases, so too will the pressure gradient for return of blood to the heart, which in turn elevates the cardiac output.

Since the relationship between the "size" of the vascular compartment and the "volume" which is contained in this compartment is an important determinant of the cardiac output and blood volume status in hypertension, it is useful to digress at this point to consider this issue. The vascular compartment is normally filled to a point where increasing or decreasing the volume within the system will change the stress on the vascular walls. It is apparent that pressure within a vascular compartment can be changed either by maintaining the size constant and changing its volume, or by keeping the volume constant and changing the vascular size or the compliance of the vascular walls. The "degree of fullness" of the vascular system can be represented by a pressure which is obtained by rapidly stopping the heart and quickly bringing arterial and venous pressures into equilibrium.[46] This must be achieved quickly before reflex changes can alter the vascular tone and is normally done by rapid pumping of the blood from the arterial to the venous side through a large fistula. Since most of the blood volume is contained in the compliant veins, as seen in Figure 6, the venous size and compliance are the major determinants of this pressure value. The average pressure in the vascular system obtained experimentally in this way has been termed the "mean circulatory filling pressure" and represents the degree of fullness of the vascular system. Although this "mean circulatory filling pressure" cannot be directly measured in man, it is important to understand the concept of "fullness of the vasculature" since the mathematical difference between the "mean circulatory filling pressure" and the right atrial pressure determines the rate of return of blood to the heart at any given resistance to flow. Thus the measurement of blood volume alone provides only half of the information needed to predict observed changes in cardiac output, a point generally ignored in clinical studies. It is only the volume with respect to the size of the vascular container that can effect a change in cardiac output which is therefore often called the "effective volume."

Application to Clinical Situations

The sequence of events leading to hypertension which has just been described has been observed in anephric men whose volumes were expanded over one month by ultrafiltration during 13 dialysis periods.[47]

In contrast, other investigators have obtained variable results in anephric or end-stage renal disease patients, which have led them to question the validity of the aforementioned theories.[48] It must be remembered, however, that these patients exhibit a host of complex alterations which are known to be capable of altering the sequence of mechanisms seen under normal conditions. Alterations of red cell mass, plasma albumin concentration and increased capillary permeability will affect the tissue blood flow requirements and distribution of body fluids and alter the apparent responses of the local "intrinsic" flow mechanisms. Interstitial tissue compliance changes, various degrees of heart failure, and alterations of circulating hormone levels, to name just a few, will also complicate the sequence of events experimentally observed in normal animals. Many of these changes frequently observed in anephric patients or end-stage renal hypertensive patients can alter the distribution of fluid volumes and the blood flow requirements of peripheral tissues, and thereby mask predicted changes in these variables. Application of normal physiologic mechanisms to explain the observed changes must be performed with caution under such circumstances.

It should be recognized that in other forms of hypertension which may not be specifically volume induced, it is certainly possible to initiate the hypertensive state solely by an initial increase in total peripheral resistance if it includes resistance changes in the renal circulation as well. In this case, blood volume expansion may not be observed, cardiac output may be normal, elevated or even depressed, and there may be no need for tissue autoregulation to participate in the hypertensive process.

Several important concepts emerge from the model of salt and water induced hypertension with reduced renal mass. First, the sequence of observed events during the development of the volume induced hypertension clearly shows that the arterial pressure elevation comes first and is in itself the cause of the elevated peripheral resistance. Second, we can now understand why it would be possible, in the course of a volume-induced type of hypertension, to observe either normal or elevated body fluid volumes or cardiac output. If a circulating vasoconstrictor factor was also involved in the hypertensive process even a subnormal level of blood volume or cardiac output could be observed, provided that the total size or compliance of the venous vascular compartment was reduced.

Third, in any form of hypertension, it is essential to evaluate the data in terms of the proper time frame, with reference to the "time frame" capabilities of the variously related homeostatic control systems. Only then is it possible to know how the system got to where it stands when you view it, and where you can expect it to be when you view it at a later time.

Extension of Concepts to Other Forms of Hypertension

Elevations of cardiac output have been observed at the onset of many experimental and clinical forms of hypertension. An early increase in cardiac output in renal hypertension was first observed by Ledingham and Cohen in rats[49] and has since been reported in dogs.[50, 51] Young, labile, borderline hypertensives exhibit an elevation in cardiac output that is nearly 20 percent higher than that of normotensives of comparable age.[52] Young, spontaneously hypertensive rats (SHR) exhibit a similar elevation in cardiac output.[53]

There is no reason, however, to believe that the phenomenon of increased cardiac output and peripheral autoregulation need occur in all forms of hypertension. Even in some forms of hypertension in which increased cardiac output is observed, it does not mean that the development of hypertension is dependent on this event. Hypertension develops in weanling spontaneously hypertensive rats despite a 20 percent reduction in cardiac output associated with chronic pharmacologic beta-adrenergic inhibition of cardiac function throughout the growth period.[53]

Different patterns in both blood volume and cardiac output should be expected depending upon the initiating factors in each case. For example, elevations of cardiac output with no alteration of total blood volume could be observed if some factor decreased the total size of the vascular compartment. This would elevate the "mean circulatory filling pressure," and for a certain period of time the cardiac output and arterial pressure. If the same factor caused vasoconstriction of renal afferent and/or efferent arterioles the arterial pressure could be chronically sustained. Such may be the case in hypertension induced by the continuous administration of small doses of angiotensin.[12, 54] Similar mechanisms probably are present in patients with pheochromocytoma who develop hypertension despite a large reduction of blood volume.[55]

The Final Common Pathway in Hypertension: Alteration of Renal Function

There appears to be a common thread that runs through every known type of hypertension, that is, alterations of renal function. Clinically, nephrologists are keenly aware that many types of renal dysfunction lead to hypertension. Experimentally and clinically the uniqueness of the renal circulation is illustrated by the well-known observation that it is the only circulatory bed, with the possible exception of the brain, in which it is certain that primary alterations in its circulation can initiate a chronic state of hypertension. The experimental Goldblatt model of hypertension resulting from constriction of a renal artery has received enormous attention since it was first reported in 1934.[56] The importance of this model is that in large measure it has stimulated for the past 50 years much of the interest in the state of the renal circulation in hypertension. Unfortunately, there are only a small total number of cases (approximately 5 percent of the hypertensive population) in which this can be demonstrated to be the cause of hypertension, but since Goldblatt's first experiments there have been persistent efforts to link the kidney with essential hypertension. These efforts have led to the accumulation of significant evidence which points toward a central role of altered renal function in all types of hypertension.

Morphology of the Renal Circulation in Hypertension

Clinically, sclerosis of the renal arterioles has been evident in chronic hypertensive patients since the late nineteenth century. Sclerosis of the media, thickening of the intima, muscular hypertrophy with increased wall to lumen ratios, hyaline degeneration, hyalinization of glomeruli, and fibrosis of the interstitial tissue and arterial wall characterize nearly every established form of hypertension studied by biopsy or necropsy.[57] In man, severity and extent of the nephrosclerosis at necropsy are directly correlated with the severity of the hypertension,[57] and similar findings are observed in the renal morphology of the spontaneously hypertensive rat, the contralateral kidney of unilateral renal artery stenosis, unilateral hydronephrosis, unilateral pyelonephritis, and unilateral perinephritis in rats.[58]

Since the time that these vascular changes have been observed, the question has been asked as to whether the renal vascular changes precede or follow the onset of hypertension. This cause and effect relationship remains unanswered by morphologic studies but it is thought by most investigators that the observed changes result from exposure of vessels to high blood pressure. Several lines of indirect evidence support this belief. For example, when hypertension is produced in rats by constriction of one renal artery with the opposite kidney left *in situ,* the hypertension is not usually abolished when the clip is removed.[59] This residual hypertension is increased if the previously constricted kidney is removed, but it is abolished if the contralateral unconstricted kidney is removed instead. Similarly, a persistence of hypertension is seen after removal of the primary cause in DOCA plus salt hypertension after cessation of exposure to deoxycorticosterone.[60] Another example is the "Dahl strain" of rats which become hypertensive only with salt loading, but do not return to normal if salt loading is stopped.[61] Studies by Folkow and associates have shown that the peripheral vascular beds of rats protected from high pressure during Goldblatt hypertension by application of ligatures to the femoral arteries did not exhibit vascular alterations seen in the unprotected vessels.[62]

Vascular changes in hypertensive animals treated with antihypertensive drugs are reversible, again suggesting that high pressure damages the vasculature.[63] This reversal of vascular damage is also suggested by early studies of Byrom and Dodson who observed that release of renal artery constriction to a single remaining kidney reversed hypertension completely, regardless of its duration.[64] Similar results have been reported clinically by Tracy, who observed that the renal vasculature of chronic hypertensive patients exhibiting a fall in arterial pressure before death (associated with coronary vascular disease or cancer) exhibited nephrosclerosis at a severity strongly associated with the lower level of pressure.[65] These studies contradicted the belief that permanent changes in the cardiovascular system would perpetuate hypertension.

Thus, the evidence suggests that hypertension leads to structural and functional systemic and renal vascular changes but that the process in many cases is reversible, although it is perhaps less so in the kidney. However, morphologic studies in man will probably not provide the answer to the questions of causation of essential hypertension. Fixed vascular lesions may not need to be observed to cause hypertension. There are probably initial alterations in the *functional state* of the renal vasculature undetectable in terms of organic changes which could readily alter the ability of the kidney to maintain fluid volume balance at normal levels of arterial pressure. This then brings us to a brief review of the status of the functional state of the kidney in hypertension.

16

Renal Alterations Expected to Produce Hypertension

The functional state of the kidney can be altered in numerous ways, some of which would be theoretically expected to lead to hypertension and others which would not. The dysfunctions most likely to cause hypertension are those which shift glomerulotubular balance so that net absorption of fluids is favored. Evidence indicates that the most common cause of fluid retention and hypertension is those situations in which glomerular filtration is impeded. This includes *renal artery constriction* which is associated with a variety of conditions (atherosclerotic lesions, fibromuscular dysplasia, emboli, perinephric compression, allergic vasculitis, nephrosclerosis, and collagen vascular diseases such as polyarteritis nodosa). Glomerular disease in which filtration is impeded has the same effect, as observed in hypertension associated with acute and chronic glomerulonephritis. These diseases that interfere with filtration are associated with the most severe hypertensive states. Excess tubular absorption of fluids, as occurs in primary aldosteronism, is also associated with hypertension, but of a milder nature.[66]

Other forms of renal disease need not result initially in hypertension but may instead cause uremia. These forms are especially associated with situations in which there is a reduction of the total number of functioning nephrons. When sufficiently advanced, however, excess salt and water intake leads to hypertension in the manner described in the previous section.

Observed Renal Functional Changes in Hypertension

The functional state of the renal circulation has been evaluated in various ways. In man, clearance studies were used to demonstrate in the 1940s that essential hypertension is associated with increased renal vascular resistance.[67] More recently, dye dilution has been utilized and studies have indicated a reduction in renal flow in essential hypertension.[68, 69] Diffusible radioactive washout techniques (zenon, krypton) have also indicated a reduction in renal flow with the dominant abnormality in the cortical flow component.[70] Renal blood flow has been reported by most investigators to be reduced,[67, 71] but there is a great deal of variability in the data. Since arterial pressure is elevated, even normal blood flow indicates a large increase of renal vascular resistance. Glomerular filtration rate remains normal even when blood flow is reduced, resulting in an increased fraction of filtered blood. Thus, the predominant site of increased vascular resistance appears to be in the postglomerular vessels.

Both renal blood flow and glomerular filtration rate fall progressively below normal with increasing severity of hypertension, as both afferent and efferent arteriolar constriction begin to contribute to the hypertensive process.

These renal changes need not be primary in their origin but could result from a variety of extrinsic influences. In certain experimental laboratory models of hypertension primary changes in the renal circulation precede the hypertensive process. Goldblatt hypertension is certainly one such instance. Jaffe and associates, using Dahl's strain, reported that during normal salt intake and before hypertension they observed "a mild nonuniform focal constriction of the early afferent arterioles."[61] When the rats were given salt, the focal lesions caused even greater narrowing of the afferent arterioles. Other strains of spontaneously hypertensive rats, however, have not shown morphologic abnormalities, but evidence is beginning to emerge which relates a primary change in renal function to this spontaneous form of hypertension. Some of this evidence suggests that *extrinsic* influences upon the kidney via the sympathetic nervous system could lead to depressed renal function. In the Okomoto strain of spontaneously hypertensive rats, direct nerve recording shows that splanchnic nerve activity was five times that in control rats, suggesting that sympathetic activity to the kidney is also affected more than the general vasculature.[72] Recently, Campbell and coworkers reported that stimulation of the posterior hypothalamus of spontaneously hypertensive rats results in greater increases in splanchnic nerve activity than in control rats.[73]

In man, evidence of increased renal sympathetic tone in patients with benign essential hypertension was reported by Hollenberg and Adams who found that alpha-adrenergic blockage with phentolamine had no effect on renal blood flow in fifteen normal people, but increased renal flow in six of nine essential hypertension patients.[74] It has recently been demonstrated in dogs that the chronic infusion of norepinephrine directly into the renal artery results in a chronic state of hypertension at doses in which no effect is seen with systemic intravenous infusions.[75]

Alternatively, *intrinsic* or inherent changes in renal function preceding hypertension have also received support recently from two separate laboratories which found that when the kidneys of genetically hypertensive rats were transplanted to control rats, hypertension was transferred to the normal rats. Conversely, hypertensive rats became normotensive with control rat kidneys.[76, 77]

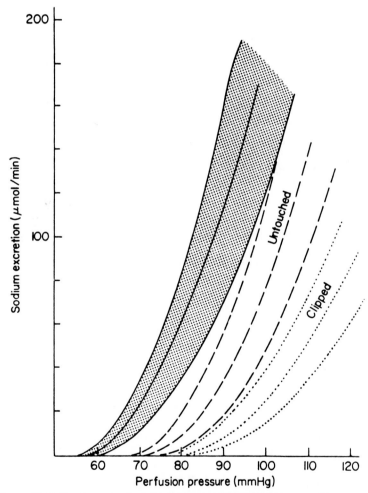

Figure 10. Effects of Goldblatt hypertension upon the acute relationship between sodium excretion and renal perfusion pressure in the untouched contralateral kidney (untouched) and the kidney with a clipped renal artery (clipped).

Renal vascular reactivity in essential hypertension patients studied during renal arteriography has been reported to exhibit increased sensitivity to low doses of angiotensin II infused into the renal artery.[74] Evidence also suggests that patients with mild essential hypertension may have variable or labile increases in renal vascular tone.

Two new experimental approaches have recently been applied in an effort to evaluate the functional state of the kidney in hypertension. Both of these approaches are designed to evaluate the sodium and water excretory ability of the kidney over a wide range of renal arterial perfusion pressure loads. In one instance, this relationship was studied acutely in renal hypertensive rabbits 3 to 6 weeks after clipping a single artery. At this time both kidneys were removed and perfused with a lightly anesthetized donor rabbit. The results seen in Figure 10 demonstrate that the functional ability of the kidneys to excrete sodium and water over a wide range of pressures has been significantly altered in both kidneys.[78] The utility of this type of analysis is demonstrated by the fact that at approximately normal arterial pressure levels, the discrepancy between salt and water excretion is not nearly as apparent as that which is seen at higher levels of renal perfusion.

Another method has recently been utilized to study the chronic steady-state relationship between arterial pressure and sodium and water excretion in conscious dogs. In these studies the arterial pressure level at which salt and water intake comes into balance with salt and water loss is determined over a wide range of controlled intakes as described in Figure 8. Each point represents the steady state pressure obtained after 5 days of the indicated daily sodium intake. When circulating angiotensin levels are chronically elevated by a continuous intravenous infusion, salt and water balance in the body can occur only at an elevated level of arterial pressure.[12, 54]

Thus, the relationships between arterial pressure and renal excretory function are presently being quantitatively determined. It is apparent that even though angiotensin has direct peripheral vasoconstrictor actions, it also directly or indirectly alters the renal arterial pressure required to maintain body sodium and water balance. The chronic influence of other extrinsic and intrinsic factors on this relationship remains undetermined.

SUMMARY

Present understanding of the physiology of arterial pressure regulation indicates that the renal-body fluid volume system determines the level at which the mean pressure resides over long periods of time. The relationships between blood volume, and size and compliance of the entire vascular system, and intrinsic regulation of tissue blood flow determine the sequence of observed changes in cardiac output and total peripheral resistance.

Current evidence is compatible with the concept that functional changes in the renal vasculature or tubular system, either intrinsic or extrinsic in origin, reflect the final common pathway in the genesis of all forms of experimental and human hypertension. At the present time the nature of these renal changes appears to alter the fundamental relationships between renal perfusion pressure and sodium and water excretion. One of the major challenges in the field of hypertension today is to test the hypothesis that changes in renal function, either extrinsic or intrinsic in form, are involved in all forms of hypertension.

REFERENCES

1. HEYMANS, C., AND NEIL, E.: *Reflexogenic Areas of the Cardiovascular System.* Little, Brown and Co., Boston, 1959.

2. MANCIA, G., LORENZ, R. R., AND SHEPHARD, J. T.: *Reflex control of circulation by heart and lungs,* in GUYTON, A. C., AND COWLEY, A. W., JR. (EDS.): *International Review of Physiology. Cardiovascular Physiology II,* Vol. 9. University Park Press, Baltimore, 1976, pp. 111.

3. SCHER, A. M., AND YOUNG, A. C.: *Servoanalysis of carotid sinus reflex effects on peripheral resistance.* Circ. Res. 12:152, 1963.

4. SAGAWA, K., AND WATANABE, K.: *Summation of bilateral carotid sinus signals in the barostatic reflex.* Am. J. Physiol. 209:1278, 1965.

5. CLEMENT, D. L., PELLETIER, L. C., AND SHEPHERD, J. T.: *Control of high and low blood pressure in the dog by aortic and sinus nerve.* Clin. Sci. Mol. Med. 48:257, 1975.

6. COWLEY, A. W., JR., LIARD, J. F., AND GUYTON, A. C.: *Role of the baroreceptor reflex in daily control of arterial pressure and other variables in dogs.* Circ. Res. 32:564, 1973.

7. ONESTI, G., FERNANDES, M., AND KIM, K. E. (EDS.): *Regulation of Blood Pressure by the Central Nervous System.* Grune & Stratton, New York, 1976, p. 81.

8. KEZDI, P., AND WENNEMARK, J.: *Baroreceptor and sympathetic activity in experimental renal hypertension.* Circulation 17:785, 1958.

9. KREIGER, E. M.: *Time course of baroreceptor resetting in acute hypertension.* Am. J. Physiol. 218:486, 1970.

10. COWLEY, A. W., JR., AND GUYTON, A. C.: *Baroreceptor reflex effects on transient and steady-state hemodynamics of salt-loading hypertension in dogs.* Circ. Res. 36:536, 1975.

11. LIARD, J. F., COWLEY, A. W., JR., McCAA, R. E., ET AL.: *Renin, aldosterone, body fluid volumes, and the baroreceptor reflex in the development and reversal of Goldblatt hypertension in conscious dogs.* Circ. Res. 34:549, 1974.

12. COWLEY, A. W., JR., AND DeCLUE, J. W.: *Quantification of baroreceptor influence on arterial pressure changes seen in primary angiotensin induced hypertension in dogs.* Circ. Res. 39:779, 1976.

13. DALY, M. DEB., AND UNGER, A.: *Comparison of the reflex responses elicited by stimulation of the separately perfused carotid and aortic body chemoreceptors in the dog.* J. Physiol. (Lond.) 182:379, 1966.

14. SAGAWA, K.: *Analysis of the CNS ischemic feedback regulation of the circulation,* in GUYTON, A. C., AND REEVES, A. A. (EDS.): *Physical Bases of Circulatory Transport Regulation and Exchange.* W. B. Saunders, Philadelphia, 1967, p. 129.

15. COWLEY, A. W., JR., MILLER, J. P., AND GUYTON, A. C.: *Open-loop analysis of the renin-angiotensin system in the dog.* Circ. Res. 28:568, 1971.

16. GUTMANN, F. D., TAGAWA, H. L., HABER, E., ET AL.: *Renal arterial pressure, renin secretion, and blood pressure control in trained dogs.* Am. J. Physiol. 224:66, 1973.

17. BROUGH, R. B., JR., COWLEY, A. W., JR., AND GUYTON, A. C.: *Quantitative analysis of the acute response to haemorrhage of the renin-angiotensin-vasoconstrictor feedback loop in areflexic dogs.* Cardiovasc. Res. 9:772, 1975.

18. LARAGH, J. H., AND SEALEY, J. E.: *The renin-angiotensin-aldosterone hormonal system and regulation of sodium, potassium, and blood pressure homeostasis,* in ORLOFF, J., BERLINER, R. W., AND GEIGER, S. R. (EDS.): *Handbook of Physiology.* American Physiological Society, New York, 1973, p. 831.

19. SAUCHO, J., RE, R., BURTON, J., ET AL.: *The role of the renin-angiotensin-aldosterone system in cardiovascular homeostasis in normal human subjects.* Circulation 53:400, 1976.

20. COLEMAN, T. G., COWLEY, A. W., JR., AND GUYTON, A. C.: *Angiotensin and hemodynamics of chronic salt deprivation.* Am. J. Physiol. 229:167, 1975.

21. COWLEY, A. W., JR., MONOS, E., AND GUYTON, A. C.: *Interaction of vasopressin and the baroreceptor reflex system in the regulation of arterial blood pressure in the dog.* Circ. Res. 34:505, 1974.

22. ROCHA, E., SILVA, J. M., AND ROSENBERG, M.: *The release of vasopressin in response to haemorrhage and its role in the mechanism of blood pressure regulation.* J. Physiol. 202:535, 1969.

23. PRATHER, J. W., TAYLOR, A. E., AND GUYTON, A. C.: *Effect of blood volume, mean circulatory pressure and stress relaxation on cardiac output.* Am. J. Physiol. 216:467, 1969.

24. SELKURT, E. E.: *Effects of pulse pressure and mean arterial pressure modification on renal hemodynamics and electrolyte and water excretion.* Circulation 4:541, 1951.

25. THURAU, K., AND DEETZEN, P.: *Diuresis in arterial pressure increases.* Pfluegers Arch. 274:567, 1962.

26. FOURCADE, J. C., NAVAR, L. G., AND GUYTON, A. C.: *Possibility that angiotension resulting from unilateral kidney disease affects contralateral renal function.* Nephron 8:1, 1971.

27. COWLEY, A. W., JR., AND McCAA, R. E.: *Acute and chronic dose-response relationships for angiotensin, aldosterone, and arterial pressure at varying levels of sodium intake.* Circ. Res. 39:788, 1976.

28. GUYTON, A. C., COLEMAN, T. G., AND GRANGER, H. J.: *Circulation: overall regulation.* Ann. Rev. Physiol. 34:13, 1972.

29. GUYTON, A. C., COLEMAN, T. G., COWLEY, A. W., JR., ET AL.: *Systems analysis of arterial pressure regulation and hypertension.* Ann. Biomed. Eng. 1:254, 1972.

30. GUYTON, A. C., COLEMAN, T. G., COWLEY, A. W., JR., ET AL.: *A systems analysis approach to understanding long-range arterial blood pressure control and hypertension.* Circ. Res. 35:159, 1974.

31. CHANUTIN, A., AND FERRIS, E. B.: *Experimental renal insufficiency produced by partial nephrectomy.* Arch. Intern. Med. 49:767, 1932.

32. KOLETSKY, S., AND GOODSITT, A. M.: *Natural history and pathogenesis of renal abolition hypertension.* Arch. Pathol. 69:654, 1960.

33. DOUGLAS, B. H., GUYTON, A. C., LANGSTON, J. B., ET AL.: *Hypertension caused by salt loading: II. Fluid volume and tissue pressure changes.* Am. J. Physiol. 207:669, 1964.

34. COLEMAN, T. G., AND GUYTON, A. C.: *Hypertension caused by salt-loading in the dog: III. Onset transients of cardiac output and other circulatory variables.* Circ. Res. 25:153, 1969.

35. NORMAN, R. A., JR., COLEMAN, T. G., WILEY, T. L., JR., ET AL.: *Separate roles of sodium ion concentration and fluid volumes in salt-loading hypertension in sheep.* J. Physiol. 229:1068, 1975.

36. MANNING, R. D., JR., COLEMAN, T. G., MCCAA, R. E., ET AL.: *Experimental hypertension—a model with expanded fluid volumes and hyponatremia.* Physiologist 18:303, 1975.

37. JOHNSON, P. C.: *The microcirculation and local and humoral control of the circulation,* in GUYTON, A. C., (ED.): *International Review of Physiology* Vol. 1. University Park Press, Baltimore, 1974, p. 163.

38. STAINSBY, W. N.: *Local control of regional blood flow.* Ann. Rev. Physiol. 35:151, 1973.

39. GRANGER, H. J., AND GUYTON, A. C.: *Autoregulation of the total systemic circulation following destruction of the central nervous system in the dog.* Circ. Res. 25:379, 1969.

40. LIEDTKE, A. J., URSCHEL, C. W., AND KIRK, E. S.: *Total systemic autoregulation in the dog and its inhibitions by baroreceptor reflexes.* Circ. Res. 32:673, 1973.

41. FOLKOW, B., HALLBACK, M., LUNDGREN, Y., ET AL.: *Background of increased flow resistance and vascular reactivity in spontaneously hypertensive rats.* Acta Physiol. Scand. 80:93, 1970.

42. DOLLERY, C. T., HENKIND, P., PATTERSON, J. W., ET AL.: *Ophthalmoscopic and circulatory changes in focal retinal ischemia.* Br. J. Ophthalmol. 50:285, 1966.

43. LANDAU, J., AND DAVIS, E.: *Capillary thinning and high capillary blood pressure in hypertension.* Lancet 1:1327, 1957.

44. BYROM, F. B.: *The pathogenesis of hypertensive encephalophy and its relation to the malignant phase of hypertension.* Lancet 2:201, 1954.

45. HUTCHINS, P. M.: *Microcirculatory dimensions in spontaneously hypertensive rats.* Microvasc. Res. 4: 325, 1972.

46. GUYTON, A. C., POLIZO, D., AND ARMSTRONG, G. G.: *Mean circulatory filling pressure measured immediately after cessation of heart pumping.* Am. J. Physiol. 179:261, 1954.

47. COLEMAN, G. G., BOWER, J. D., LANGFORD, H. G., ET AL.: *Regulation of arterial pressure in the anephric state.* Circulation 42:509, 1973.

48. KIM, K. E., ONESTI, G., SCHARTZ, A. B., ET AL.: *Hemodynamics of hypertension in chronic end-stage renal disease.* Circulation 46:456, 1972.

49. LEDINGHAM, J. M., AND COHEN, R. S.: *Changes in the extracellular fluid volume and cardiac output during the development of experimental renal hypertension.* Can. Med. Assoc. J. 90:292, 1964.

50. BIANCHI, G., TENCONI, L. T., AND LUCCA, R.: *Effect in the conscious dog of constriction of the renal artery to a sole remaining kidney on hemodynamics, sodium balance, body fluid volumes, plasma renin concentration, and pressor responsiveness to angiotensin.* Clin. Sci. 38:741, 1970.

51. FERRARIO, C. M., PAGE, I. H., AND MCCUBBIN, J. W.: *Increased cardiac output as a contributory factor in experimental renal hypertension in dogs.* Circ. Res. 27:799, 1970.

52. BIRKENHAGER, W. H., SCHALEKAMP, M. A. D. H., KRAUSS, X. H., ET AL.: *Consecutive hemodynamic patterns in essential hypertension.* Lancet 1:560, 1972.

53. PFEFFER, M. A., FROHLICH, E. D., PFEFFER, J. M., ET AL.: *Pathophysiological implications of the increased cardiac output of young spontaneously hypertensive rats.* Circ. Res. 34 (I):235, 1974.

54. DECLUE, J. W., COWLEY, A. W., JR., COLEMAN, T. G., ET AL.: *Influence of long-term low dosage infusions of angiotensin II on arterial pressure, plasma aldosterone concentration, and renal sodium excretion.* Physiologist 19:165a, 1976.

55. TARAZI, R. C., DUSTAN, H. P., FROHLICH, E. D., ET AL.: *Plasma volume and chronic hypertension: relationship to arterial pressure levels in different hypertensive diseases.* Arch. Intern. Med. 125:835, 1970.

56. GOLDBLATT, H., LYNCH, J., HANZEL, R. F., ET AL.: *Studies on experimental hypertension.* J. Exp. Med. 59:347, 1934.

21

57. TRACY, R. E.: *Correlation of lengthy hospital records of blood pressure with nephrosclerosis.* Arch. Pathol. 82:526, 1966.

58. LEDINGHAM, J. M.: *Experimental renal hypertension.* Clin. Nephrol. 4:127, 1975.

59. FLOYER, M. A.: *The effect of nephrectomy and adrenalectomy upon the blood pressure in hypertensive and normotensive rats.* Clin. Sci. 10:405, 1951.

60. FRIEDMAN, S. M., FRIEDMAN, C. L., AND NAKASHIMA, M.: *Sustained hypertension following administration of deoxycorticosterone acetate.* J. Exp. Med. 93:361, 1951.

61. JAFFE, D., SUTHERLAND, L. E., BARKER, D., ET AL.: *Effects of chronic excess salt ingestion: morphological findings in kidneys of rats with different genetic susceptibilities to hypertension.* Arch. Pathol. 90:1, 1970.

62. FOLKOW, B., GUREVICH, M., HALLBACK, M., ET AL.: *The hemodynamic consequences of regional hypotension in spontaneously hypertensive and normotensive rats.* Acta Physiol. Scand. 82:A9, 1971.

63. KOJIMAHARA, M., SEKIYA, K., AND OONEDA, G.: *Studies on the healing of arterial lesions in experimental hypertension.* Virchows Arch. Abt. A. Pathol. Anat. 354:150, 1971.

64. BYROM, F. B., AND DODSON, L. F.: *The mechanism of the vicious circle in chronic hypertension.* Clin. Sci. 8:1, 1949.

65. TRACY, R. E., AND TOCA, V. T.: *Nephrosclerosis and blood pressure. II. Reversibility of proliferative arteriosclerosis.* Lab. Invest. 30:30, 1974.

66. CONN, J. W.: *Presidential address: Primary aldosterone, a new clinical syndrome.* J. Lab. Clin. Med. 45: 3, 1955.

67. Wesson, L. G., JR.: *Physiology of the Human Kidney.* Grune & Stratton, New York, 1969, p. 130.

68. LOGAN, A. G., VELASQUEZ, N. T., AND COHN, J. N.: *Renal cortical blood flow, cortical fraction, and cortical blood volume in hypertensive subjects.* Circulation 67:1306, 1973.

69. LOWENSTEIN, J. STEINMETZ, P. R., EFFROS, R. M., ET AL.: *The distribution of intrarenal blood flow in normal and hypertensive man.* Circulation 35:250, 1967.

70. HOLLENBERG, N. K., EPSTEIN, M., BASCH, R. I., ET AL.: *"No man's land" of the renal vasculature.* Am. J. Med. 47:845, 1969.

71. KOLSTERS, G., SCHALEKAMP, M. A. D. H., BIRKENHAGER, W. H., ET AL.: *Renin and renal functions in benign essential hypertension: evidence for a renal abnormality,* in *Pathophysiology and Management of Arterial Hypertension.* Proc. of Copenhagen Conference, Astra Pharmaceutical, Goteborg, 1975, p. 54.

72. OKAMOTO, K., NOSAKO, S., YAMORI, Y., ET AL.: *Participation of neural factor in the pathogenesis of hypertension in the spontaneously hypertensive rat.* Jap. Heart J. 8:168, 1967.

73. CAMPBELL, J. C., ROBINSON, D. S., AND WHITEHORN, D.: *Differences in central nervous system regulation of blood pressure in spontaneously hypertensive and matched control rats.* Physiologist 19:147, 1976.

74. HOLLENBERG, N. K., AND ADAMS, D. F.: *The renal circulation in hypertensive disease.* Am. J. Med. 60: 773, 1976.

75. KATHOLI, R. E., CAREY, R. M., AYERS, C. R., ET AL.: *Production of sustained hypertension with chronic intrarenal norepinephrine infusion in conscious dogs.* Circ. Res. 40 (Suppl. I): 118, 1977.

76. BIANCHI, G., FOX, U., DI FRANCESCO, G., ET AL.: *The hypertensive role of the kidney in spontaneously hypertensive rats.* Europ. J. Clin. Invest. 3:213, 1973.

77. RAPP, J. P., KNUDSEN, K. D., IWAI, J., ET AL.: *Genetic control of blood pressure and corticosteroid production in rats.* Circ. Res. 32(I): 139, 1973.

78. THOMPSON, J. M. A., AND DICKINSON, C. J.: *The relation between the excretion of sodium and water and the perfusion pressure in the isolated, blood perfused rabbit kidney, with special reference to changes occurring in clipped-hypertension.* Clin. Sci. Molec. Med. 50:223, 1976.

Clinical Significance and Management of Systolic Hypertension*

Robert C. Tarazi, M.D., and Ray W. Gifford, Jr., M.D.

The challenge of systolic hypertension has only recently been recognized as an important therapeutic problem. Part of the neglect of systolic blood pressure levels in the evaluation and management of patients was due to the assumed insignificance of these levels. They were thought to be much more labile and much less significant than the diastolic pressure which was said to represent "the real load on the heart". These impressions have persisted despite factual and theoretical evidence to the contrary.

As early as 1931, Ayman[1] demonstrated that diastolic blood pressure levels were as variable as systolic pressure. More recently, epidemiologic investigations like the Framingham study,[2] confirmed earlier impressions[3, 4] regarding the pathogenetic importance of systolic hypertension. Cardiac enlargement,[5, 6] heart failure,[7] coronary arterial disease,[2] and strokes[8] were all more closely related to systolic than to diastolic levels. Cardiac response to antihypertensive therapy, as judged by the electrocardiogram, was also shown in two different studies[9, 10] to be better correlated with changes in systolic than in diastolic pressure. The bases for these correlations are not difficult to find; they are deeply rooted in cardiovascular physiology. However, their full implications regarding patient management are only now being slowly envisioned; systolic hypertension is obviously *not* a benign entity but the problem is that it is difficult (some would even say dangerous) to control.

DEFINITION

Various definitions have been given for systolic hypertension.[3, 11, 12] Easiest to recognize are those with systolic blood pressure (SBP) higher than 150 or 160 mm. Hg[3] and diastolic blood pressure (DBP) consistently 90 mm. Hg or lower; these are patients with pure or isolated systolic hypertension. However, this definition is unduly restrictive; patients with diastolic hypertension (DBP > 90 mm. Hg) may also have inappropriate elevations of systolic pressure which can markedly alter their clinical picture and response to therapy.[13, 14]

A rise in diastolic pressure is normally associated with a commensurate rise in systolic pressure which can be mathematically defined if no pathologic alteration in aortic wall distensibility develops with the hypertension.[11, 12] However, such is not the rule; empirical formulae have been developed to define the upper limit of the "appropriate"

*Studies on which this manuscript is based were supported in part by a grant of the National Heart, Lung, and Blood Institute (HL 6835).

23

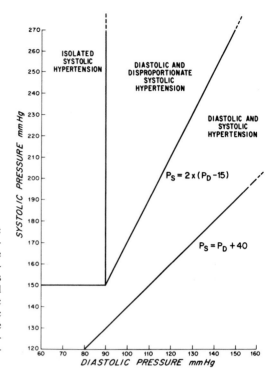

Figure 1. Relation between systolic and diastolic blood pressure. Isolated systolic hypertension refers to the combination of systolic blood pressure greater than 150 mm. Hg and diastolic blood pressure (DBP) ≤ 90 mm. Hg. However, the diagnosis of disproportionate systolic hypertension should not be restricted to patients with normal diastolic pressure. Koch-Weser[13] has shown that systolic levels higher than (DBP − 15) × 2 are inappropriate for the diastolic level and justify a diagnosis of systolic hypertension in a patient with elevated diastolic blood pressure (From Koch-Weser, J.[13])

systolic pressure for any diastolic level. In older textbooks, the systolic pressure was expected to equal 3/2 DBP.[15] More recently, Koch-Weser[13] defined systolic hypertension as:

$$SBP > [(DBP - 15) \times 2].$$

This definition is particularly useful in that it allows recognition of undue systolic elevations whatever the diastolic pressure, and prevents the unwarranted restriction of the term only to patients with isolated systolic hypertension. (Fig. 1).

PATHOPHYSIOLOGIC BASIS

Hemodynamic Mechanisms

Systolic hypertension has usually been subdivided into two hemodynamic types: one related to increased stroke volume and the other due to diminished aortic distensibility.[16] It is widely held that the first type occurs usually in younger subjects and that the second is characteristic of older patients. Although superficially attractive, this view seems unduly simplistic in our opinion. Investigation of patients with various types of systolic hypertension (age range 16 to 72 years) has shown that the hemodynamic mechanism cannot always be deduced from the age, arterial pressure level or other clinical characteristics of the patient.[14] Further, more than one pathological mechanism is usually involved in the systolic hypertension in any age group.

In younger patients (below 40 years) with essential hypertension, systolic hypertension is indeed often associated with some increase in stroke volume, as found in two different studies.[14, 17] However even in these patients, a closer look at aortic distensibility has shown a significant increase of the ratio of pulse pressure to stroke volume (PP/SV mm. Hg/ml. ejected),[14, 18] suggesting increased aortic rigidity.[11, 14, 19] A study of 26 patients with isolated systolic hypertension by Adamopoulos and coworkers[20] concluded that patients younger than 35 years had a higher cardiac output than older patients, and related their hypertension to a hyperkinetic circulation. However neither the cardiac output nor the stroke volume of these younger patients was significantly different from normal, implying therefore that some reduction in aortic distensibility must have contributed in part to their wide pulse pressure. The reduction of aortic distensibility in many patients with borderline hypertension is consistent with the increased collagen reported in the aorta of very young spontaneously hypertensive rats.[21]

Similarly, not all patients above 40 years with systolic hypertension have a reduced aortic distensibility as determined by an increased PP/SV ratio, although many do. Statistically "significant" differences between group averages often hide marked overlaps in individual values. The stroke volume of older patients with systolic hypertension is not necessarily reduced and may even be high enough in some to contribute to the wide pulse pressure.

Thus, aortic distensibility cannot always be predicted on the basis of age or any single hemodynamic factor (heart rate, systolic or diastolic pressure). Both in older as well as in younger individuals, determination of some index of aortic distensibility is needed for a comprehensive hemodynamic evaluation of their hypertension. A detailed discussion of available indexes is not within the scope of this presentation; various methods have been outlined by Wiggers,[11] Burton,[12] Conway,[22] Abboud and Huston,[23] and Tarazi and coworkers.[14] We found the PP/SV ratio a valuable index of aortic rigidity, provided it is judged in relation to the many factors that may be expected to influence aortic distensibility (Fig. 2). Differentiation of systolic hypertension according to the predominant hemodynamic mechanism might prove of importance in the prognosis of the disorder and may lead to rational selection of therapy in difficult cases.

Cardiovascular Consequences

As has been mentioned, cardiac involvement in hypertension is more closely related to systolic than to diastolic levels.[2, 5-10] This is not surprising since cardiac work (CW) is really a function of systolic pressure:

$$CW = SV \times HR \times \overline{SBP}$$

where SV = stroke volume, HR = heart rate, and $\overline{SBP}$ = mean pressure during systole.

In more precise terms, the increased resistance to left ventricular ejection in hypertension is not accurately described by the diastolic pressure, mean arterial pressure or total peripheral resistance alone.[14, 24] Impedance to left ventricular ejection includes both a resistive and a compliant component; changes in the first are determined primarily by the cross-sectional area of the arterioles, whereas changes in the latter are dominated by aortic compliance to ejected blood.[25] Increased aortic rigidity may thus impose a load on the left ventricle that may not be fully evaluated by consideration of diastolic or mean arterial pressure alone. Systolic blood pressure is more directly relevant in this context, and evaluations of resistance to ventricular ejection might be more appropriately based on mean systolic pressure and flow ($\overline{SBP}$/SF) rather than on the classical formula for total peripheral resistance (TPR = MAP/CO).[14]

These physiologic considerations have important clinical implications. An increased load due to a higher pressure is costlier to the heart in terms of myocardial oxygen requirements than a volume overload.[26] The higher cost of increased pressure demands,

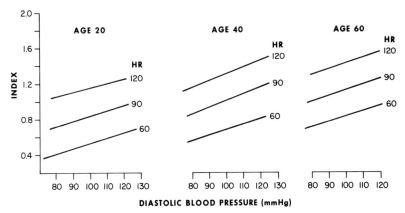

Figure 2. An index of aortic distensibility can be obtained from the ratio of pulse pressure to stroke volume, or PP/SV mm. Hg pressure rise per ml. of blood ejected.[14] Aortic distensibility is influenced by many factors including heart rate (HR), diastolic pressure (DBP) and age, and this dependence is reflected in the highly significant (p < 0.001) correlation of this index with these variables (r = 0.731). PP/SV = 0.0069 age (years) + 0.0048 DBP (mm. Hg.) + 0.009 HR − 0.64 standard error of estimate = 0.178. This nomogram is based on the equation defined above from a study of 76 subjects.[14] (From Tarazi, et al.[14])

therefore, an accurate definition of the pressure being considered. The relationship between diastolic pressure levels and cardiac enlargement or cardiac performance, although significant, is not close.[24] Taking into account the characteristics of the large vessels and systolic pressure levels[14] may help define better the therapeutic goals in individual patients.

Although the links between hypertension and atherosclerosis are incontrovertible,[26] there is no special self-evident relation between systolic blood pressure and atherosclerosis. It seems reasonable, however, to think that the high tension imposed during systole could be as damaging, although relatively short-lived, as the more sustained but lower tension during diastole. It appears clinically that strokes and coronary arterial disease are both more closely related to systolic than to diastolic arterial pressure.[2, 7, 8]

THERAPEUTIC PROBLEMS

The relative neglect of systolic hypertension did not stem entirely, in our opinion, from the variability of systolic levels and their assumed greater dependence on cardiac response to transient stresses. It also reflects a common clinical observation, i.e., the disorder is difficult to control. Also important, and always brought up in discussion periods, is an understandable concern stemming from anecdotal experiences of vascular or renal complications related to attempts at lowering systolic hypertension. No statistics are available to substantiate that fear, but conversely the value of treating isolated systolic hypertension has not been conclusively proved either. For combined systolic and diastolic hypertension, the evidence is clear that adequate blood pressure control leads to diminished morbidity and mortality. In both conditions, isolated systolic hypertension or combined systolic and diastolic hypertension, failure to evaluate adequately the inappropriately high systolic levels can lead either to incomplete control or to problems in management.

These therapeutic problems can be discussed as: (1) wide fluctuations in systolic blood pressure during antihypertensive therapy, (2) dangers of hypotension, and (3) reduced baroceptor reflexes in older patients.[27]

Fluctuations in Systolic Blood Pressure

Patients with diminished aortic distensibility may experience wider variations in systolic pressure than other hypertensives for equivalent changes in diastolic pressure (Fig. 3). The reason is that diminished aortic distensibility leads to a steeper pressure-volume relationship, as can be determined experimentally;[28] in clinical terms this is revealed by a steeper slope in the relationship between systolic and diastolic arterial pressure.[13] Since rapid and marked reductions in blood pressure are not usually well tolerated, especially in older patients (see below), the practical corollary is to use a careful drug approach with small dosages initially. This effect of reduced distensibility of the large vessels (windkessel) is one of the reasons for the unusual sensitivity of these patients to antihypertensive measures; it is *not* however the only reason. Others include the frequent finding of elevated peripheral resistance and low plasma volume in these older patients.[14, 20] Tarazi and Dustan[28] have shown that this hemodynamic pattern is associated with increased depressor response to acute ganglionic blockade.

Dangers of Hypotension

The concept that increased arterial pressure is somehow needed to force blood through narrowed atherosclerotic vessels is outdated.[29] The presence of uncontrolled

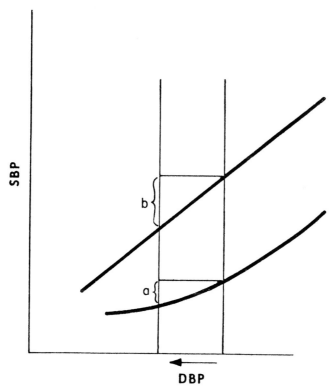

Figure 3. Relation between systolic (SBP) and diastolic (DBP) blood pressure levels under conditions of normal aortic distensibility (lower line) and of reduced distensibility (upper line). For the same reduction in DBP, the drop in SBP is much greater when the aorta is more rigid (less distensible), i.e., b > a. (From Tarazi, et al.[14])

hypertension in a patient with ischemic heart disease is certainly more detrimental to the heart than the unproven risk of response to a drug which lowers blood pressure. There is *no* evidence that myocardial infarction is precipitated by antihypertensive therapy;[30] similarly, even during the heroic period of ganglionic blockade, permanent neurologic damage was extremely rare in patients who had repeated fainting episodes. Antihypertensive therapy is not contraindicated in patients with a history of cerebrovascular accidents; on the contrary, all available evidence indicates its value to prevent the occurrence or recurrence of strokes, whether hemorrhagic or thrombotic.[31, 32]

On the other hand, one must take into account the element of *time* when considering the effects of lowering arterial pressure. A gradual reduction of pressure allows time for many adaptation processes, whereas an abrupt reduction may strain the limits of autoregulation and lead to reduction of cerebral blood flow in proportion to the lowering of arterial pressure.[33] The influence of the speed or time course of pressure reduction may explain to a large degree the contrast between the benefits reported by most large scale trials[31, 32] and the occasionally alarming symptoms observed by clinicians.

In summary, the difficulties in control of systolic hypertension, either isolated or associated with diastolic hypertension, should *not* be taken as a reason to abandon attempts at careful therapy. These are particularly warranted in our opinion when there is evidence of target organ disease; in such cases, dysfunction of the kidneys, brain or heart may be favorably influenced. This implies careful followup and proper choice of drugs.

Baroceptor Reflexes in Older Patients

Systolic hypertension is especially common in older patients, and hence the need to consider the effectiveness of their baroceptor reflexes and its constraints on the choice of antihypertensive therapy. It has been repeatedly shown that the effectiveness of baroceptor reflexes is diminished by age.[27, 34] Sharpey-Shafer,[35] and Appenzeller and Descarries[36] demonstrated that the blood pressure rebound after its dip during a Valsalva maneuver is markedly reduced and sometimes absent in older patients and in patients with cerebrovascular disease, hence the frequency of dizzy spells or fainting in these patients during straining for coughing, defecating or micturition. It stands to reason, therefore, that neural blockers that interfere with baroceptor mechanisms would be dangerous in patients with borderline baroceptor compensation. These include such drugs as ganglion blockers, sympatholytics or alpha-blockers; however, beta adrenergic blockers do not lead to orthostatic hypotension.[37]

Therapy may therefore be initiated with diuretics in less than maximum dosage. If need be, hydralazine in combination with propranolol or other beta blockers, may be a second step of treatment. Although older patients may be suspected of having greater tendency to cardiac dysfunction, Eisalo and associates[38] found that propranolol was effective in lowering the blood pressure of hypertensives age 60 years or older without greater incidence of complications than that reported for younger subjects. It has been suggested that hydralazine may be tolerated by many older hypertensives without need for beta blockade, because of their diminished baroceptor sensitivity and hence lesser tendency to reflex tachycardia. In our experience, methyldopa in small or moderate doses has been effective in many patients with isolated systolic or combined systolic and diastolic hypertension. Although it is a sympatholytic, methyldopa does not frequently lead to postural hypotension, possibly because of its central rather than peripheral effect at lower dosage levels.[39]

REFERENCES

1. AYMAN, D.: *Essential hypertension: the diastolic blood pressure; its variability.* Arch. Intern. Med. 48: 89, 1931.
2. KANNEL, W. B., GORDEN, T., AND SCHWARTZ, M. J.: *Systolic versus diastolic blood pressure and risk of coronary heart disease: the Framingham study.* Am. J. Cardiol. 27:335, 1971.
3. GUBNER, R. S.: *Systolic hypertension: a pathogenic entity. Significance and therapeutic considerations.* Am. J. Cardiol. 9:773, 1962.
4. COLANDREA, M. A., FRIEDMAN, G. D., NICHAMAN, M. Z., ET AL.: *Systolic hypertension in the elderly: an epidemiologic assessment.* Circulation 41:239, 1970.
5. RAMIREZ, E. A., AND PONT, P. H. G.: *Relation of arterial blood pressure to the transverse diameter of the heart in compensated hypertensive heart disease.* Circulation 31:542, 1965.
6. KANNEL, W. B., GORDON, T., AND OFFUTT, D.: *Left ventricular hypertrophy by electrocardiogram: Prevalence, incidence, and mortality in the Framingham study.* Ann. Intern. Med. 71:89, 1969.
7. KANNEL, W. B., CASTELLI, W. P., McNAMARA, P. M., ET AL.: *Role of blood pressure in the development of congestive heart failure.* N. Engl. J. Med. 287:782, 1972.
8. KANNEL, W. B., WOLF, P. A., VERTER, J., ET AL.: *Epidemiologic assessment of the role of blood pressure in stroke.* JAMA 214:301, 1970.
9. GEORGE, C. F., BRECKENRIDGE, A. M., AND DOLLERY, C. T.: *Value of routine electrocardiography in hypertensive patients.* Br. Heart. J. 34:618, 1972.
10. IBRAHIM, M. M., TARAZI, R. C., DUSTAN, H. P., ET AL.: *Electrocardiogram in evaluation of resistance to antihypertensive therapy.* Arch. Intern. Med. 137:1125, 1977.
11. WIGGERS, C. J.: *Physiology in Health and Disease.* Lea and Febiger, Philadelphia, 1949, pp. 587–591.
12. BURTON, A. C.: *Physiology and Biophysics of the Circulation.* Year Book Medical Publishers, Chicago, 1966, pp. 72–83, 152–158.
13. KOCH-WESER, J.: *Correlation of pathophysiology and pharmacology in primary hypertension.* Am. J. Cardiol. 32:499, 1973.
14. TARAZI, R. C., MAGRINI, F., AND DUSTAN, H. P.: *The role of aortic distensibility in hypertension,* in MILLIEZ, P., AND SAFAR, M. (EDS.): *Recent Advances in Hypertension.* Laboratories Boehringer Ingelheim, France, 1975, pp. 133–142.
15. SAVY, P.: *Traité de Thérapeutique Clinique.* Masson et Cie., Paris, 1948, pp. 1378–1380.
16. PICKERING, G.: *High Blood Pressure.* Grune & Stratton, Inc., New York, 1968, pp. 22–27.
17. FINKIELMAN, S., WORCEL, M., AND AGREST, A.: *Hemodynamic patterns in essential hypertension.* Circulation 31:356, 1965.
18. TARAZI, R. C., AND DUSTAN, H. P.: *The hemodynamics of labile hypertension,* in STRAUSS, J. (ED.): *Pediatric Nephrology.* Plenum Press, New York, 1976, p. 97.
19. HAMILTON, W. F., AND REMINGTON, J. W.: *The measurement of the stroke volume from the pressure pulse.* Am. J. Physiol. 148:14, 1947.
20. ADAMOPOULOS, P. N., CHRYSANTHAKOPOULIS, S. G., AND FROHLICH, E. D.: *Systolic hypertension: nonhomogeneous diseases.* Am. J. Cardiol. 36:697, 1975.
21. BRIGGS, T., SCOTT, F. R., AND MORRISON, E. S.: *Cell proliferation and bio-energetics in aorta and myocardium of spontaneously hypertensive rats.* Circulation 48:IV-149, 1973.
22. CONWAY, J., AND SMITH, K. S.: *Aging of arteries in relation to hypertension.* Circulation 15:827, 1957.
23. ABBOUD, F. M., AND HUSTON, J. H.: *Measurement of arterial aging in hypertensive patients.* J. Clin. Invest. 40:1915, 1961.
24. TARAZI, R. C., FERRARIO, C. M., AND DUSTAN, H. P.: *The heart in hypertension,* in GENEST, J., KOIW, E., AND KUCHEL, O. (EDS.): *Hypertension: Physiology and Treatment.* McGraw-Hill, New York, 1977, pp. 738–754.
25. COHN, J.: *Vasodilator therapy for heart failure: the influence of impedance on left ventricular performance.* Circulation 48:5, 1973.
26. DUSTAN, H. P.: *Atherosclerosis complicating chronic hypertension.* Circulation 50:871, 1974.
27. PICKERING, T. G., GRIBBIN, B., AND OLIVER, D. O.: *Baroreflex sensitivity in patients on long-term hemodialysis.* Clin. Sci. 43:645, 1972.
28. TARAZI, R. C., AND DUSTAN, H. P.: *Neurogenic participation in essential and renovascular hypertension. Correlation with hemodynamic indices and intravascular volume.* Clin. Sci. 44:197, 1973.

29. TARAZI, R. C., AND GIFFORD, R. W., JR.: *Drug treatment of hypertension,* in *Drugs in Cardiology.* Stratton Intercontinental Medical Book Corporation, New York, 1975, pp. 1–41.

30. BOCK, K. D., AND KREUZENBECK, W.: *Spontaneous blood pressure variations in hypertension; the effect of antihypertensive therapy and correlations with the incidence of complications,* in *Antihypertensive Therapy, An International Symposium.* New York, 1966, pp. 224–238.

31. MARSHALL, J.: *A trial of long-term hypotensive therapy in cerebrovascular disease.* Lancet 1:10, 1964.

32. CARTER, A. B.: *Hypotensive therapy in stroke survivors.* Lancet 1:485, 1970.

33. STRANDGAARD, S., OLESEN, J., SKINHOJ, E., ET AL.: *Autoregulation of brain circulation in severe arterial hypertension.* Br. Med. J. 3:507, 1973.

34. BRISTOW, J. D., HONOUR, A. J., PICKERING, G. W., ET AL.: *Diminished baroreflex sensitivity in high blood pressure.* Circulation 39:48, 1969.

35. SHARPEY-SHAFER, E. P.: *Effect of Valsalva maneuver on the normal and failing circulation.* Br. Med. J. 1:693, 1955.

36. APPENZELLER, O., AND DESCARRIES, L.: *Circulatory reflexes in patients with cerebrovascular disease.* N. Engl. J. Med. 271:820, 1964.

37. TARAZI, R. C., DUSTAN, H. P., AND BRAVO, E. L.: *Haemodynamic effects of propranolol in hypertension: a review.* Postgrad. Med. J. 52 (Suppl. 4):92, 1976.

38. EISALO, A., HEINO, A., AND MUNTER, J.: *The effect of alprenolol in elderly patients with raised blood pressure.* Acta Med. Scand. Suppl. 554:23, 1974.

39. HENNING, M.: *Studies on the mode of action of α-methyldopa.* Acta Physiol. Scand. Suppl. 322, 1969.

Borderline Hypertension: Significance and Management

Stevo Julius, M.D., Sc.D.

The term "labile hypertension" is commonly used to describe patients whose blood pressure is neither fully normal nor clearly hypertensive. This term underscores the difference from "established" hypertension, where the blood pressure is always and undeniably elevated. It is frequently misconstrued that "labile" also denotes excessive blood pressure oscillations. There is no good evidence that in an average patient with "labile" hypertension, blood pressure fluctuates more than in established hypertension or in normotensive subjects.[1] The notion of excessive blood pressure variability in "labile" hypertension has been extended into pathophysiology to assume that hypertension stems from multiple and repetitive pressor episodes which eventually induce changes in the vascular wall and lead to permanent hypertension. This assumption has not been critically tested. Attempts to predict the development of future hypertension from increased blood pressure responsiveness to various pressor stimuli in "labile" hypertension have failed.[1] In animal experiments, excessive blood pressure variability induced by removal of arterial baroreceptors[2] does not lead to permanent hypertension. Furthermore, it has been shown by Sokolow and coworkers[3] that the highest values or the range of blood pressure variability obtained by multiple readings in hypertensive patients do not relate to the future vascular damage; hypertensive complications are a direct consequence of the *average* blood pressure to which the blood vessels are exposed.

Because of the unwarranted and misleading connotation of excessive blood pressure lability in "labile" hypertension, we prefer to use the more descriptive term, borderline hypertension. Borderline hypertension is best defined by setting the limits for normotension and hypertension and by interpolating between these limits a zone of borderline elevated readings. Thus, a patient has borderline hypertension if the average of his multiple readings falls into the borderline range, regardless of whether individual readings are found to be occasionally in the normotensive or sometimes in the hypertensive range. The following limits for adults appear to be reasonable:

> *Normotension* — age 17 to 40, blood pressure <140/90; age 41 to 60, blood pressure <150/90; age over 60, blood pressure <160/90.
> *Hypertension* — age 17 to 60, blood pressure > 160/100; age over 60, blood pressure > 170/100.
> *Borderline Hypertension* — readings between the hypertensive and normotensive range.

SIGNIFICANCE

Borderline hypertension is a frequent clinical problem. It is estimated that over 18 million people in the United States have borderline blood pressure readings.[4]

Practicing physicians almost daily must decide how much diagnostic workup is needed and whether treatment is indicated in individual patients with borderline hypertension. Unfortunately the medical literature provides very little guidance for practical management of patients with borderline hypertension. Consequently, the approach to such patients varies a great deal and ranges from extreme concern to total neglect.

The purpose of this chapter is to develop a rational approach to the management of borderline hypertension. The basis for this approach is in the assessment of the clinical significance of borderline hypertension. After reviewing the literature, the following picture of the significance of borderline hypertension emerges: (1) borderline hypertension carries an increased risk for future established hypertension (Table 1); (2) mortality in borderline hypertension is increased (Fig. 1); but (3) the absolute level of the risk is not overwhelming. For example, it is true that previous borderline hypertensive patients later develop established hypertension three times as frequently as their normotensive counterparts but it is also true that only a minority of the whole group will in fact develop the disease (Table 1).

These facts are at the root of the clinical dilemma of borderline hypertension. Should one consider an increased risk of morbidity, regardless of how high the risk is, as sufficient ground for medical intervention? Or, would it be appropriate to disregard the slightly increased risk? There are no authoritative answers to these questions, but one

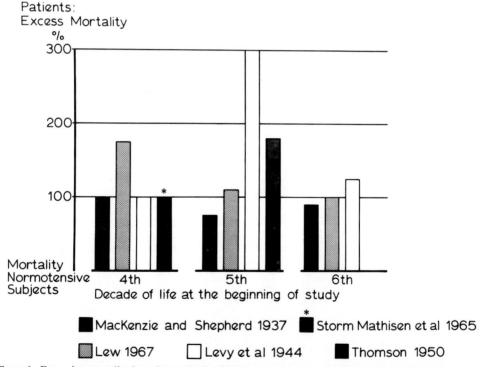

Figure 1. Excessive mortality in patients with borderline hypertension in various studies. Patients' mortality is compared to the age-adjusted mortality of the general population. (Courtesy of The American Journal of Cardiology.[15])

Table 1. Development of sustained hypertension in patients with borderline hypertension

| Study | Initial pressure | | Final pressure ("Hypertension") | Average length of followup (years) | Average initial age (years) | Percent hypertensive | |
	Normal	Borderline				Initially normal	Initially borderline
Males[5]	Systolic <140 Diastolic <79	Systolic 140–149 Diastolic 90–99	Doctor diagnosed high blood pressure	22–31	19	7.3	20.2
Males[6]	Systolic <140 Diastolic <90	Systolic 140–159 Diastolic 90–94	Clinical essential hypertension Diastolic >95	10+	20–24	1.0 2.3	5.0 7.5
Males[7]	Diastolic <90	Diastolic >90	Diastolic >95 at age 50	20–30	20–30	9.5	24.6
Males[8]	Always <150/<90	Systolic >150 or diastolic >90 followed by ≤ 150 or ≤ 90	Systolic >150 or diastolic >90, sustained	5 5 5 5	25 35 45 55	0.05 0.17 0.57 1.49	0.24 0.56 2.20 4.80
Males[9]	<140/<90	>140/>90	Systolic >150 and/or diastolic >90 at age 40	20	20	12.0	26.0
Males[10]	<139/89	140/90 to 159/94	>160/95	15–20	15–29 30–44	6.1 12.8	10.8 25.5

HYPERTENSION

can arrive at some reasonable projections. Figure 2 is based on the proven efficacy of treatment of mild hypertension in the VA Cooperative Study[16] and on the average incidence of established hypertension in patients with previous borderline hypertension.[1] It can be seen in the figure that over five years only 10 of 100 patients with borderline hypertension would develop hypertension. Only in these 10 would the prevalence of cardiovascular complications be similar to the VA study; consequently, only in them could we expect a similar efficacy of treatment as described in the VA study. It follows that the treatment would be effective in only 4 out of 100 patients. Ninety-six percent of all treated patients would not benefit from the medication. It is obvious that the yield is too low and that unrestricted treatment of all patients with borderline hypertension is not justified. The deductions in Figure 2 are simplifed; the actual situation is more complex. Thus, some morbidity may occur in patients who remain borderline and antihypertensive treatment could conceivably be of some value also in these patients. On the whole, however, the projection in Figure 2 is weighted in favor of treatment. It is assumed that all 10 potential hypertensive patients will develop the disease in the first year and thus benefit from five full years of treatment. The problem of compliance with the treatment has been disregarded; in a general population of asymptomatic patients, the patient compliance could not conceivably approach the levels achieved in the VA study. In the VA study, potentially uncompliant patients have been removed from the study; a whole logistic apparatus to secure patients' cooperation was developed and the patients were highly motivated.

In summary, projections in Figure 2 speak against introduction of antihypertensive treatment in all patients with borderline hypertension. An attempt must be made to

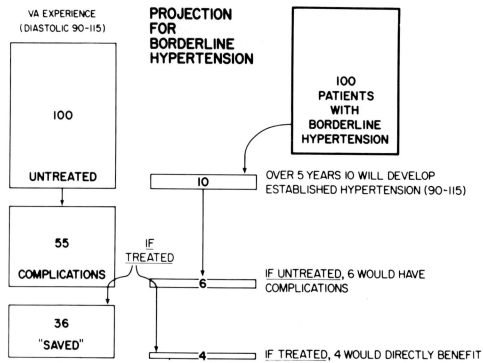

Figure 2. A graphic presentation of the experience of the Veterans Administration Study [16] on effects of treatment in mild hypertension (left panel). The Veterans Administration data are used in the right panel to project the effectiveness of treatment in borderline hypertension.

34

uncover those individual patients who are at the highest risk for development of hypertension and its cardiovascular complications. In these individuals the treatment may be warranted.

IDENTIFICATION OF THE HIGH-RISK PATIENTS

High risk in borderline hypertension can be defined as risk for atherosclerotic cardiovascular changes and the risk for future sustained hypertension. The risk factors for atherosclerosis are well-studied and their importance is generally accepted. The exact relationship between all the atherosclerosis risk factors and borderline hypertension is not clear. In some instances, addition of risk for atherosclerosis to borderline hypertension results in excessive morbidity. For example, in a patient with borderline hypertension who also has elevated cholesterol, the risk for coronary heart disease exceeds the risk which could be expected from simple addition of cholesterol and the borderline hypertension risks.[17] A similar relationship may exist between other risk factors for atherosclerosis (elevated triglycerides, elevated blood sugar, high uric acid, and smoking) and borderline hypertension. A combination of borderline hypertension with risk factors for atherosclerosis, therefore, should be considered as one of the indications for treatment of borderline hypertension.

The other indication for treatment in borderline hypertension is the presence of risk factors for development of established hypertension. Only a few specific risk factors for the development of future hypertension are recognized. These are blood pressure levels,[18] family history,[19] race,[20] overweight,[7] and tachycardia.[5, 21] Of these, blood pressure levels and tachycardia deserve further comment.

BLOOD PRESSURE LEVELS. Even within the range of borderline blood pressure readings, a higher blood pressure level significantly increases the chances of development of future hypertension. It has been shown that individuals whose blood pressure is in the upper range of normal show a steeper increase of blood pressure with age.[18] It is therefore very important to obtain reliable blood pressure readings. For purposes of better classification of borderline hypertension, it is advisable to obtain an average of a number of repeated blood pressure readings. We teach the subjects to take their own blood pressure two times daily over seven consecutive days. When these readings are averaged, a patient with borderline hypertension can be better described.[22] About 30 percent of patients will have values exceeding two standard deviations above the mean of the normotensive subjects. It stands to reason that these "hypertensive at home" patients have a more serious form of borderline hypertension and may progress to later established hypertension. Another 30 percent of patients with borderline hypertension have "borderline" readings at home; their average value is between one and two standard deviations above the mean of control subjects. The rest of the patients will have normal blood pressure readings at home. In spite of various blood pressure levels at home, all patients with borderline hypertension appeared rather similar. Thus during the clinical examination,[22] average systolic and diastolic blood pressures taken in the clinic on three different days, and the patient's weight and heart rate were similar in those who at home were normotensive or hypertensive. Repeated home blood pressure readings, therefore, provided an independent tool for further classification of patients with borderline hypertension. What might happen if repeated blood pressure readings are not taken, and only spot readings are obtained, is shown in Figure 3. In this study,[23] casual blood pressures were taken every second year on three different occasions. Roughly one third of patients who initially had borderline hypertension "developed" hypertension two years later. Two years after this second measurement, the percentage of hypertension was the same but the "hypertensive" group now consisted of different individuals. Half of the subjects who were hypertensive at the second examination did

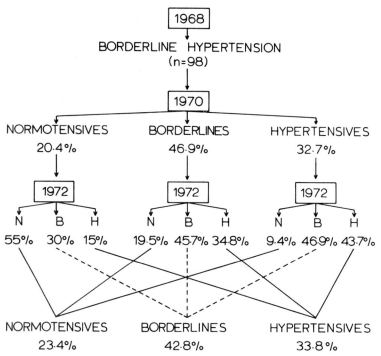

Figure 3. Experience with three blood pressure measurements performed in the same individuals over a period of four years in East Berlin.[23] Lowest of two sitting casual readings is reported. Borderline hypertension = systolic of 140–158 and/or diastolic of 90–94; hypertension = blood pressure ≥160/96. (Courtesy of Dr. K. H. Günther.)

not show "hypertension" during the third examination. It can be seen in Figure 3 that during the final examination a large crossover occurred also among those who at the second examination were described as "normotensive" or borderline.

HEART RATE. The presence of tachycardia in patients with borderline hypertension is usually thought to be a benign sign. It is assumed that if a subject has a rapid heart rate in the office, he is "only anxious" and his blood pressure is "falsely" elevated. The fact that with prolonged rest the blood pressure of such a patient may become normal is usually seen as proof of a particularly good prognosis. Smirk's assumption that the lowest so-called "basal" blood pressure level to which the blood pressure may decrease determines the patient's prognosis is erroneous.[24] In the study by Sokolow and coworkers,[3] the lowest blood pressure reading bore no relationship to an individual's prognosis; complications were a result of the prevailing *average* blood pressure. Consequently, even if it were proven that patients with tachycardia tend to have a normal blood pressure at rest, this in itself would not be indicative of a favorable prognosis.

Contrary to the popular belief, tachycardia is in fact an independent risk factor for development of future hypertension.[5, 17, 21] This is well-illustrated in Figure 4.[21]

In this study the development of sustained hypertension over five years of observation was related to the initial heart rate and blood pressure. It is shown that subjects with transient tachycardia but normal blood pressure tend to develop more future hypertension than normotensive subjects. The level of risk from tachycardia is similar to the risk from transient blood pressure elevation. When transient tachycardia and transient hypertension occurred in the same individual, the risk for future hypertension dramatically increased.

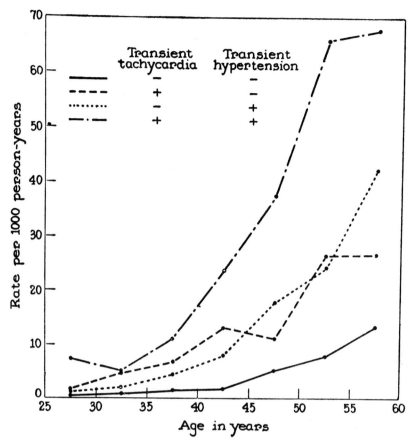

Figure 4. Rates of developing sustained hypertension by age according to the presence or absence of transient tachycardia and transient hypertension. Each age group was followed for five years. (Courtesy of J AMA.[21])

CLINICAL APPROACH TO BORDERLINE HYPERTENSION

The approach to a patient with borderline hypertension must rely on the available evidence about the natural history of borderline hypertension. The evidence of abnormally high morbidity and mortality in borderline hypertension cannot be disregarded. However, it must also be recognized that the level of risk is not sufficiently high to warrant antihypertensive treatment in *all* patients with borderline hypertension. The following principles are proposed.

1. Every patient with borderline hypertension requires continuous medical management.

2. Treatment may be desirable in some patients with borderline hypertension.

3. Treatment should be continued only if a good blood pressure response can be achieved with moderate amounts of medication and without side effects.

Management

OBSERVATION OF BLOOD PRESSURE TRENDS. It is very important to obtain numerous blood pressure levels to establish the patient's baseline. Use of home blood pressure self-determination is convenient but not mandatory. Obtaining an average of repeated

37

readings by trained observers is sufficient but the condition of measurements must be standardized, the number of readings should be sizable and the readings obtained on different days over a reasonably short period of time. It should be possible to repeat these readings at a later date under these same circumstances.

Repeat "baseline" readings should be taken annually in patients under 35 years of age and semi-annually above that age. An increase of the baseline reading of 10 mm. Hg (diastolic or systolic) over one year, or a steady increase of 5 mm./year in two consecutive years is considered significant.

PATIENT EDUCATION. Patients should be informed about the significance of borderline hypertension. Contrary to the prevailing practice, it should be made clear that indeed *there is a problem*. The patient should understand why medical attention is needed but treatment may not be necessary. The patient should record or memorize his baseline blood pressure readings. We make it a practice to point out to the patient that attitudes toward borderline hypertension vary a great deal. In our highly mobile society, the patient is likely to get confused when he encounters various physicians and receives contradictory advice. Knowledge about previous blood pressure levels under these circumstances is very useful to the patient.

CORRECTION OF RISK FACTORS. Many of the risk factors can be corrected. Overweight is frequently present and lends itself to dietary modification. Abnormal serum lipids should be corrected with specific diet and in extreme cases with the appropriate medication. Patients with chemical diabetes must be educated and put on a low-carbohydrate diet. Smoking should be discouraged in all patients with borderline hypertension.

High sodium intake has not been recognized as a prospective risk factor for hypertension. However, studies of populations with very low sodium intakes[25] indicate that chronic extreme sodium depletion is not harmful. The total absence of hypertension in such populations is impressive. Since moderate sodium restriction is not harmful and may have some preventive value against future hypertension, low-sodium diet is routinely recommended. The best approach is to identify in a patient the areas for correction, such as routine addition of salt before tasting, use of canned soups, crackers, pickles and similar gross dietary indiscretions. Removal of these, rather than a rigid but unenforceable diet, is the primary goal.

Physical exercise is of no proven value in borderline hypertension, but it may be helpful in weight control and may contribute to the patient's general feeling of well being.

Treatment

The objective of treatment in borderline hypertension is to achieve a blood pressure lowering of at least 10 mm. Hg (diastolic or systolic). This will bring the blood pressure close to the median blood pressure of the normotensive population.

Certain principles must be developed as a guide for treatment. First, the treatment of borderline hypertension should not be aggressive. The expected benefit is too low to use the system of increasing dosages and multiple medications usually applied in established hypertension. A single drug regimen in moderate doses is preferred. The term "moderate doses of medication" is used advisedly; the choice of medication will very much depend on the physician's preference. In the University of Michigan's Hypertension Clinic, either chlorthalidone, 50 mg./day, or propranolol, up to 120 mg./day, is preferred. If the treatment causes subjective side effects or substantial biochemical changes, it should not be applied. Second, a trial period must be instituted to evaluate the effectiveness and side effects. The possible outcome must be explained to the patient in advance so that he does not perceive the discontinuation of treatment after the trial period as treatment failure or conversely as "cure" of his hypertension. The third therapeutic principle relates to the continuity of the treatment. Once past the trial period the patient should be maintained on medication for years; the treatment aims to prevent complications which develop slowly over a long period of time. The fourth therapeutic principle calls for periodic reassessment. Since borderline hypertension does not uniformly lead to hypertension, and spontaneous regression of the blood pressure toward lower values can be expected, it is reasonable to discontinue the treatment every second year and reevaluate the management program on these occasions. The criteria for selection for treatment are given in Table 2.

The proposed regimen takes into consideration the following elements: (1) complications in borderline hypertension and rate of progression to essential hypertension depend on the severity of the initial blood pressure elevation; (2) there is no evidence that patients with late-onset borderline hypertension are more morbidity-prone; (3) complications are a function of time; and (4) risk factors contribute to the severity of complications. Consequently three groups of severity of borderline hypertension are recognized. In the group with highest readings (> 140/90) treatment should be attempted. In the intermediate group (140–130/80–90) the treatment is considered at a younger age (since the life expectancy is sufficiently long to anticipate complications). Presence of risk factors in these patients enters into the therapeutic decision. In the very mild group (<130/80) special procedures for assessment of the baseline are recommended. In our opinion the use of home blood pressures in these cases is indispensable.

Table 2. Flow sheet for treatment of borderline hypertension

Step I
a. Physical examination
Funduscopy
Signs of left ventricular hypertrophy
b. Laboratory examination
ECG
Chest x-ray
Urine, creatinine
Lipids, FBS
c. Obtain home blood pressure readings seven
days, each morning and evening

Step II	
Attempt Treatment	*Observe BP Trends One a Year If . . .*
a. Average home BP >140/90	a. Average home BP <130/80
b. Average home BP 130–140/80–90	b. Average home BP 130–140/80–90
Patient under age 50	Patient over 50 years of age
Family history positive, *or*	
Family history negative but	
two other risk factors	

Step III	
a. If no side effects and BP −10 mm.	a. If after a year BP up 10 mm. Hg,
−continue for two years	attempt treatment
−reassess	
b. If no response or side effects,	b. If after a year BP up 5 mm. Hg,
follow semi-annually; if BP	repeat readings in six months
up 5 mm. Hg, treat more vigorously	

Consideration must also be given to signs of pressure-related target organ involvement. Signs of cardiac hypertrophy, grade I – II retinopathy, and/or slight depression of renal function mandate treatment at any blood pressure level.

CONCLUSIONS

The management and treatment of borderline hypertension must reflect our knowledge of the natural history of the condition. Patients with this condition are at a higher risk for hypertension-related morbidity and mortality. The risk, however, is not sufficient to warrant treatment in every individual. In view of the absence of clear results about the effectiveness of treatment in these patients, an active but not overly aggressive approach is proposed. The cornerstone of this approach is the physician's responsibility to continuously monitor all patients and the need to apply the treatment to a selected minority of patients who are at highest risk or to those individuals who have shown signs of progression of the disease.

REFERENCES

1. JULIUS, S., AND SCHORK, M. A.: *Borderline hypertension—A critical review.* J. Chronic Dis. 23:723, 1971.
2. COWLEY, S. W., JR., LIARD, J. F., AND GUYTON, A. C.: *Role of the baroreceptor reflex in daily control of arterial blood pressure and other variables in dogs.* Circ. Res. 32:564, 1973.
3. SOKOLOW, M., WEDEGAR, D., KAIN, H. K., ET AL.: *Relationship between level of blood pressure measured casually and by portable recorder, and severity of complications in essential hypertension.* Circulation 34:279, 1966.
4. JULIUS, S.: *Borderline hypertension: definitions and treatment.* Cardiovasc. Med. 1:77, 1976.
5. PAFFENBARGER, R. S., JR., THORNE, M. C., AND WING, A. L.: *Chronic disease in former college students—VII. Characteristics in youth predisposing to hypertension in later years.* Am. J. Epidemiol. 88: 25, 1968.
6. KOOPERSTEIN, S. I., SCHIFRIN, A., AND LEAHY, T. J.: *Level of initial blood pressure and subsequent development of essential hypertension: A 10 and 15 year follow-up study.* Am. J. Cardiol. 10:416, 1962.
7. STAMLER, J., LINDBERG, H. A., BERKSON, D. M., ET AL.: *Epidemiological analysis of hypertension and hypertensive disease in the labor force of a Chicago utility company.* Proc. Coun. High Blood Press. Res. 7:23, 1958.
8. LEVY, R. L., HILLMAN, C. C., STROUD, W. D., ET AL.: *Transient hypertension: Its significance in terms of later development of sustained hypertension and cardiovascular diseases.* JAMA 126:829, 1944.
9. JULIUS, S., HARBURG, E., MCGINN, N. F., ET AL.: *Relation between casual blood pressure readings in youth and at age 40: A retrospective study.* J. Chronic Dis. 17:397, 1964.
10. MATHEWSON, F. A.: *Blood pressure in Canadian aviators: A fifteenth year report.* Trans. Ass. Life Insur. Med. Dir. 50:219, 1966.
11. MATHISEN, H. S., LOKEN, H., BROX, D., ET AL.: *The prognosis in essential hypertension.* Scand. J. Clin. Lab. Invest. 17 (Suppl. 84):257, 1965.
12. LEW, E. A.: *Blood pressure and mortality—Life insurance experience,* in STAMLER, J., STAMLER, R., AND PULLMAN, T. N. (EDS.): *The Epidemiology of Hypertension: Proceedings of an International Symposium,* Grune & Stratton, New York, 1967, p. 392.
13. MACKENZIE, L. F., AND SHEPHERD, P.: *The significance of past hypertension in applicants later presenting normal average blood pressure.* Proc. Ass. Life Insur. Med. Dir. Am. 24:157, 1937.
14. THOMSON, K. J.: *Some observations on the development and course of hypertensive vascular disease.* Proc. Ann. Meet. Med. Sec. Am. Life Convention 38:85, 1950.
15. JULIUS, S., AND ESLER, M.: *Autonomic nervous cardiovascular regulation in borderline hypertension.* Am. J. Cardiol. 36:685, 1975.
16. VETERANS ADMINISTRATION COOPERATIVE STUDY GROUP ON ANTIHYPERTENSIVE AGENTS: *Effects of treatment on morbidity in hypertension. II. Results in patients with diastolic blood pressure averaging 90 – 114 mm. Hg.* JAMA 213:1143, 1970.
17. STAMLER, J., BERKSON, D. M., DYER, A., ET AL.: *Relationship of multiple variables to blood pressure,* in

PAUL, O. (ED.): *Epidemiology and control of Hypertension*, Symposia Specialists, Miami, 1975, p. 307.

18. HARLAN, W. R., OSBORNE, R. K., AND GRAYBIEL, A.: *Longitudinal study of blood pressure*. Circulation 26:530, 1962.

19. THOMAS, C. B., ROSS, D. C., AND HIGGENBOTTOM, C. Q.: *Precursors of hypertension and coronary disease among healthy medical students. Discriminant function analysis II using parental history as the criterion*. Bull. Johns Hopkins Hosp. 115:245, 1964.

20. NATIONAL CENTER FOR HEALTH STATISTICS: *Blood pressure of adults by race and area, United States, 1960–1962, Vital and Health Statistics*. PHS Pub. No. 1000–Series 11, No. 5. Public Health Service, Washington, D.C., July, 1964.

21. LEVY, R. L., WHITE, P. D., STROUD, W. D., ET AL.: *Transient tachycardia: Prognostic significance alone and in association with transient hypertension*. JAMA 129:585, 1945.

22. JULIUS, S., ELLIS, C. N., PASCUAL, A. V., ET AL.: *Home blood pressure determination: Value in borderline ("labile") hypertension*. JAMA 229:663, 1974.

23. LINSS, G., GÜNTHER, K. H., AND BÖTHIG, S.: *Normotension or hypertension, part 3*. (German) Dtsch. Gesundheitsw. 29:635, 1964.

24. SMIRK, F. H.: *High Arterial Pressure*. Oxford, Blackwell, 1957.

25. FREIS, E. D.: *Salt, volume and the prevention of hypertension*, Circulation 53:589, 1976.

Low-Renin Hypertension: Classification, Mechanisms and Therapy*

Gordon P. Guthrie, Jr., M.D., Jacques Genest, M.D., Otto Kuchel, M.D., Wojciech Nowaczynski, D.Sc., and Roger Boucher, Ph.D.

In the continuing effort to identify pathogenic mechanisms in patients with essential hypertension, attention has been focused on subgroups defined by characteristic features. One such feature is plasma renin activity (PRA)[1,2] which is low and unresponsive to the stimulus of sodium restriction or depletion. Patients with low-renin hypertension (synonymous with hyporeninemic hypertension or a suppressed or hyporesponsive PRA) have a renin secretion resistant to stimulatory maneuvers similar to patients with primary aldosteronism,[3] and this resemblance is one reason for the interest in this subgroup. Other reasons stimulating study are suggestions that therapy for the hypertension might be specifically tailored to this group, and that the low-renin classification may have implications for morbidity or mortality. All these areas remain controversial and unsettled, perhaps related in part to the problems of defining low renin hypertension.

CLASSIFICATION

Since it is difficult to identify low-renin hypertensive subjects in the basal state on a normal sodium intake, most investigators employ some form of stimulation to renin secretion, and the wide variety of maneuvers used to define this subgroup has led to some problems in comparing the low-renin patients of different reports. The most commonly employed stimulation is a low-sodium diet, normally about 10 mM. per day for 3 to 5 days, combined with 3 to 4 hours of upright posture prior to the PRA determination, as used by our group.[4] Because of the inconvenience, time and expense of prolonged in-hospital dietary sodium restriction, more convenient methods are usually used, often involving diuretics. Such protocols involve oral furosemide with an upright PRA measured several hours after either one dose of the drug (e.g., 60 mg. as described by Wallach, et al.[5]) or several doses (e.g., 40 mg. every 6 hours × 3 as described by Carey, et al.[6]). Another method recently reported by Kaplan and coworkers[7] uses 40 mg. of intravenous furosemide with the PRA measured 30 minutes later. This timing is based on previous observation that furosemide administered intravenously in this dose, attains a maximum effect after approximately 30 minutes.[8] The intravenous furosemide test shows apparently good correlation of the PRA and identifies the low-renin subgroup compared to subsequent standard dietary sodium restriction, although intravenous furosemide may be an unreliable stimulus if the PRA is measured much

*This work was supported by the group grant of Medical Research Council of Canada to the multidisciplinary research group in hypertension.

beyond 2 hours.[9] Another renin-stimulating agent is chlorthalidone (100 mg. daily) given for several days[10, 11] which again correlates well with the dietary technique. While it appears to have a lower incidence of adverse effects than oral furosemide, it does not always identify precisely the same low renin patients as the other techniques.[10]

A key element in the identification of low-renin essential hypertensive patients is the comparison group used to define the normal range for the stimulated PRA value. The technique of "renin-sodium indexing"[12] (using the corresponding PRA and 24 hour urinary sodium excretion) is often insufficiently discriminating, especially at levels of sodium intakes above 100 mM./day. Also important is the matching of the control (comparison) group for age, sex and race, all of which may influence the PRA, as discussed below. Of the variables affecting interpretation of the PRA, the factors of sodium and volume and of sympathetic nervous system activity are probably the most important and usually the least well controlled.

Using diets or diuretics, most investigators have found that approximately 20 to 30 percent of essential hypertensive patients may be classified as having low-renin hypertension, with several qualifications. The incidence of low-renin hypertension increases with age,[13-16] varying from around 7 percent in the patients in their 20s to nearly 40 percent in those in their 50s.[4, 13] Also, many reports have found the incidence of low renin hypertension to be higher both in women,[17] possibly reflecting lower mean PRA values in normotensive women, and in blacks,[7, 18] also possibly related to the subresponsiveness of normotensive blacks.[7] The most disturbing observation in the interpretation of studies of low-renin hypertension, however, is that this classification may not be consistent. The circadian rhythm of renin secretion,[18] prior drug therapy,[20] or simply the passage of time[21, 22] may change the classification of a patient from a low to normal renin subgroup. With strict criteria, the incidence of low-renin hypertension does not usually exceed 5 to 9 percent of all essential hypertensive patients.[22] Since the chosen technique may affect the reproducibility of classification (with renin-sodium indexing apparently the least reliable[23]), reported observations of tailored therapeutic responses or effects on morbidity should be interpreted cautiously, especially in view of the apparent ability of patients to shift subgroups.

DIFFERENTIAL DIAGNOSIS

Although low-renin essential hypertension comprises a substantial albeit small fraction of patients with essential hypertension, a number of important syndromes characterized by excessive adrenal corticosteroid secretion possess this marker. These syndromes, however, usually differ from low-renin essential hypertension by other biochemical and clinical correlates of mineralocorticoid excess, especially hypokalemia.

Primary aldosteronism is the most common secondary low-renin hypertension (incidence of about 1 percent of the hypertensive population) and usually appears in one of two forms: an aldosterone-producing adrenal adenoma (75 percent of cases) or bilateral adrenal hyperplasia (25 percent of cases). These two varieties of primary hyperaldosteronism cannot be reliably distinguished by clinical criteria and both are characterized by a low PRA associated with an elevated aldosterone secretory or excretory rate or a plasma aldosterone level not suppressible by saline or exogenous mineralocorticoid treatment.[24] Although both types may be medically treated with spironolactone and/or thiazide therapy, usually only adrenal adenomas respond well to surgery,[25] and thus preoperative differentiation is important. Bilateral adrenal vein catheterization with aldosterone measurements and adrenal venography are currently the most reliable tools, with adrenal scanning using [131]I-19-iodocholesterol, a promising new noninvasive technique.[26] Much rarer cases of primary aldosteronism include "glucocorticoid-suppressible" forms and those induced by malignancies.

Other less common forms of mineralocorticoid excess causing low-renin hypertension include the congenital adrenocortical enzymatic deficiencies, i.e., congenital adrenal hyperplasia. Deficiency of 17α-hydroxylase causes hypertension with elevated plasma levels of deoxycorticosterone (DOC), corticosterone and 18-hydroxycorticosterone and is associated with primary amenorrhea in the female or pseudohermaphrodism in the male.[27] Deficiency of 11β-hydroxylase[28] causes excessive DOC and 11-deoxycortisol production, with virilization of the affected children. Glucocorticoid therapy of both varieties of enzymatic deficiencies cures the hypertension and electrolyte disturbances by suppressing the excessive ACTH drive to these mineralocorticoids.

Isolated adrenal overproduction of DOC specifically in low-renin hypertension has been reported by some groups[29] but not by others,[30] as has secretion of the weak mineralocorticoid (1/70 the sodium-retaining potency of aldosterone) 18-OH-DOC.[31] But since both secretory rates[32] and plasma levels[33] of the latter steroid are higher than normal in normal renin essential hypertensive patients as well, the precise relation of 18-OH-DOC to low-renin hypertension is unclear.

POSTULATED MECHANISMS

Mineralocorticoid Excess

Interest in the low-renin subgroup originates in part from the possibility that the suppressed PRA may result from a mineralocorticoid excess, either aldosterone or some other unidentified steroid. The published evidence for this hypothesis is inconclusive and often contradictory. The indirect positive evidence includes some reports of increased extracellular fluid volume,[34] exchangeable sodium space[30] and blood volume[35] in low-renin hypertension, although a review of all data fails to uniformly support volume expansion in such patients,[1] certainly not to the same degree as in primary aldosteronism. The reports of decreased salivary sodium to potassium ratios,[36] favorable therapeutic responses to nonspecific inhibition of adrenocorticoid biosynthesis,[30] or competitive antagonism to mineralocorticoid receptors[37] are further indirect support, as is a demonstrated mutual positive correlation of 18-OH-DOC, DOC and corticosterone secretory rates only in low-renin hypertension,[38] suggesting a fundamental alteration in adrenal pathways and in mineralocorticoid synthesis in this subgroup.

Efforts to directly identify excessive excretion of new mineralocorticoids in low-renin hypertension have yielded mixed results. Sennett and colleagues[39] isolated a novel steroid, 16β-OH-dehydroepiandrosterone, from the urine of such patients and found it to possess mineralocorticoid activity in adrenalectomized rats,[40] an effect not confirmed by other workers. Furthermore, this compound has been noted[41] to lack the ability to bind to mineralocorticoid receptors of kidney slices. Recent work suggests that this steroid originates from hepatic 16β-hydroxylation of circulating dehydroepiandrosterone.[42]

As already mentioned, some low-renin hypertensive patients secrete excessive quantities of 18-OH-DOC and some studies suggest that a hydroxylated metabolite of this compound, 16α-18-dihydroxy-DOC, may act as a "positive allosteric factor,"[43] amplifying the mineralocorticoid effect of other steroids such as aldosterone. The latter concept, however, has not been confirmed.[44]

The search for "cryptic mineralocorticoid" has been kept alive by the occasional reporting of cases of low-renin hypertension (usually in children) with overt evidence of mineralocorticoid excess in which no measurable steroid seems responsible.[45]

Some evidence suggests that the postulated mineralocorticoid excess of low-renin hypertension is in fact a mild inappropriate hyperaldosteronism. Aldosterone secretion in such patients does not normally decrease with sodium loading[46] or appropriately increase after volume depletion,[13] and mean plasma aldosterone levels are slightly but significantly higher in this group (Fig. 1). Some workers feel that low-renin hypertension is in fact a variant form or early phase of primary aldosteronism,[47] supported by the high incidence of adrenal abnormalities found in such patients.[48] That the secretion of aldosterone is either normal or only slightly lower in the face of marked suppression of the PRA[49, 50] supports the possibility of either relative autonomy or another trophic factor to aldosterone secretion in low-renin hypertensive patients. In fact, some apparent evidence for a cryptic mineralocorticoid can be interpreted as supporting a primary role for aldosterone in the pathogenesis of low-renin hypertension. For example, the favorable response to aminoglutethimide[30] has been found to correlate only with inhibition of aldosterone secretion,[51, 52] the secretion rates of other steroids being maintained despite the inhibitor by a compensatory ACTH increase.

Evidence against a hypermineralocorticoid state from a cryptic steroid includes the failure to detect increased *in vitro* mineralocorticoid activity in the plasma of such patients by a renal receptor radioassay.[52] In addition, low-renin patients who become normotensive on high dose spironolactone therapy do not have changes in measurements of mineralocorticoid activity (e.g., total body potassium) different from low-renin patients not responding to this drug.[53]

Thus, evidence for a state of excess mineralocorticoid activity in low-renin hyper-

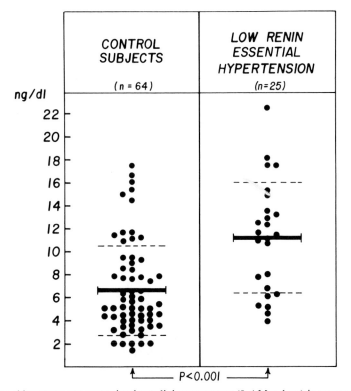

Figure 1. Plasma aldosterone concentration by radioimmunoassay (9 AM values) in normotensive controls and patients with low renin essential hypertension. The solid horizontal bars denote the means and hatched lines, ± 2 S.D. n = number of subjects. Low renin essential hypertensive patients are those who have a PRA value <0.6 ng./ml./hr. in upright posture after 3 days of sodium restriction (10 mM./day).

tension, whether from aldosterone or another steroid, is unclear. That the adrenal cortex is in some way involved in essential hypertension not specifically subclassified in the renin subgroup[4] is illustrated by a recent study of the response of eight steroids to an ACTH infusion (25 units over 8 hours) in 10 hypertensive patients and 8 normals.[54] The patients had significantly greater plasma aldosterone, DOC and 11-deoxycortisol plasma levels and 18-OH-DOC secretory rates and lower corticosterone levels than the normals after ACTH. Analysis of relative adrenal hydroxylation efficiencies by intermediate steroid ratios, specifically the corticosterone/DOC ratio as an estimate of 11β-hydroxylation and the 17-OH-progesterone/progesterone ratio, to estimate 17α-hydroxylation (Fig. 2) indicates relative impairment of both hydroxylation steps in both low and normal renin subgroups compared to normals.[54] Whether these relative abnormalities in adrenal function in essential hypertension during supraphysiologic ACTH stimulation are primary or secondary is not established.

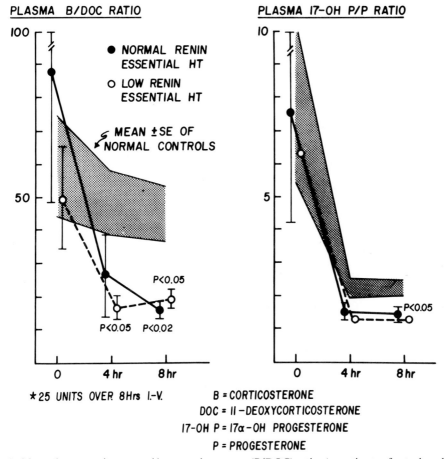

Figure 2. Mean plasma corticosterone/deoxycorticosterone (B/DOC) ratios (an estimate of net adrenal 11β-hydroxylation efficiency) and 17-OH progesterone/progesterone (17-OH P/P) ratios (an estimate of 17α-hydroxylation efficiency) in patients with essential hypertension before and 4 and 8 hours after an infusion of ACTH. The hypertensive patients are subclassified into low (open circles) and normal (solid circles) renin subgroups, and the grey areas denote the mean ± one standard error of these ratios in control subjects. All subjects in whom 17-ON P/P ratios were calculated were male, and a single low-renin patient is shown.

Sympathetic Hyporeactivity

The sympathetic nervous system, including the adrenal medulla and circulating catecholamines, has an important influence on renin release.[55, 56] Another hypothesis for the cause of low-renin hypertension is a lower sympathetic drive to renin secretion.[57] Two reports have noted in low-renin patients a blunted rise in timed urinary norepinephrine excretions[58, 59] thought to be a reflection of a general sympathetic hypoactivity, although others have not noted consistent abnormalities in catecholamine metabolites.[1] Lower mean serum dopamine β-hydroxylase levels, a biosynthetic enzyme released with norepinephrine from sympathetic neuronal vesicles, has been reported in patients with low-renin hypertension,[60] which is supporting evidence for a lower net sympathetic tone. The findings by Lowder and associates[61] of lower circulating cyclic AMP levels during insulin-provoked hypoglycemia in low-renin patients also suggest a blunted adrenergic responsiveness. Our group, using a sensitive radioenzymatic assay for plasma and urinary catecholamines, has noted[62] lower basal and furosemide-stimulated plasma catecholamine levels in low renin patients (Fig. 3). Furthermore, a relatively high basal fractional catecholamine clearance is found, indicating net addition of free catecholamines to the urine in these same low-renin patients. Assuming this higher fractional clearance reflects active tubular secretion or leakage of catecholamines into the urine from peritubular sympathetic nerve terminals, this suggests that in the basal state low-renin patients have a relatively high *focal* renal sympathetic discharge. Whether this seemingly high renal sympathetic tone concurrent with a general sympathetic hypoactivity is a primary or secondary event is not clear. The reported lower proportion of favorable therapeutic responses in these patients to high-dose propranolol[63, 64] might be related to the proposal that higher doses of propranolol lower the blood pressure by a central inhibition of sympathetic outflow.[65]

Secondary Renal Abnormality

Some workers believe that neither adrenal nor sympathetic mechanisms account for low-renin hypertension, but that renin release is suppressed as a consequence of prolonged exposure of the kidney to an elevated blood pressure.[66] Support for this hypothesis is the lack of any evidence for a distinct subpopulation with low-renin levels[67] and lack of the normal feedback relation between blood pressure and renin in hypertensive subjects.[68] The multiple confirmations that the PRA declines with age in patients with essential hypertension,[7, 11, 13-16, 67] in contrast to normotensive subjects,[13, 68] support this point (although other studies have found the PRA decreases with age in normal subjects as well).[14, 15, 69]

None of these hypotheses alone fully accounts for the low-renin essential hypertensive state,[1] and quite probably such patients are a heterogenous group.

THERAPY

The clinical value of the peripheral plasma renin determination is as controversial as the pathogenesis of low-renin hypertension.[70] Opinions are mixed concerning its usefulness as a tool to facilitate the detection of secondary or low-renin hypertension among the large number of hypertensive patients. Some reports observe that up to 40 percent of patients with renovascular hypertension may have a normal peripheral PRA[71, 72] in the recumbent position and without any stimulation by posture or sodium restriction, and that it poorly predicts postoperative prognosis. Others, however, have demonstrated the value of stimulated PRA in both detection[5] and prediction of cure[73-77] of renovascular hypertension. Its usefulness in the detection of primary aldosteronism is some-

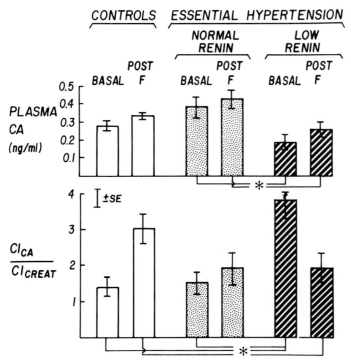

Figure 3. Mean plasma catecholamine (CA) concentrations (the sum of norepinephrine and epinephrine) and fractional clearance of CA ($Cl_{CA}/Cl_{creatinine}$) following 40 mg. of intravenous furosemide (post F) while supine in control subjects and essential hypertensive patients with normal and low plasma renin activity. $^*p < 0.05$.

what more securely established, since virtually all patients with this disorder have a low PRA.[1] The problem with PRA as a screening procedure lies in the differentiation of the large false positive group, i.e., those with low-renin essential hypertension.

Several years ago, Laragh and associates[12, 78] proposed that the renin profiling of patients with essential hypertension bore important prognostic implications. They hypothesized that the major vascular complications of essential hypertension, i.e., stroke and myocardial infarction, were related to these subgroups, with the low-renin patients at the least risk. Examination of this hypothesis in the study of large numbers of patients by other investigators has failed to support their proposal.[79, 80] In addition, the recurring point made by many investigators is that reduction of blood pressure is the goal in the treatment of hypertensive patients, regardless of their renin subgroups classification, as well as the best means of preventing cardiovascular complications.

Vigorous diuresis has been proposed as specific therapy for low-renin hypertension.[81] The bases for this rationale are the alleged expanded extracellular fluid volumes in such patients and the greater percentage of favorable responses to diuretics in low-renin patients. As has been mentioned, however, the evidence for volume-mediated hypertension in such individuals is not consistent, and all hypertensive patients, including those with renin-dependent hypertension, usually respond at least partially to diuretics.

Also, low-renin hypertension has been treated with moderate to high doses of spironolactone alone. This agent, however, has no clear advantage over other diuretics,[82, 83] and in fact has the drawbacks of greater cost and higher incidence of side effects, notably gynecomastia in males.

In summary, the detection of a consistently low renin in a hypertensive patient, when achieved in a standardized manner, can be a useful piece of diagnostic information which may prompt an indepth evaluation of adrenal steroids, especially aldosterone, but the practical impact upon therapy remains limited and doubtful. Measurement of PRA does not appear to have any value in predicting the occurrence of severe cardiovascular complications.

REFERENCES

1. DUNN, M. J., AND TANNEN, R. L.: *Low-renin hypertension.* Kidney Int. 5:317, 1974.

2. GUNNELLS, J. C., JR., AND McGUFFIN, W. L., JR.: *Low renin hypertension.* Annu. Rev. Med. 26:259, 1975.

3. CONN, J. W., COHEN, E. L., AND ROVNER, D. R.: *Suppression of plasma renin activity in primary aldosteronism: Distinguishing primary from secondary aldosteronism in hypertensive disease.* JAMA 190: 213, 1964.

4. GENEST, J., NOWACZYNSKI, W., KUCHEL, O., ET AL.: *The adrenal cortex and essential hypertension.* Recent Prog. Horm. Res. 32:377, 1976.

5. WALLACH, L., NYARAI, I., AND DAWSON, K. G.: *Stimulated renin: A screening test for hypertension.* Ann. Intern. Med. 82:27, 1975.

6. CAREY, R. M., DOUGLAS, J. G., SCHWEIKERT, R., ET AL.: *The syndrome of essential hypertension and suppressed plasma renin activity. Normalization of blood pressure with spironolactone.* Arch. Intern. Med. 130:849, 1972.

7. KAPLAN, N. M., KEM, D. C., HOLLAND, O. B., ET AL.: *The intravenous furosemide test: A simple way to evaluate renin responsiveness.* Ann. Intern. Med. 84:639, 1976.

8. ROSENTHAL, J., BOUCHER, R., NOWACZYNSKI, W., ET AL.: *Acute changes in plasma volume, renin activity, and free aldosterone levels in healthy subjects following furosemide administration.* Can. J. Physiol. Pharmacol. 46:85, 1968.

9. GENEST, J.: Unpublished data.

10. DRAYER, J. I. M., KLOPPENBORG, P. W. C., AND BENRAAD, T. J.: *Detection of low-renin hypertension; evaluation of out-patient renin-stimulating methods.* Clin. Sci. Mol. Med. 48:91, 1975.

11. WOODS, J. W., PITTMAN, A. W., PULLIAM, C. C., ET AL.: *Renin profiling in hypertension and its use in treatment with propranolol and chlorthalidone.* N. Engl. J. Med. 294:1137, 1976.

12. BRUNNER, H. R., NEWTON, M. A., GOODWIN, F. T., ET AL.: *Essential hypertension: Renin and aldosterone, heart attack and stroke.* N. Engl. J. Med. 286:441, 1972.

13. TUCK, M. L., SULLIVAN, J. M., AND DLUHY, R. G.: *Relation of age, diastolic pressure and known duration of hypertension to presence of low renin essential hypertension.* Am. J. Cardiol. 32:637, 1973.

14. SAMBHI, M. P., CRANE, M. G., AND GENEST, J.: *Essential hypertension: New concepts about mechanisms.* Ann. Intern. Med. 79:411, 1973.

15. HAYDUK, K., KRAUSE, D. K., KAUFMANN, W., ET AL.: *Age-dependent changes of plasma renin concentration in humans.* Clin. Sci. Mol. Med. 45 (suppl.):273, 1973.

16. GUTHRIE, G. P., JR., GENEST, J., NOWACZYNSKI, W., ET AL.: *Dissociation of plasma renin activity and aldosterone in essential hypertension.* J. Clin. Endocrinol. Metab. 43:446, 1976.

17. MROCZEK, W. J., FINNERTY, F. A., AND CATT, K. J.: *Lack of association between plasma renin and history of heart attack or stroke in patients with essential hypertension.* Lancet 2:464, 1973.

18. GRIM, C., WINNACKER, J., PETERS, T., ET AL: *Low renin, "normal" aldosterone and hypertension: Circadian rhythm of renin, aldosterone, cortisol and growth hormone.* J. Clin. Endocrinol. Metab. 39:247, 1974.

19. MODLINGER, R. S., AND GUTKIN, M.: *Normal plasma renin activity in low renin hypertension.* J. Clin. Endocrinol. Metab. 40:380, 1975.

20. LOWDER, S. C., AND LIDDLE, G. W.: *Prolonged alteration of renin responsiveness after spironolactone therapy. A case of false-negative testing for low-renin hypertension.* N. Engl. J. Med. 291:1243, 1974.

21. CRANE, M. G., HARRIS, J. J., AND JOHNS, V. J., JR.: *Hyporeninemic hypertension.* Am. J. Med. 52:457, 1972.

22. GENEST, J., NOWACZYNSKI, W., BOUCHER, R., ET AL.: *Aldosterone and renin in essential hypertension.* Can. Med. Assoc. J. 113:421, 1975.

23. LOWDER, S. C., AND LIDDLE, G. W.: *Interpretation of low renin profile.* N. Engl. J. Med. 292:1350, 1975.

24. HORTON, R.: *Aldosterone: Review of its physiology and diagnostic aspects of primary aldosteronism.* Metabolism 22:1525, 1973.

25. Melby, J. C.: *Solving the adrenal lesions of primary aldosteronism.* N. Engl. J. Med. 294:441, 1976.

26. Hogan, M. J., McRae, J., Schambelan, M., et al.: *Location of aldosterone-producing adenomas with* ^{131}I-*19-iodocholesterol.* N. Engl. J. Med. 292:410, 1976.

27. Biglieri, E. G., Herron, M. D., and Brust, N.: *17α-hydroxylation deficiency in man.* J. Clin. Invest. 45:1946, 1966.

28. Biglieri, E. G., Stockigt, J. R., and Schambelan, M.: *Adrenal mineralocorticoids causing hypertension.* Am. J. Med. 52:623, 1972.

29. Brown, J. J., Ferriss, J. B., Fraser, R., et al.: *Apparently isolated excess deoxycorticosterone in hypertension: A variant of the mineralocorticoid excess syndrome.* Lancet 2:243, 1972.

30. Woods, J. W., Liddle, G. W., Stant, E. G., Jr., et al.: *Effect of an adrenal inhibitor in hypertensive patients with suppressed renin.* Arch. Intern. Med. 123:366, 1969.

31. Melby, J. C., Dale, S. L., and Wilson, T. E.: *18-hydroxy-deoxycorticosterone in human hypertension.* Circ. Res. 28 & 29 (Suppl. 2):143, 1971.

32. Nowaczynski, W., Kuchel, O., and Genest, J.: *Aldosterone, deoxycorticosterone, 18-hydroxydeoxycorticosterone and progesterone in benign essential hypertension,* in Paul, O. (ed.): *Epidemiology and Control of Hypertension.* Symposia Specialists, Miami, 1976, p. 265.

33. Williams, G. H., Bradley, L. M., and Underwood, R. H.: *The regulation of plasma 18-hydroxydeoxycorticosterone in man.* J. Clin. Invest. 58:221, 1976.

34. Jose, A., Crout, J. R., and Kaplan, N. M.: *Suppressed plasma renin activity in essential hypertension.* Ann. Intern. Med. 72:9, 1970.

35. Helmer, O. M., and Judson, E. W.: *Metabolic studies on hypertensive patients with suppressed plasma renin activity not due to hyperaldosteronism.* Circulation 38:965, 1968.

36. Adlin, E. V., Channick, B. J., and Marks, A. D.: *Salivary sodium-potassium ratio and plasma renin activity in hypertension.* Circulation 39:685, 1969.

37. Crane, M. G., and Harris, J. J.: *Effect of spironolactone in hypertensive patients.* Am. J. Med. Sci. 260:311, 1970.

38. Messerli, F. H., Kuchel, O., Nowaczynski, W., et al.: *Mineralocorticoid secretion in essential hypertension with normal and low plasma renin activity.* Circulation 53:406, 1976.

39. Sennett, J. A., Brown, R. D., Island, D. P., et al.: *Evidence for a new mineralocorticoid in patients with low-renin essential hypertension.* Circ. Res. 36 (Suppl. 1):2, 1975.

40. Komanicky, P., and Melby, J. C.: *Production of hypertension by 16β-dehydroepiandrosterone in the rat.* Clin. Res. 24:273A, 1976.

41. Funder, J. W., Robinson, J. A., Feldman, D., et al.: *16β-Hydroxydehydroepiandrosterone: the dichotomy between renal receptor binding and urinary electrolyte activity.* Endocrinology 99:619, 1976.

42. Nowaczynski, W., Messerli, F. H., Kuchel, O., et al.: *Origin of urinary 16β-hydroxy-dehydroepiandrosterone in essential hypertension.* J. Clin. Endocrinol. Metab. 44:629, 1977.

43. Melby, J. C., and Dale, S. L.: *Adrenal steroidogenesis in "low renin" or hyporeninemic hypertension.* J. Steroid Biochem. 6:761, 1975.

44. Fuller, P. J., Pressley, L., Adam, W. R., et al.: *16α-18-dihydroxydeoxycorticosterone and the binding of aldosterone to mineralocorticoid receptors in kidney of adrenalectomized rats.* J. Steroid Biochem. 7:387, 1976.

45. Sann, L., Revol, A., Zachmann, M., et al.: *Unusual low plasma renin hypertension in a child.* J. Clin. Endocrinol. Metab. 43:265, 1976.

46. Collins, D. R., Weinberger, M. H., Dowdy, A. J., et al.: *Abnormally sustained aldosterone secretion during salt loading in patients with various forms of benign hypertension: Relation to plasma renin.* J. Clin. Invest. 49:1415, 1970.

47. Grim, C. E.: *Low renin "essential" hypertension: A variant of classic primary aldosteronism?* Arch. Intern. Med. 135:347, 1975.

48. Gunnells, J. C., Jr., McGuffin, W. L., Robinson, R. R., et al.: *Hypertension, adrenal abnormalities, and alterations in plasma renin activity.* Ann. Intern. Med. 73:901, 1970.

49. Laragh, J. H., Sealey, J., and Brunner, H. R.: *The control of aldosterone secretion in normal and hypertensive man: Abnormal renin-aldosterone patterns in low renin hypertension.* Am. J. Med. 53:649, 1972.

50. Bühler, F. R., Laragh, J. H., Sealey, J., et al.: *Plasma aldosterone-renin interrelationships in various forms of essential hypertension.* Am. J. Cardiol. 32:554, 1973.

51. Mancheno-Rico, E., Kuchel, O., Nowaczynski, W., et al.: *A dissociated effect of amino-glutethimide on the mineralocorticoid secretion in man.* Metabolism 22:123, 1973.

52. BAXTER, J. D., SCHAMBELAN, M., MATULICH, D. T., ET AL.: *Aldosterone receptors and the evaluation of plasma mineralocorticoid activity in normal and hypertensive states.* J. Clin. Invest. 58:579, 1976.

53. HOFFBRAND, B. I., EDMONDS, C. J., AND SMITH, T.: *Spironolactone in essential hypertension: Evidence against its effect through mineralocorticoid antagonism.* Br. Med. J. 1:682, 1976.

54. HONDA, M., NOWACZYNSKI, W., GUTHRIE, G. P., JR., ET AL.: *Response of several adrenal steroids to ACTH stimulation in essential hypertension.* J. Clin. Endocrinol. Metab. 44:264, 1977.

55. VANDER, A. J.: *Effect of catecholamines and the renal nerves on renin secretion in anesthetized dogs.* Am. J. Physiol. 209:659, 1965.

56. BUNAG, R. D., PAGE, I. H., AND McCUBBIN, J. W.: *Neural stimulation of release of renin.* Circ. Res. 19: 851, 1966.

57. KUCHEL, O., FISHMAN, L. M., LIDDLE, G. W., ET AL.: *Effect of diazoxide on plasma renin activity in hypertensive patients.* Ann. Intern. Med. 67:791, 1967.

58. COLLINS, R. D., WEINBERGER, M., GONZALES, C., ET AL.: *Catecholamine excretion in low renin hypertension.* Clin. Res. 18:167, 1970.

59. ESLER, M. D., AND NESTEL, P. J.: *Renin and sympathetic nervous system responsiveness to adrenergic stimuli in essential hypertension.* Am. J. Cardiol. 32:643, 1973.

60. NOTH, R. H., AND MULROW, P. J.: *Serum dopamine β-hydroxylase as an index of sympathetic nervous system activity in man.* Circ. Res. 38:2, 1976.

61. LOWDER, S. C., HAMET, P., AND LIDDLE, G. W.: *Contrasting effects of hypoglycemia on plasma renin activity and cyclic adenosine 3',5'-monophosphate (cyclic AMP) on low renin and normal renin essential hypertension.* Circ. Res. 38:105, 1976.

62. GUTHRIE, G. P., JR., KUCHEL, O., BUU, N. T., ET AL.: *Catecholamine responses to furosemide in low and normal renin essential hypertension.* (abstr.) Circulation 54(Suppl. 2):96, 1976.

63. BÜHLER, F. R., LARAGH, J. H. BAER, L., ET AL.: *Propranolol inhibition of renin secretion: A specific approach to diagnosis and treatment of renin-dependent hypertensive diseases.* N. Engl. J. Med. 287: 1209, 1972.

64. HOLLIFIELD, J. W., SHERMAN, K., VANDER ZWAGG, R., ET AL.: *Proposed mechanisms of propranolol's antihypertensive effect in essential hypertension.* N. Engl. J. Med. 295:68, 1976.

65. MYERS, M. G., LEWIS, P. J., REID, J. L., ET AL.: *Brain concentration of propranolol in relation to hypotensive effect in the rabbit with observations on brain propranolol levels in man.* J. Pharmacol. Exp. Ther. 192:327, 1975.

66. BROWN, J. J., LEVER, A. F., AND ROBERTSON, J. I. S.: *Renal abnormality of essential hypertension.* Lancet 2:320, 1974.

67. PADFIELD, P. L., BROWN, J. J., AND LEVER, A. F.: *Is low-renin hypertension a stage in the development of essential hypertension or a diagnostic entity?* Lancet 1:548, 1975.

68. SCHALEKAMP, M. A. D. H., KRAUSS, X. H., AND SCHALEKAMP-KUYKEN, M. P. A.: *Studies on the mechanism of hypernatriuresis in essential hypertension in relation to measurements of plasma renin concentration, body fluid compartments and renal function.* Clin. Sci. 41:219, 1971.

69. CRANE, M. G., AND HARRIS, J. J.: *Effect of aging on renin activity and aldosterone excretion.* J. Lab. Clin. Med. 87:947, 1976.

70. GUTHRIE, G. P., JR., GENEST, J., AND KUCHEL, O.: *Renin and the therapy of hypertension.* Ann. Rev. Pharmacol. Toxicol. 16:287, 1976.

71. DEL GRECO, F., SIMON, N. M., GOODMAN, S., ET AL.: *Plasma renin activity in primary and secondary hypertension.* Medicine (Baltimore) 46:475, 1967.

72. COHEN, E. L., ROVNER, D. R., AND CONN, J. W.: *Postural augmentation of plasma renin activity — importance in diagnosis of renovascular hypertension.* JAMA 197:973, 1966.

73. MARKS, L. S., AND MAXWELL, M. H.: *Renal vein renin — value and limitations in the prediction of operative results.* Urol. Clin. North Amer. 2:311, 1975.

74. GUNNELLS, J. C., JR., McGUFFIN, W. L., JR., JOHNSRUDE, J., ET AL.: *Peripheral and renal venous plasma renin activity in hypertension.* Ann. Intern. Med. 71:555, 1969.

75. STRONG, C. G., HUNT, J. C., SHEPS, S. G., ET AL.: *Renal venous renin activity — enhancement of sensitivity of lateralization by sodium depletion.* Am. J. Cardiol. 27:602, 1971.

76. GENEST, J.: *The renin-angiotensin-aldosterone system. Physiopathology,* in BREST, A. N., AND MOYER, J. H. (EDS.): *Cardiovascular Diseases.* F. A. Davis, Philadelphia, 1968, p. 144.

77. TREMBLAY, G. Y., VEYRAT, R., DE CHAMPLAIN, J., ET AL.: *Criteria for success of surgery in patients with hypertension associated with renal artery stenosis.* Trans. Assoc. Am. Physicians 77:201, 1964.

78. BRUNNER, H. R., SEALEY, J. E., AND LARAGH, J. H.: *Renin as a risk factor in essential hypertension: more evidence.* Am. J. Med. 55:295, 1973.

52

79. KAPLAN, N. M.: *The prognostic implications of plasma renin in essential hypertension.* JAMA 231:167, 1975.

80. GENEST, J., BOUCHER, R., KUCHEL, O., ET AL.: *Renin in hypertension—How important as a risk factor?* Can. Med. Assoc. J. 109:475, 1973.

81. KOCH-WESER, J.: *Correlation of pathophysiology and pharmocotherapy in essential hypertension.* Am. J. Cardiol. 32:499, 1973.

82. ADLIN, E. V., MARKS, A. D., AND CHANNICK, B. J.: *Spironolactone and hydrochlorothiazide in essential hypertension. Blood pressure response and plasma renin activity.* Arch. Intern. Med. 130:855, 1972.

83. DOUGLAS, J. G., HOLLIFIELD, J. W., AND LIDDLE, G. W.: *Treatment of low-renin essential hypertension: Comparison of spironolactone and a hydrochlorothiazide-triamterene combination.* JAMA 227:518, 1974.

Significance of Renin and Angiotensin in Hypertension

Jehoiada J. Brown, M.D., Robert Fraser, Ph.D.,
Brenda Leckie, Ph.D., Anthony F. Lever, M.D.,
James J. Morton, Ph.D., Paul L. Padfield, M.D.,
Peter F. Semple, M.D., and J. Ian S. Robertson, M.D.

INTRODUCTION*

The enzyme renin, formed and stored mainly, although not exclusively, in the kidney, is released into both renal venous blood and into renal lymph. Renin reacts with a substrate (angiotensinogen) in the alpha-2 globulin fraction of plasma, to form a largely inactive decapeptide, angiotensin I. Angiotensin I is then converted within the circulation, and especially in transit across the lungs,[14-17] into the octapeptide angiotensin II. Angiotensin II is the principal active component of the renin-angiotensin system in man.[8, 18] Further degradation forms a heptapeptide, sometimes known as angiotensin III,[19-21] which is an effective stimulus to aldosterone secretion,[22-24] although having less pressor effect (only 15 to 50 percent) than angiotensin II. Further degradation, into largely inactive peptide fragments, is brought about by various peptidases ("angiotensinases") within the circulation and in transit through tissues.

ASSAY OF COMPONENTS OF RENIN-ANGIOTENSIN SYSTEM

Practicable assays for all the main components of the renin-angiotensin system are available.

Renin Assay

Since 1962, when renin assays began to be employed clinically on a wide scale, two rather divergent approaches have been adopted.

Plasma Renin Concentration

In assays of plasma renin concentration,[25, 26] the enzyme is extracted from a sample of plasma (or serum), freed, so far as possible, from endogenous renin-substrate and from angiotensinases, and then allowed to incubate under controlled conditions with a prepared substrate. The rate at which angiotensin is generated in such a system gives a measure of the concentration of renin in the incubation mixture, and, after calibration against the standard renin preparation, the concentration of renin in the original sample can be determined.

---

*This article is purposely concerned mainly with aspects of which we have practical experience in this department. For wider views, and more extensive bibliography, the reader is referred to several recent books and review articles.[1-13]

An alternative method for measuring plasma renin concentration involves the addition of an excess concentration of exogenous renin-substrate to the sample before incubation, thus eliminating variations in the rate of angiotensin generation due to differences in substrate concentration.[27]

Plasma Renin Activity

Measurements of what has come to be called, by contrast, plasma renin activity,[25, 29, 30] involve the inactivation, by one means or another, of angiotensinases in the sample. These are then incubated, renin reacting with the endogenous substrate, and the rate of generation of angiotensin determined. It will be apparent that with methods for measuring plasma renin activity, the result depends not only on the concentration of renin, but also on the concentration of renin-substrate in the specimen. It is known that the variations in the concentration of renin-substrate encountered in physiological and clinical circumstances in man are within a range which will impose an important influence on the rate of generation of angiotensin I;[25, 28, 31] hence the quantitative information given by assay of plasma renin activity is essentially different from that of plasma renin concentration measurement. Several methods have been devised for assessing the effect of variations in renin-substrate concentration, and so deriving a measure of plasma renin concentration from plasma renin activity.[25, 29, 31] Such procedures are not, however, routinely employed in clinical practice.

Renin Standard: International Reference Preparation

A considerable handicap to progress has been the lack, until very recently, of an internationally accepted renin standard.[25, 32-34] Thus, there was no common currency in terms of which results of renin assays might be expressed. In 1974, however, the World Health Organization established an International Reference Preparation of Human Renin.[25, 35] This preparation has been shown to be stable on storage in the dried form, and not susceptible to further activation on acidification. Thus it is now possible to express renin assay results in the same terms internationally.

Active and Inactive Renin

A particularly exciting recent development has been the recognition that both in the kidney and in blood, renin exists partly in an inactive form of molecular weight around 55,000.[36-42] Inactive renin can be converted to a smaller active enzyme with a molecular weight around 37,000 by various procedures such as acidification to pH 3.0 (Fig. 1), or treatment with trypsin. Some renin assay methods, which employ acidification to lower pH, will give a measure of both active and inactive renin together in the sample; others, which do not employ such acidification, will estimate active renin only. The mean proportion of inactive renin in normal subjects is 56 percent $\pm$ 2 percent S.E.M.[44] Significantly higher proportions of inactive renin are found in normal pregnancy.[40, 41, 44]

Comparison of Renin Assay Methods

With such a wide diversity of renin assay procedures, considerable conflict between the results reported from different laboratories might be expected. Surprisingly, there have been remarkably few areas of qualitative (as distinct from quantitative) disagreement, at least in samples obtained in steady-state conditions. This was accentuated in the recently reported International Collaborative Study of Renin Assay in which 17 different laboratories in various parts of the world, employing very diverse renin assay

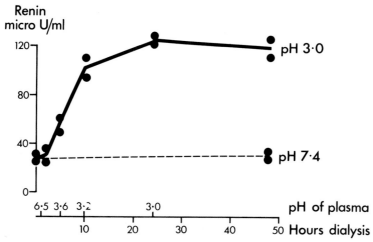

Figure 1. Activation of inactive renin in human plasma. Aliquot of plasma dialyzed at pH 3.0 shows activation of inactive renin, which is maximal at 24 hr. Aliquot not acidified maintains its initial plasma renin concentration. Dialysis at +4°C.

methods, reported on the renin content of seven plasma specimens.[25] Despite the very wide range of absolute values returned for these specimens by the different laboratories, there was very little important disagreement on the ranking order of renin content. Such agreement may not hold for samples obtained after acute stimulation or suppression of renin release.

Renin-Substrate Assay

Numerous methods have been described for estimating plasma renin-substrate concentration, most of these being based on the principle of adding a large quantity of exogenous renin, and incubating so as to convert all available substrate to angiotensin, which is then assayed.[29, 41, 45, 46] It is assumed that one molecule of angiotensin is formed from one molecule of substrate. Important increases in renin-substrate concentration occur in pregnancy[41, 47, 48] and in women taking the estrogen-progestagen oral contraceptive;[49, 50] conversely substrate concentration may be lowered in, for example, the nephrotic syndrome.[51] The administration of angiotensin II has been shown to elevate renin-substrate levels in rat and dog.[52, 53]

Angiotensins: Assays and Antagonists

Assays for the various forms of angiotensin have been greatly facilitated with the introduction of radioimmunoassay procedures.[8]

Angiotensin I

The application of such assays to the measurement of angiotensin I concentration has been mainly directed to *in vitro* systems concerned with the estimation of renin concentration,[28] renin activity[54-56] or renin-substrate.[46] A good deal less attention has been paid to actual circulating levels of angiotensin I *in vivo* although a practicable technique has been used in this laboratory[57] and has been employed to demonstrate, for example, that there is a fall in the blood concentration of angiotensin I across the pulmonary circulation with a corresponding increase in the concentration of plasma angiotensin II.[17] This work provided direct evidence confirming earlier experiments implicating the lung as an important site of conversion of angiotensin I to angiotensin II.[14-16]

Angiotensin II

Angiotensin II is the main active component of the renin-angiotensin system in blood in man, and thus angiotensin II assays[8] are most immediately relevant to any assessment of the overall importance of the renin-angiotensin system in any given circumstance. Furthermore, since angiotensin II is available in pure synthetic form, it can be infused intravenously in man with reasonable safety and, thus, it is possible to construct dose-response curves of, for example, aldosterone or blood pressure to angiotensin II in various conditions.[58-63] These approaches have given great impetus to a properly quantitative evaluation of the renin-angiotensin system, especially since there is no major problem in expressing the results of angiotensin II assays in universally accepted absolute terms. This is an area of especially rapid development at present, and as will be seen, has very important connotations when considering the role of angiotensin II in the pathogenesis of various forms of hypertension.

Synthetic Antagonists to Angiotensin II

The need to consider changes in the position and shape of dose-response curves to angiotensin II is underlined by the availability of synthetic analogues and antagonists to angiotensin II. One such antagonist which has been widely used clinically in recent years is Saralasin, which has sarcosine substituted in position one and alanine in position eight of the angiotensin II molecule.[64, 65] Saralasin competes with angiotensin II for receptor sites, while it is a much less potent agonist than is angiotensin II. Thus the effect of Saralasin administration in circumstances when circulating levels of angiotensin II are high will be to antagonize the actions of angiotensin II. Conversely, if Saralasin is given when endogenous angiotensin II is low, its agonist effect will be more apparent.[65-68] Understanding of the action of Saralasin in a given circumstance will be further facilitated with knowledge of the shape of and position on the dose-response curve to angiotensin II of the effect under examination.[66]

Angiotensin III

In peripheral arterial and venous plasma in man, angiotensin III is present in comparatively low concentrations, and seems therefore not to be an important circulating hormone.[18] This is in contrast to certain other species, such as the rat, in which the molar proportion of angiotensin III is at least equivalent to that of angiotensin II.[19, 20]

Relationship between Renin and Angiotensin II in Vivo

Effect of Substrate

It has been emphasized that variations in renin-substrate concentration have an important bearing on the quantity of angiotensin II formed by a given concentration of renin. For example, when a small group of patients with the nephrotic syndrome were studied and compared with a group of control subjects, although the peripheral plasma renin concentrations covered a similar range in the two groups, and although the concurrent values for renin concentration and angiotensin II in peripheral plasma were closely correlated in the patients and in the normal subjects, the slopes of the regressions relating renin to angiotensin II were quite different in the patients and the controls.[51] We attributed this difference to the lower renin-substrate concentrations in the nephrotic patients.

Active and Inactive Renin

A method for the assay of plasma renin concentration which we have used extensively estimates both active and inactive renin together.[26, 40, 44] Although in many circumstances, below, within, and above the physiological range, plasma renin concentration measurements correlate well with concurrent estimations of plasma angiotensin II,[8-10, 40, 51, 62, 69-75] the relationship becomes closer if active renin only is considered.[40, 44]

In some circumstances, the ratio between active and inactive renin is altered. Normal pregnancy is one instance in which the proportion of inactive renin is much increased (mean 66 percent ± 3 percent S.E.M.).[40, 41, 44] In pregnancy the relationship between total renin and angiotensin II is no longer apparent.[47]

The relationship between total renin and angiotensin II may also be lost during acute changes. Thus acute stimulation of renin release by the administration of isoprenaline or diazoxide, or by tilting, has been observed to increase active renin but to reduce inactive renin.[39] Saralasin administration can raise active plasma renin concentration while leaving inactive renin levels unaltered[44, 75] (Fig. 2). The qualitative agreement

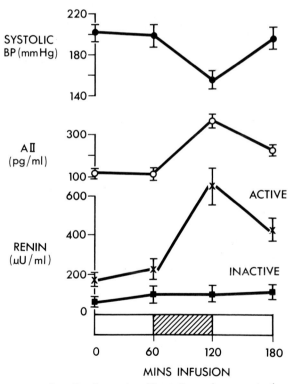

Figure 2. Increase in concentration of active renin without change in concentration of inactive renin during Saralasin infusion (10 μg./kg./min.) for 1 hr., as shown by shaded block. Mean values ±S.E.M. in 5 hypertensive patients sodium-depleted at time of study. Saralasin causes fall in systolic blood pressure with a concomitant rise in active renin and in plasma angiotensin II. Inactive renin is unaltered.

between widely different renin assay methods applied to a variety of physiological and pathological states has been mentioned. The previous lack of a system of units for renin measurement has favored such agreement and has concealed marked quantitative discrepancies. It must be emphasized that estimations of plasma renin concentration, activity and angiotensin II, while often correlating well with one another,[9, 25] cannot be equated in magnitude.

Factors Influencing the Renin-Angiotensin System

Evaluation of the renin-angiotensin system in hypertension involves an appreciation of the various influences on the system likely to be encountered clinically.

Physiological and Pathophysiological Influences[77, 89]

The renin-angiotensin system is stimulated by sodium depletion, and suppressed by sodium loading.[76] Potassium depletion[78] or dehydration[80] also have a stimulant effect on the renin-angiotensin system, although in most clinical circumstances these are much less powerful than the effects of sodium. Conversely, loading with potassium[78] or water[8] suppresses renin. Severe hemorrhage[79] leads to clear increases in circulating levels of renin and angiotensin II in man, although usually, with bleeds of up to 500 ml.,[8, 79, 81] no changes are discernible. Renin and angiotensin II are increased by ambulation or the adoption of the upright posture; levels also tend to be slightly but distinctly higher by day than by night.[77] Peripheral blood levels of renin and of angiotensin II are systematically higher in the luteal phase of the menstrual cycle.[77, 82] Very marked increases in renin and of angiotensin II occur in normal pregnancy.[8, 41, 47, 48]

Influence of Drugs

A wide variety of drugs affect the renin-angiotensin system.[185] Prominent among these are the natriuretic diuretics, including the thiazides,[11, 77, 89] the powerful diuretics acting on the loop of Henle, and the potassium-conserving diuretics, amiloride,[83, 187] spironolactone,[85, 86] and triamterene.[84] The non-diuretic thiazide, diazoxide, can cause very marked elevation of renin.[39, 87] So, also, can a variety of adrenergic hormones.[88] The renin-angiotensin system is activated by some antibiotics, notably gentamicin, viomycin and capreomycin.[90] Estrogen-progestagen oral contraceptives have a complex effect on the renin-angiotensin system, leading to a marked increase in the concentration of renin-substrate,[49, 50] with a compensatory fall in plasma renin concentration and a rather variable effect on plasma renin activity and plasma angiotensin II levels. Among the drugs which suppress renin, either by an action on the kidney, or, less directly, via a mineralocorticoid effect, are licorice,[92] carbenoxolone,[11] methyldopa, most beta-blockers[89] and the recently-introduced compound with both alpha- and beta-adrenergic blocking actions, labetalol.[93]

Precautions Needed on Blood Sampling for Renin or Angiotensin Assay

The foregoing observations on factors influencing the renin-angiotensin system indicate the care needed to standardize the conditions under which blood samples are taken for renin and angiotensin II assay if the maximum amount of useful information is to be obtained. It is our current practice to allow at least three months for the effects of oral contraceptives or carbenoxolone to wear off, and at least four weeks for that of diuretics. We recommend a two-week period off other hypotensive agents. Should this prolonged untreated period be unacceptable, however, some compromise is necessary. In these circumstances we employ bethanidine treatment alone, withdrawing this drug a few days before sampling. These recommendations are somewhat arbitrary; more detailed knowledge of the duration of the effects of various drugs on the renin-angiotensin system is needed. In women of reproductive age, the date of the last menstrual period should be recorded when taking samples for renin or angiotensin assay.

Considerable information can often be obtained from samples taken under outpatient circumstances with the patient recumbent for 30 minutes beforehand. Where more exact information is required, however, our own routine procedure is to place the subject on a fixed known and normal intake of sodium and potassium for at least three days, taking off blood samples between 8:30 and 9:30 a.m. after overnight recumbency and fasting. Whenever possible, in patients who have been admitted to the metabolic ward, we also obtain during the same admission measurements of total exchangeable (or total body) sodium and potassium.

The "Sodium Index"

A variety of other procedures have been adopted for renin sampling, particular attention having been paid to the state of sodium balance. Laragh and his colleagues[4] have particularly recommended the estimation of sodium output in a 24-hour collection of urine obtained concurrently with the sample for renin assay. As already mentioned, renin is elevated by sodium depletion and depressed by sodium loading and therefore one can readily demonstrate an inverse relationship between urinary sodium output, which is low when plasma renin is high, and vice versa. Laragh and his associates have suggested that by employing a nomogram relating plasma renin activity to concurrent urinary sodium output, the need to admit the patient and control dietary sodium intake can be avoided. Other workers have stated, however,[94, 95] that provided the urinary sodium output is within the normal range (approximately 75 to 200 mEq./day), very little relationship with plasma renin activity can be discerned between renin and urinary sodium, and it is almost equally valid to define the broad normal limits of renin values.

Our own data provide some support for both viewpoints. We have found that in normal subjects with a urinary sodium output of 75 mEq./24 hour and higher that, although there is an inverse relationship between urinary sodium output and both plasma renin concentration and plasma angiotensin II, the slope of the regression line relating these variables differs only very slightly from horizontal (Fig. 3). Thus, provided one can be sure that the dietary sodium intake is within the normal range, there seems very little advantage in relating measurements of renin or of angiotensin II to urinary sodium output, rather than to broad "normal" limits. Measurements of urinary sodium output might be helpful in detecting undeclared aberrations of diet, but this theoretical advantage is outweighed by the practical difficulties of obtaining accurate 24-hour urinary collections in outpatients. We concur with the views of Maxwell[96] and of Woods and his colleagues,[97] who have suggested that if measurements of renin (or angiotensin II) are to be related to 24-hour urinary sodium output, the relation is best expressed graphically with logarithmic axes, which transforms the overall relationship to a rectilinear one. This greatly facilitates interpretation as compared with the rectangular hyperbolic relationship found when the axes are plotted linearly (Fig. 4).

Relation to Exchangeable Sodium Measurement

An approach which we consider potentially more revealing, albeit more elaborate, in considering the pathogenesis of various forms of hypertension, is to relate measurements of plasma renin or angiotensin II concentrations to the total exchangeable sodium. Total exchangeable sodium might be expanded and remain so, being largely unin-

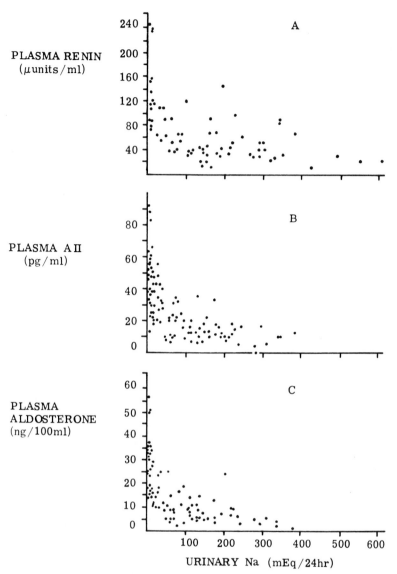

Figure 3. Normal subjects in varied sodium status. Relationship between 24-hour urinary sodium output and concurrent plasma concentrations of renin, angiotensin II and aldosterone. With urinary sodium of 75 mEq./day or more, plasma renin concentration was not significantly related to UNaV (r = −0.19; p > 0.05); plasma angiotensin II and aldosterone concentrations showed weak negative correlations (r = −0.333; p < 0.05 and r = −0.397; p < 0.05 respectively). With UNaV < 10 mEq./day, none of the three measurements showed a significant relationship to urinary sodium. Where estimates were made concurrently, renin and angiotensin II were significantly correlated (r = +0.67; p < 0.01). Both in turn were related to plasma aldosterone levels (respectively r = +0.48; p < 0.05, and r = +0.69; p < 0.001).

fluenced by variations in dietary sodium intake. In normotensive subjects, a significant inverse correlation can be demonstrated between plasma renin and angiotensin II concentrations and the concurrent total exchangeable sodium,[98-100] the latter expressed in terms of the "leanness index." This relationship having been established for normotensive subjects, it is then possible to observe whether or not in a hypertensive patient,

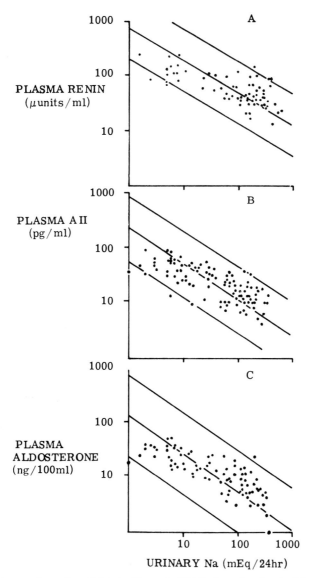

Figure 4. Logarithmic transformation of data in Figure 3. Middle line of each set of three is the calculated regression (±2 S.D. also shown).

there is a disproportion between circulating angiotensin II and the concurrent level of exchangeable sodium. It appears to us likely that any such disproportion would be likely to have immediate relevance to the pathogenesis of hypertension.

ACTIONS OF ANGIOTENSIN II

Renin, by way of angiotensin II, has a wide array of actions in man.[1-13] Of these, there are three which seem of particular importance in clinical hypertension. These are the blood pressure-raising effect; the stimulant effect on aldosterone secretion; and the direct renal action. The first two of these three have been the most extensively studied to

63

date. Again, in considering these effects clinically, it is necessary to emphasize the importance of studying the dose-response curves to angiotensin II. It has been shown that in normal subjects, sodium depletion, while lowering the pressor dose-response curve to angiotensin II, elevates and steepens the aldosterone dose-response curve.[58-60] As will be seen, these dose-response curves are altered in very different fashions in hypertension.

RENIN AND ANGIOTENSIN IN HYPERTENSION

Clinically, assays of renin and of angiotensin II are most obviously relevant to those forms of hypertension which are associated with hyperaldosteronism.[9-11] Aldosterone excess in hypertension falls into two broad groups: the so-called "secondary" forms of aldosterone excess, where renin and angiotensin II levels are high and the excessive aldosterone secretion appears to be due largely, if not entirely, to stimulation by the renin-angiotensin system. These syndromes are in sharp contrast to the "primary" varieties of aldosterone excess where overproduction of aldosterone is associated with suppression of the renin-angiotensin system. The most typical example of the latter is the aldosterone-secreting adenoma of the adrenal cortex (Conn's syndrome). A similar pattern is seen with bilateral nodular hyperplasia of the adrenal cortices (the so-called "idiopathic" or "pseudo-primary" aldosteronism).

Hypertension with Secondary Aldosterone Excess

Renin-secreting Tumor

The most straightforward example of hypertension with secondary aldosterone excess is provided by the rare patients with a renin-secreting renal tumor.[102-104] Tumors of this sort are usually benign and consist of juxtaglomerular cells. The tumors produce an excess of renin, apparently largely autonomously, and since they are usually small, there is no appreciable renal ischemia. Hypertension is associated with very high peripheral plasma levels of renin, angiotensin II and aldosterone; on renal venous sampling, elevated levels of renin and of angiotensin II are detected in blood coming from the affected side. Removal of the tumor restores the peripheral levels of renin, angiotensin II and aldosterone to normal and relieves the hypertension. This condition is of great theoretical importance since we can here, with reasonable certainty, attribute the hypertension and hyperaldosteronism solely to excess secretion of renin.

Renal Artery Stenosis

An analogous but, in several important respects, different syndrome is hypertension due to renal artery stenosis. This condition is of special interest as the clinical counterpart of the "Goldblatt" model of experimental hypertension in laboratory animals. A patient with severe unilateral renal artery stenosis will have hypertension which is usually, though not invariably, associated with high concentrations of renin, angiotensin II and aldosterone in peripheral plasma.[105-107] Renal venous plasma drawn from the affected kidney will have clearly higher levels of renin and of angiotensin II than arterial plasma; conversely the unaffected kidney may be disposing of renin and angiotensin II being delivered to it in renal arterial blood in that there will be lower levels of these substances in renal venous plasma on that side than in arterial plasma. Surgical management of renal artery stenosis may correct these various biochemical abnormalities and restore blood pressure to normal.

Other Unilateral Renal Lesions

A wide variety of unilateral parenchymal renal lesions can be responsible for hypertension with very similar biochemical characteristics to those outlined for renal artery stenosis and relieved by unilateral nephrectomy. Such afflictions include hydronephrosis, pyelonephritis, renal tuberculosis and renal carcinoma. It seems likely that the common element in these diverse disorders is that they all, like main renal artery stenosis, produce unilateral renal ischemia.[108]

Inactive Renin and Renal Carcinoma

Some renal carcinomas appear to secrete an excess of inactive renin.[109] In one such patient of ours, a 64-year-old male with hypertension, peripheral plasma contained 94 μU./ml. active renin (range in 11 normal males, 32 to 93 μU./ml.) and 1221 μU./ml. inactive renin (range in 11 normal males, 45 to 125 μU./ml.). After removal of the kidney containing a renal carcinoma, the respective levels of active and inactive renin were 32 and 95 μU./ml.; 37 and 12 μU./ml.; and 19 and 20 μU./ml. on the 3rd, 22nd and 34th postoperative days respectively. Thus the gross excess of inactive renin disappeared following excision of the renal carcinoma.

Renin and Angiotensin II Assay in Renal Venous Blood

Both in patients with renin-secreting tumors and in those with unilateral renal artery stenoses, comparison of the concentrations of renin in plasma drawn simultaneously from the two renal veins is an important diagnostic procedure.[9, 107] There are nevertheless marked quantitative differences between the two diseases in this respect.[107] In unilateral renal artery stenosis, four distinct components contribute to the renal vein-renin ratio. These are: increased renin secretion on the affected side; reduced renal blood flow on the affected side; suppression of renin secretion on the contralateral side; and disposal, on the contralateral side, of renin arriving in the renal arterial plasma.[110]

In a series of 24 patients with hypertension and unilateral arteriographic renal artery stenosis (or occlusion), plasma renin concentration was higher in the affected renal vein than on the unaffected side in 22 cases. In fourteen, plasma renin concentration was lower in the unaffected renal vein than in plasma drawn simultaneously from the inferior vena cava below the renal veins, indicating that the kidney with a normal renal artery was responsible for a net extraction of renin from blood. This pattern was more consistent and more pronounced in the 12 patients with the more severe stenoses, and in whom, at ureteric catheterization studies, renal plasma flow (assessed by PAH clearance) was less than 100 ml. per minute on the affected side.

In this series there was a close correlation between renin and angiotensin II concentrations in renal venous plasma (r = +0.9; n = 93; p < 0.001). Plasma angiotensin II levels showed a similar pattern to renin concentration, being higher in renal venous plasma on the affected side than in lower vena caval plasma, while on the unaffected side there was evidence of net extraction of angiotensin II across the kidney.

This pattern was emphasized in a 45-year-old hypertensive female (B.P. 186/134 mm. Hg) with right renal artery occlusion studied more recently. Plasma angiotensin II concentrations (pg./ml.) in successive concurrent samples were:

Sample No.	Femoral artery	Right renal vein	Left renal vein
1	31	83	19
2	28	96	19
3	28	117	16

In patients with a unilateral renin-secreting tumor there are present only three of the four components contributing to the renal vein renin and angiotensin II ratio in renal artery stenosis; renal blood flow is not reduced on the affected side. Thus the differential may be less obvious.[9, 104, 107] In a patient with a renin-secreting tumor studied by us there was evidence of net extraction of both renin and angiotensin II from peripheral blood by the normal kidney.[104]

Intractable Hypertension during Regular Hemodialysis

A third syndrome of secondary hyperaldosteronism with hypertension is encountered in patients on regular dialysis for chronic renal failure who have severe hypertension intractable to drug therapy. In the majority of patients on regular hemodialysis, blood pressure is readily controlled by weight-losing hemodialysis, combined with salt and water restriction between dialysis, with the addition of antihypertensive drugs if necessary.[111, 112] In a small proportion of cases, however, the blood pressure is not controlled in this way, being very resistant to antihypertensive therapy. Patients of this latter kind have, in our experience, very high levels of renin, angiotensin II, and aldosterone in peripheral blood, and these levels are driven higher by vigorous dialysis. Massive therapy with a wide variety of antihypertensive agents has frequently failed to bring the blood pressure down, and we have often recommended early bilateral nephrectomy. This rapidly reduces renin, angiotensin II, and aldosterone to low levels, and subsequently blood pressure is readily controlled by hemodialysis alone.[111, 112] There have been reports from other centers that in a proportion of patients of this variety, renin may be lowered by beta-blocking agents such as propranolol.[113, 114] When effective, propranolol has the advantage that the kidneys remain; hence erythropoetin is not reduced and anemia is less of a problem. It is not, however, as reliable in lowering renin as is bilateral nephrectomy.[115] More recent experience with minoxidil suggests that this drug may be a useful alternative to nephrectomy.[115, 188]

Malignant Phase Alone

Fourthly, secondary hyperaldosteronism may be seen in association with the malignant phase of hypertension *per se* in the absence of any radiologically-demonstrable lesion of either kidney or the main renal artery. In such cases adequate control of the blood pressure alone may lead to resolution of the retinal abnormalities of the malignant phase and to restoration of the very high levels of renin, angiotensin II, and aldosterone to normal.[11, 116-118] The mechanism of the secondary aldosterone excess in this syndrome is not clearly understood. It is known from renal biopsy studies that the retinal hemorrhages and exudates of the malignant phase are very commonly accompanied by fibrinoid arterial and arteriolar lesions in the kidney[118, 119] and it seems probable that these might act as multiple renal artery stenoses. With control of the malignant phase and healing of these arterial lesions, the stimulus to renin is removed.

An alternative or additional explanation for the high levels of renin, angiotensin II, and aldosterone, is relative sodium depletion in the malignant phase.[106] However, the disproportionately high plasma angiotensin II levels in relation to exchangeable sodium[98-100] suggest this cannot be the sole cause; if it were, the angiotensin levels, though high, would be proportionate to the fall in exchangeable sodium.

McAllister and his colleagues[117] have drawn attention to a dissociation between the fall of renin and of aldosterone on treatment of the malignant phase, and have suggested that relative hypertrophy of the zona glomerulosa may lead to persistence of high aldosterone secretion after renin, and hence angiotensin II, have been lowered.

Relationship between Renin, Angiotensin II, and Exchangeable Sodium in Hypertension with Secondary Aldosterone Excess

Having, as described earlier, established the relationship in normotensive subjects between plasma renin and angiotensin II concentrations of peripheral blood and the total exchangeable sodium,[98, 99] it was of interest to examine this relationship in patients with various forms of secondary hyperaldosteronism with hypertension.[98-100] We found that in patients with malignant phase or renal hypertension, including hypertension associated with chronic renal failure, circulating levels of angiotensin II in peripheral blood were inappropriately high in relation to total exchangeable sodium (Fig. 5). This disproportion appeared to be due mainly to abnormally elevated peripheral levels of angiotensin II; whereas in the patients with chronic renal failure the disproportion was due rather to expansion of exchangeable sodium. Since the pressor effect of a given circulating level of angiotensin II is enhanced by sodium loading and depressed by sodium depletion,[58-60] a distorted relationship such as this could very well provide an explanation for the raised blood pressure. When blood pressure was not raised in patients with chronic renal failure, the relationship between total exchangeable sodium on the one hand, and renin and angiotensin II on the other, was normal. We suggested[99] that in those patients with chronic renal failure on regular hemodialysis in whom the blood

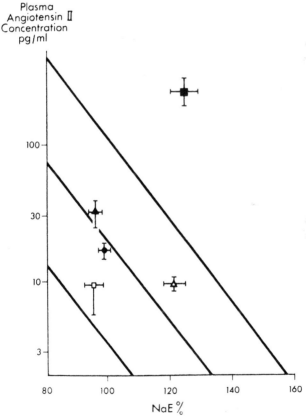

Figure 5. Relationship between exchangeable sodium and plasma angiotensin II concentrations. Diagonal lines indicate mean ±2 S.D. for normotensive subjects. For each hypertensive group mean ± S.E.M. plotted thus: renal and malignant *(solid square)*; primary aldosterone excess before *(open triangle)* and after *(closed triangle)* treatment; normal renin *(closed circle)* and low renin *(open square)* essential hypertension.

pressure was readily controlled, the renin-releasing mechanisms were relatively insensitive to sodium depletion. Thus if there were initially a disproportionate elevation of angiotensin II in peripheral blood for total exchangeable sodium, removal of excess sodium by hemodialysis would not result in undue stimulation of renin release and hence the disproportion between circulating angiotensin II and exchangeable sodium would be corrected and blood pressure would fall. By contrast in the minority of patients in whom removal of sodium was not followed by correction of blood pressure, the renin-releasing signals in the diseased kidneys were supposed to be extremely sensitive. In these latter circumstances, the removal of sodium would cause further renin release and drive peripheral blood levels of angiotensin II even higher. In this way the disproportion between angiotensin II and arterial pressure would remain or be exacerbated and blood pressure would not be lowered until the diseased kidneys were removed or renin release was suppressed in some other way.

Relationship between Angiotensin II and Arterial Pressure in Hypertension with Secondary Aldosterone Excess

A further aspect of interest was an examination of the relationships of circulating angiotensin II to arterial pressure and to plasma aldosterone in renal hypertension and particularly those forms of renal hypertension associated with secondary hyperaldosteronism. We had earlier,[58, 59] in normal subjects, constructed dose-response curves under controlled conditions, giving infusions of angiotensin II for one hour (Fig. 6). The relationships found in established renal hypertension were very different. A series of patients with hypertension and renal lesions, or in the malignant phase, was studied under similar conditions to the infused normal volunteers, although in the patients, basal samples only were obtained; they were not infused with angiotensin II.[9, 10, 63, 72, 120, 121] It was observed that in the hypertensives, although there was a range of peripheral plas-

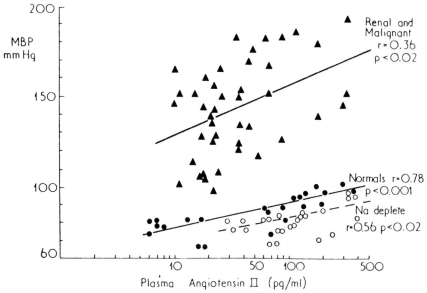

Figure 6. Relationship between plasma angiotensin II and mean arterial pressure. Lower part of graph shows data from normal subjects sodium replete *(solid circles)* and sodium deplete *(open circles)* before and during 1 hour infusions of angiotensin II. *Triangles* show data obtained in untreated hypertensives with renal lesions and/or malignant phase hypertension, not infused with angiotensin; throughout the range, blood pressure is higher for a given angiotensin II level than in normals infused to give comparable angiotensin II levels.

68

ma angiotensin II concentrations similar to that obtained in the normal subjects before and during angiotensin II infusions, throughout this range of angiotensin II levels blood pressure was very much higher for a given angiotensin II level than in the normal subjects (Fig. 6). Obviously, at the lower levels of angiotensin II this was simply a question of definition; in a hypertensive subject with a plasma angiotensin II level within the normal range, it must follow that blood pressure is higher for that angiotensin II level than in a normal subject. However, the same enhanced relationship was seen in hypertensive patients with elevated levels of angiotensin II. Infusion of angiotensin into normal subjects in normal sodium balance achieved similar elevated angiotensin II values to those found in the patients with renal hypertension, but the height of blood pressure was very much less in the subjects receiving the acute infusions. If, therefore, in renal and malignant hypertension the elevated circulating levels of angiotensin II are responsible for the high blood pressure, chronic exposure to these high levels has in some way changed the relationship between the plasma angiotensin II concentration and arterial pressure.

Relationship between Angiotensin II and Aldosterone in Hypertension with Secondary Aldosterone Excess

The patients with renal and malignant hypertension similarly showed an altered plasma aldosterone relationship to angiotensin II as compared with acutely infused normal subjects who were in normal sodium balance. In the hypertensives, the regression of plasma aldosterone on plasma angiotensin II was similar to that of sodium depleted normal subjects (Fig. 7 and Fig. 9), although in the latter, blood pressure response to angiotensin II was, conversely, suppressed.

Significance of Enhanced Pressor and Aldosterone-stimulant Effect of Angiotensin II in Renal Hypertension

In established secondary hyperaldosteronism with hypertension, therefore, both the arterial pressure and plasma aldosterone concentration were higher for a given level of

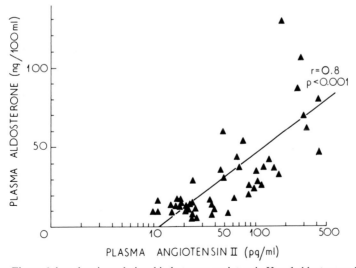

Figure 7. As for Figure 6, but showing relationship between angiotensin II and aldosterone. Renal hypertensives show a steeper regression than do sodium-replete normals, and similar to the steep relationship of sodium-deplete normals (see Fig. 9).

69

plasma angiotensin II than in normal subjects acutely infused with angiotensin II. This was most clearly seen in a patient with a renin-secreting tumor, which might be regarded as the most straightforward clinical example of prolonged overexposure to high levels of renin and hence of angiotensin II. This patient had some of the highest circulating levels of angiotensin II in the whole series before operation and these were matched only by the very highest rates of angiotensin II infused in normal subjects. In the patients with the renin-secreting tumor, both the blood pressure and the plasma aldosterone concentration were very much higher for these levels of angiotensin II than for the acutely-infused normal subjects (Figs. 8 and 9). However, after removal of the renin-secreting tumor and restoration of renin and angiotensin II into the normal range, both blood pressure and plasma aldosterone fell in that patient to strictly normal values. In this instance, hypertension and hyperaldosteronism could be attributed solely to excess renin secretion, and the quantitative observations are of great theoretical interest. Attribution of the abnormal features to increased renin secretion alone is less certain in other forms of renal hypertension. Nevertheless, there are evident similarities.

In a later study, in an untreated patient with a renal artery thrombosis,[121] we saw a similar disproportionately high blood pressure in relation to plasma angiotensin II as compared with acutely infused normals. In this woman we observed that when infusions of angiotensin II were given, the blood pressure increments followed the elevated regression line of established renal hypertension, that is, above, and roughly parallel to the regression line for normal subjects (Fig. 10). After removal of the abnormal kidney, with a lowering of circulating levels of renin and of angiotensin II, there was gradual resetting of the angiotensin II/blood pressure relationship towards normal. The roughly parallel shifts of these regressions are emphasized; if in this patient elevation of angiotensin II was the sole initial cause of the hypertension, then whatever the mechanism

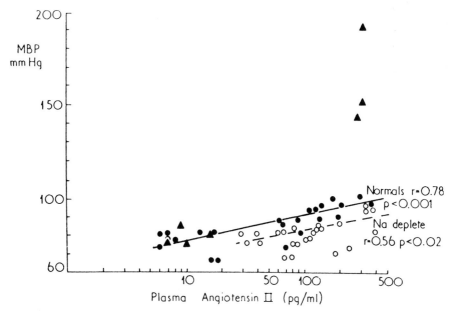

Figure 8. Relationship between mean arterial pressure and plasma angiotensin II in a patient with renin-secreting tumor before *(upper group of triangles)* and after *(lower group of triangles)* operation. Comparison with relationship in normal subjects infused for 1 hour with angiotensin II. If excess renin is the sole primary cause of the hypertension with renin-secreting tumor, then the pressor effect of angiotensin II is enhanced by prolonged administration.

70

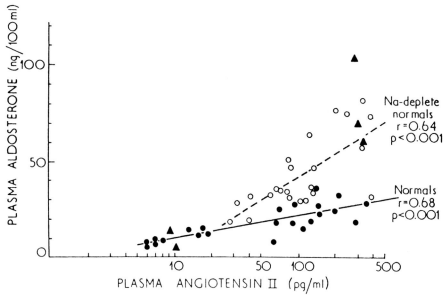

Figure 9. Relationship between plasma aldosterone and plasma angiotensin II before and after operation in patient with renin-secreting tumor. Comparison with relationship in normal subjects infused for 1 hour with angiotensin II. Symbols as in Figure 8.

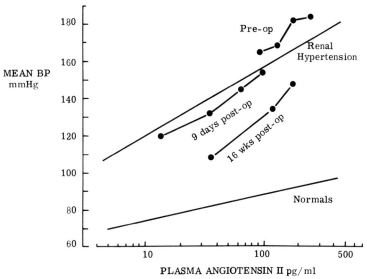

Figure 10. Patient with hypertension and unilateral renal artery thrombosis; relationship between mean arterial pressure and plasma angiotensin II before and after nephrectomy. Upper regression line is that for hypertensive patients of Figure 6; lower line is that for sodium-replete infused normals of Figure 6. In the patient, lowest point in each set is basal; incremental points are obtained during 1-hour graded infusions of angiotensin II. Before operation, basal plasma angiotensin II and blood pressure are raised, and regression during infusion follows that of other renal hypertensives. Nine days after removal of ischemic kidney, plasma angiotensin II has fallen to normal; arterial pressure, though lower, is not normal, and the relationship is still that of established hypertension. Sixteen weeks after operation blood pressure has fallen further, and the relationship is now approaching normal.

of the upward resetting of the angiotensin II/blood pressure relationship, it did not involve obvious steepening of the dose-response curve.

Role of Renin and Angiotensin II in Renal Hypertension

The evolution of renal hypertension is difficult to follow closely in man and the clinical studies have been supplemented by experimental observations in conscious dogs with renal artery stenoses. In these, we and our colleagues have found that immediately after applying renal artery constriction there is a rise in arterial pressure and an increase in circulating arterial plasma concentrations of renin and of angiotensin II.[72, 73] In the same animals, on a separate occasion, the renal artery was not constricted but similar blood pressure increments were obtained by infusing angiotensin II intravenously. It was found that the regression lines correlating arterial pressure with arterial plasma angiotensin II concentrations were almost identical in the two sets of experiments. Therefore the early rise in blood pressure which results from renal artery stenosis can be entirely explained by elevation of circulating levels of renin and hence of angiotensin II. However, with more prolonged renal hypertension in the dog, as in established renal hypertension in man, this simple straightforward relationship no longer holds and blood pressure becomes disproportionately high for a given circulating level of renin or angiotensin II.[72, 73, 123, 124] In the dog, an initially elevated plasma renin level may fall back towards normal while the blood pressure remains high. At present it is uncertain whether in man a similar sequence can occur. It is possible, but not proven, that some of the patients with hypertension and a renal lesion, but with normal plasma angiotensin II concentrations (Fig. 6) might have basically angiotensin-dependent hypertension. In both species, with established renal hypertension, there has been some form of enhancement of the relationship between arterial pressure and plasma angiotensin II concentration.

Possible Mechanisms of Alteration of the Pressor and Aldosterone Relationships to Angiotensin II in Renal Hypertension

It has been shown experimentally in normal man that prolonged infusion of angiotensin II at low concentrations will steepen the angiotensin II/aldosterone dose-response curve to further incremental doses of angiotensin II.[179] This may be due in part to a trophic action on the adrenal cortex. Such an effect occurring in high renin hypertension could explain the steep angiotensin II/aldosterone relationship. There might then be several consequences. Relative sodium and water retention induced by aldosterone might expand plasma volume and increase cardiac output;[180, 181] by autoregulation of tissue perfusion, this would then increase vascular resistance and elevate arterial pressure further. Alternatively or additionally, increased vascular sodium content might enhance the response of smooth muscle to vasoconstrictor agents.[182]

Other possibilities are that angiotensin may induce a slow increase in blood pressure via the nervous system;[183] or that exposure to high blood pressure may increase the wall/lumen ratio of blood vessels, increasing resistance and the pressor response to vasoconstrictor substances.[184] These aspects are discussed in more detail elsewhere.[101, 107]

Hypertension in Pregnancy

Hypertension in pregnancy is an exceptional variety of hypertension associated with high levels of renin, angiotensin II and aldosterone. In normal pregnancy, circulating levels of renin, angiotensin II and aldosterone are greatly elevated,[41, 47, 48] but in contrast to most physiological circumstances, there is dissociation between total renin and angiotensin II levels;[47] this is probably because the proportion of inactive renin is increased.[40, 44, 48] Since there is dissociation also between angiotensin II and aldosterone,[47] some factor other than angiotensin II must be responsible for the elevation of aldosterone. Our own findings in hypertensive pregnancy have been that, compared with normal pregnancy, there is suppression of renin, renin-substrate, angiotensin II and aldosterone.[124] Thus the hypertension appears not to be due to angiotensin II, unless the pressor effect of a given circulating concentration of angiotensin II is enhanced in pregnancy hypertension.

Hypertension Due to Oral Contraceptives

As already mentioned, the changes induced in the renin-angiotensin system by estrogen-progestagen oral contraceptives are complex, there being elevation of renin substrate, suppression of plasma renin concentration, and a variable increase in plasma renin activity and circulating levels of angiotensin II.[9-11, 49, 50] Prospective studies have shown that in nearly all women going on to the estrogen-progestagen pill, blood pressure rises perceptibly; in a small proportion this increase is marked.[125-127] We were interested in the possibility that in women showing marked hypertension on oral contraceptives, there might be, as in renal hypertension, a disproportion between total exchangeable sodium and circulating levels of angiotensin II. However, in studies conducted by us so far, no evidence of such disproportion has been found, the plasma angiotensin II levels lying towards the middle of the normal range when plotted in relation to total exchangeable sodium.[127]

Hypertension with Primary Aldosterone Excess

The various syndromes of "primary" aldosterone excess stand in sharp contrast to the forms of hypertension with secondary aldosteronism previously discussed.

Aldosterone-secreting Adenoma[85, 86, 128-130]

In primary hyperaldosteronism an adrenocortical adenoma produces, apparently autonomously, excess of aldosterone, leading to sodium retention with potassium depletion and hypertension. The sodium retention suppresses renin and hence angiotensin II. However, because of the autonomous nature of the adrenocortical lesion, the fall in angiotensin II does not lead to suppression of aldosterone, and hence in the established condition there is the very characteristic dissociation between high levels of aldosterone and the very low levels of renin and angiotensin II. Indeed, in one such series, we were able to demonstrate a significant inverse correlation between concurrent measurements of plasma aldosterone and plasma renin.[86] If the effects of the excess of aldosterone are antagonized by giving a potassium-conserving diuretic, such as spironolactone[85, 86, 128] or amiloride,[83, 187] total exchangeable sodium falls, total exchangeable potassium increases and blood pressure comes down. With a fall in total exchangeable sodium, plasma levels of renin and angiotensin II rise from low values into the normal range (Fig. 5). A similar correction of blood pressure and biochemical abnormalities follows surgical removal of the adenoma and hence correction of the aldosterone excess.[86, 128, 135]

Non-adenomatous Primary Hyperaldosteronism

It is now known that roughly a quarter of all patients presenting with hypertension, aldosterone excess and renin suppression do not have the classic single adrenocortical adenoma, but have instead bilateral nodular hyperplastic changes in the adrenal glands or, in occasional instances, no discernible adrenocortical lesion.[86, 131-135] This variety of the syndrome is sometimes known as "idiopathic aldosteronism"[133] or "pseudo-primary aldosteronism."[132] The nature of these changes has led to the supposition that an as yet unidentified trophic factor is responsible for the changes. To date none has been firmly identified, although one recent report[134] of bilateral adrenocortical hyperplasia disclosed definite evidence of a humoral aldosterone-stimulatory factor.

Differentiation of Adenomatous and Non-adenomatous Cases of Primary Aldosterone Excess: Quadric Analysis

Surgical treatment of these non-adenomatous cases of primary aldosterone excess is difficult, since extensive bilateral resection of the adrenal cortices is necessary to correct the aldosterone excess; even then there may be recurrence.[135] It is therefore important to establish, if possible, before operation, which variety of the disease, adenomatous or non-adenomatous, the patient has, the latter preferably being treated with potassium-conserving diuretics. With this aim, we did a retrospective survey[136, 137] of 31 patients with hypertension, aldosterone excess, and renin suppression, in whom the diagnosis had been verified histologically. Twenty of these had a typical adenoma; the remainder were non-adenomatous. Review of these cases showed that although the blood pressures were similar in the two groups, the biochemical abnormalities were generally more severe in the patients with adenoma. For example in the adenoma group, plasma concentrations of renin and potassium were lower and of aldosterone, sodium, and bicarbonate higher than in the patients without adenoma. However, none of these biochemical abnormalities taken alone was sufficient to separate the two groups clearly. We therefore went on to apply the statistical technique of quadric analysis to the data with the aid of a computer, assessing eight variables simultaneously. This method clearly separated the adenoma and non-adenoma groups, and formed the basis of preoperative distinction between the two forms of the disease. We have subsequently employed this technique prospectively in 40 further cases of primary aldosterone excess, and in all but 1 of the 24 receiving operative treatment, the diagnosis has been correct. However, the series will have an inevitable bias, since we now avoid operating on patients in whom we suspect there is not an adenoma, preferring to treat these definitively with a potassium-conserving diuretic. For this reason we have verified the findings at operation only four times in non-adenomatous patients. Nonetheless, this technique emphasizes a further use of renin assay. Not only is the demonstration of low renin levels in association with high aldosterone important in making the initial diagnosis of primary aldosterone excess, but precise evaluation of plasma renin is an important component in quadric analysis, helping to distinguish the two main sub-varieties of the disease. The need for similar precision of renin assay has been emphasized by other workers[138, 139] in employing statistical methods to differentiate adenomatous and non-adenomatous primary aldosterone excess.

Relationship of Renin and Angiotensin II to Exchangeable Sodium in Primary Aldosterone Excess

When plasma renin or angiotensin II levels are evaluated in primary aldosterone excess in relation to total exchangeable sodium, they are seen[73, 148] to be appropriate, in that although there is clear expansion of total exchangeable sodium, the renin and angiotensin levels in peripheral blood are reduced accordingly. When the total exchangeable sodium is corrected either by treatment with a potassium conserving diuretic, or following surgical removal of an adenoma, plasma levels of renin and angiotensin II rise accordingly and appropriately (Fig. 5).

74

Hypertension with Renin Suppression due to Excess of Other Mineralocorticoids

Deoxycorticosterone and 18-Hydroxy-Deoxycorticosterone

It might be expected that excessive production of other mineralocorticoids than aldosterone would produce a somewhat similar syndrome of hypertension with sodium retention, potassium depletion, and suppression of renin and angiotensin II. Small series have been reported in which this biochemical pattern has been found in association with excess of deoxycorticosterone[140] or 18-hydroxy-deoxycorticosterone.[141, 142] Rather surprisingly, however, in a group of patients with hypertension and apparently isolated deoxycorticosterone excess, there was no demonstrable expansion of total exchangeable sodium,[99] in sharp contrast to patients with primary aldosteronism.

17α-Hydroxylase Deficiency

An extremely interesting rare form of hypertension with mineralocorticoid excess and renin suppression is encountered in congenital 17α-hydroxylase enzyme deficiency.[6, 144, 145] In this disease there is deficient production of both androgens and of estrogens; hence genetic males present with pseudohermaphroditism, while genetic females fail to develop secondary sexual characteristics. Cortisol biosynthesis is also defective in this disease; hence the normal feedback of cortisol to ACTH fails and there is excessive ACTH secretion. This excessive output of ACTH stimulates overproduction of a number of corticosteroids with mineralocorticoid activity, including deoxycorticosterone, 18-hydroxy-deoxycorticosterone, corticosterone, and 18-hydroxy-corticosterone. The gross excess of these mineralocorticoids leads to hypertension with sodium retention and potassium deficiency, which can be clearly recognized by estimations of total exchangeable sodium and potassium. Renin and angiotensin II are consequently suppressed and aldosterone levels are low. The appropriate treatment for this disease is to suppress the ACTH excess by giving, for example, dexamethasone, as in the patient illustrated in Figures 11 and 12, recently studied in our wards.[145] Once ACTH falls, the excessive production of mineralocorticoids is stopped, total exchangeable sodium falls

Untreated		On dexamethasone	
		0.5mg BD	
Na	146 mEq/l	Na	136
K	2.8 "	K	4.4
HCO$_3$	32 "	HCO$_3$	28
Na$_E$	2801 mEq (43.6/kg)	Na$_E$	2258 mEq (34.3/kg)
K$_E$	2110 mEq (32.8/kg)	K$_E$	2489 mEq (37.8/kg)
BP	250/165 mmHg	BP	136/94

Figure 11. Patient with 17α-hydroxylase deficiency, showing changes in plasma electrolytes, exchangeable sodium and potassium, and arterial pressure, induced by 2 months of treatment with oral dexamethasone.

75

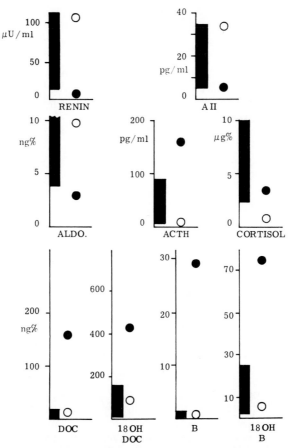

Figure 12. Same patient as in Figure 11, before *(closed circles)* and during *(open circles)* treatment with dexamethasone 0.5 mg. twice a day. Pretreatment plasma cortisol is low and ACTH is elevated; deoxycorticosterone, 18-OH-deoxycorticosterone, corticosterone and 18-OH-corticosterone in plasma are greatly elevated; while renin, angiotensin II and aldosterone levels are very low. Dexamethasone further lowers cortisol, while ACTH is suppressed. ACTH-dependent mineralocorticoids (lowest panel) return to normal, while renin, angiotensin II and aldosterone come up into their normal ranges. Vertical blocks show limits of respective normal ranges.

and total exchangeable potassium rises into the normal range and renin and angiotensin levels increase to normal. This increase in circulating angiotensin II, coupled with the changes in sodium and potassium balance, leads to a rise in aldosterone from sub-normal values into the normal range as the blood pressure comes down.

Low-Renin "Essential" Hypertension

Despite the wide variety of methods employed for assessing renin clinically, most workers agree that approximately 20 to 30 percent of all patients with apparently "essential" hypertension, have evidence of renin suppression,[6, 147] to values comparable to those seen in patients with clear mineralocorticoid excess. This has led to the not unreasonable speculation that these patients with renin suppression might have excess of an as yet unidentified mineralocorticoid responsible for their hypertension.[146, 153, 154] Studies in this department have not, however, supported such a supposition.

Renin, Angiotensin II, and Body "Space" Measurements

The frequency-distribution of renin and angiotensin II levels in unselected series of patients with hypertension shows a bell-shaped curve, spread rather more widely than in normotensive subjects, but with no evidence of a separate sub-population with low renin or angiotensin II levels.[151] Furthermore, measurements of exchangeable sodium, extracellular fluid and plasma volumes in patients with low renin "essential" hypertension, have not shown evidence of expansion of these body spaces,[148, 149] such as is clearly seen in primary aldosterone excess and 17-α-hydroxylase deficiency. When the renin and angiotensin II levels in patients with low-renin hypertension are expressed in relation to concurrent total exchangeable sodium,[148] it is seen that the renin and angiotensin values are disproportionately low for concurrent values of exchangeable sodium (Fig. 5). It follows therefore that if there is an as yet unidentified mineralocorticoid responsible for the high blood pressure in these patients, it is one whose effects differ markedly from those of, for example, aldosterone or other known mineralocorticoids. Our own current view is that renin suppression in hypertension is only occasionally due to mineralocorticoid excess; in the great majority of hypertensive patients showing renin suppression, this is part of a long-term adaptation to the raised blood pressure.[148 -152]

Response of Renin to Furosemide

One of the criteria commonly used to differentiate patients with low-renin hypertension is the failure of renin to rise appropriately folliwng the administration of a diuretic such as furosemide.[6, 147] However we and others have shown that the suppression of the acute response to furosemide is likely to be general in essential hypertension and does not appear to be restricted to those patients with initially low renin levels.[155-159, 186] It has also been shown that normal subjects excrete significantly more sodium during the first hour following intravenous furosemide than do hypertensive patients.[155]

Response of Blood Pressure to Diuretics

The generally beneficial effects of potassium-conserving natriuretic drugs in hypertension with mineralocorticoid excess raised the question of their appropriateness in patients with low-renin "essential" hypertension. There have been reports suggesting that both potassium-conserving diuretics and thiazides are more effective in patients with low-renin hypertension than in hypertensive patients with high plasma renin levels.[4, 146, 153, 154] As has been discussed, in the great majority of cases of low renin hypertension there is no evidence of expansion of exchangeable sodium or of plasma volume; hence the main premise on which this hypothesis was based may be unfounded. Nevertheless, it would be expected that a drug, such as a diuretic, which normally increases renin and angiotensin II levels, might be particularly beneficial in lowering the blood pressure if that drug could induce a natriuresis without at the same time incurring the normal rise in circulating angiotensin II. However, we have also seen[155] that the suppression of the acute renin response to diuretics may be a general phenomenon in hypertension, and not restricted solely to those patients with initially low renin levels.

Renin Assay as a Guide to Use of Beta-blockers in Treatment

A complementary therapeutic suggestion has been made, that in patients with hypertension and initially high renin levels, it is most appropriate to treat with antihypertensive agents, such as propranolol, which suppress renin release. Bühler and his colleagues[160, 161] have particularly advocated this approach, although their findings have been extensively criticized by some other workers[162, 163] who have not found that the pretreatment renin level is a particularly good guide to whether or not blood pressure will respond to a beta-blocker, or that suppression of renin, and hence angiotensin II, is a major component in the antihypertensive effect of these drugs. These controversies remain unresolved.

Renin Assay as a Guide to Prognosis in Hypertension

In 1972, Brunner and his colleagues[164] observed that patients with hypertension and elevation of plasma renin activity relative to urinary sodium excretion were especially prone to myocardial infarction and strokes; it was argued conversely that those with low renin levels were comparatively immune to these complications. This idea again has stimulated a great deal of controversy.[165-176] If the concept were valid, agents which elevate renin might be dangerous and contraindicated therapeutically; correspondingly, treatment might be less urgent in the presence of low renin levels. This contention was vulnerable to a number of criticisms. The patients with high renin levels had significantly higher diastolic pressures, a higher incidence of retinal hemorrhages and exudates, and more severe renal impairment than those with normal and low renin, all of these being features which are known to be associated with a high incidence of complications, irrespective of renin estimation. Further, the racial composition of the three groups was not similar, and thus ethnic or social factors could have had an important bearing on the results. Thirdly, these patients were studied over a period of up to ten years, during which time they were presumably treated with antihypertensive drugs which had varying effects on both renin levels and on blood pressure. In the absence of information on these points the role of renin in prognosis is difficult to evaluate. Several later reports[170-173] have failed to confirm the initial findings of Brunner and his colleagues, whereas other reports[165, 175] have supported the notion. As we have stated previously,[9] it is our view that both the protagonists and antagonists of this concept have grossly underestimated the epidemiological problems involved in evaluating a condition with so many potential variables. The assessment of one risk factor (in this case renin) among several is extremely difficult if the others change independently and continuously. In this instance it is, moreover, uncertain whether the factor under principal consideration, renin, was constant. In an updated analysis of these patients, Brunner and coworkers found that the incidence of heart attack remained lower in the low renin patients, while strokes were equally distributed among all patients, independently of renin.[177]

Effect of Saralasin in Hypertension

As mentioned previously, understanding of the action of Saralasin in a given situation is helped by an appreciation of the position and shape of the angiotensin II dose-response curve of the phenomenon being studied[66-68] and by recognition of the mild agonist effect of Saralasin. Since most of the data in this laboratory on angiotensin II dose-response curves have been obtained in recumbent subjects, we have confined studies in hypertensives similarly to recumbency.

In normal subjects in normal sodium balance, the prevailing levels of plasma angiotensin II are on a shallow part of both the aldosterone-stimulating and pressor dose-response curves.[58, 59] Hence the intravenous infusion of Saralasin in normals has little detectable effect on either arterial pressure or plasma aldosterone concentration[66-68]

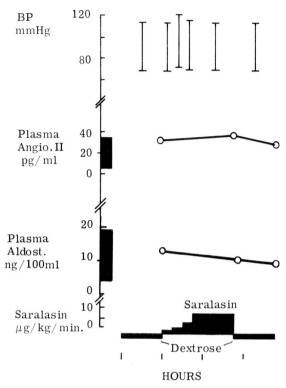

Figure 13. Effects of Saralasin infusion in a normal subject in normal sodium balance. Saralasin does not affect blood pressure or plasma aldosterone. Vertical blocks indicate normal ranges.

(Fig. 13). Sodium depletion of normal subjects elevates the endogenous plasma concentrations of angiotensin II and aldosterone; however, although the angiotensin II/aldosterone dose-response curve is steepened, the angiotensin II/pressor dose-response curve is moved roughly in parallel to the right.[58-60] Hence the infusion of Saralasin into sodium-deplete normal subjects clearly reduces the elevated plasma aldosterone concentration, while again having little detectable effect on arterial pressure (Fig. 14).[66]

In patients with essential hypertension and normal basal levels of plasma angiotensin II and aldosterone, Saralasin has little effect on either; after sodium depletion, and elevation of endogenous angiotensin II and aldosterone, Saralasin clearly reduces plasma aldosterone, while having a minor effect in reducing arterial pressure.

In hypertensive patients with initially elevated plasma angiotensin II and aldosterone levels, Saralasin infusion reduces both aldosterone and blood pressure, and these effects typically become even more marked after sodium depletion. These marked falls in blood pressure are usually accompanied by an increase in circulating renin concentration, which is due mainly to a rise in the active component, inactive renin remaining unchanged.

By contrast, in hypertensive patients with low levels of endogenous angiotensin II, the agonist action of Saralasin is most apparent. In a patient with an aldosterone-secreting adenoma for example,[66-68] we observed an increase in both arterial pressure and plasma aldosterone during Saralasin administration. This agonist effect, particularly the pressor action, is potentially dangerous; the dose of Saralasin recommended in early work, 10 μg./kg./minute, seems unnecessarily large, and we would now give no more

79

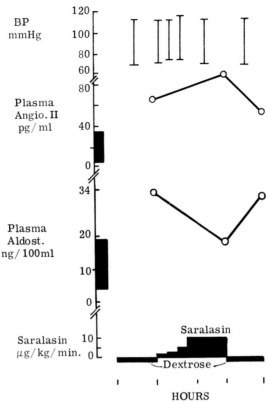

Figure 14. Effects of Saralasin infusion in the normal subject of Figure 13, sodium-deplete. Basal plasma angiotensin II and aldosterone are now elevated. Saralasin returns plasma aldosterone to normal, without lowering blood pressure. Vertical blocks indicate normal ranges.

than 2.5 μg./kg./minute, which is sufficient to antagonize concentrations of angiotensin II likely to be encountered clinically.

Overall, in patients with hypertension, the effect of Saralasin in lowering both arterial pressure and plasma aldosterone is closely related to the initial plasma concentration of angiotensin II (Figs. 15 and 16).[66-68]

PRACTICAL APPLICATIONS OF RENIN AND ANGIOTENSIN II ASSAYS IN HYPERTENSION

Assays of renin and of angiotensin II are invaluable in separating hypertension with aldosterone excess into primary and secondary varieties and, furthermore, in helping to differentiate primary aldosterone excess into cases with and without adenoma. Gross elevation of renin and angiotensin II in intractable hypertension with chronic renal failure is an indication for total nephrectomy. Bilateral renal vein renin assay is crucial to the diagnosis of renin-secreting tumor and at least very important in the evaluation of hypertension with renovascular and unilateral renal disease. Very sensitive assays are needed for the accurate assessment of subnormal values in primary hyperaldosteronism and for inclusion in quadric analysis. Similar accuracy is needed to lateralize renin-secreting tumors. A good deal less sensitivity and precision of renin assay will possibly

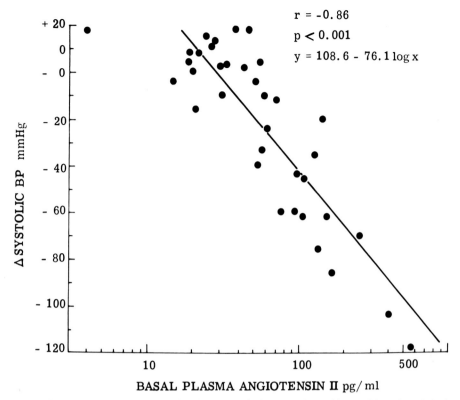

Figure 15. Effect of Saralasin on systolic blood pressure in hypertensive subjects with varied etiologies and in varied sodium status. Change in systolic pressure induced by Saralasin is closely related inversely to the pre-Saralasin plasma angiotensin II concentration.

suffice in the other situations mentioned. At present the role of renin assay in determining prognosis in hypertension, or in assessing the appropriateness of a particular form of therapy in essential hypertension, is disputed.

FUTURE DEVELOPMENTS

In the immediate future the combination of angiotensin II infusion coupled with assay of angiotensin II in peripheral plasma will permit the construction of dose-response curves in various circumstances and hence lead to more extensive and penetrating insight into the quantitative importance of angiotensin II in various physiological and clinical situations. The need for such dose-response curves has already been underlined with the availability of angiotensin II antagonists such as Saralasin. Finally, one of the most exciting areas of immediate development in this field is the recognition of inactive, large-molecular precursors of renin and the development of methods for their assay. The simultaneous measurement, in absolute terms related to a stable internationally-recognized standard, of both active and inactive forms of renin, particularly when combined with measurements of substrate concentration and of concurrent circulating plasma levels of angiotensin II, brings us, some 80 years after the initial discovery and characterization of renin by Tigerstedt and Bergman,[178] to the brink of a truly quantitative understanding of the system.

81

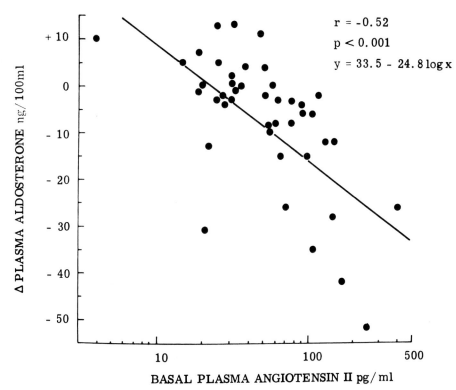

Figure 16. Effect of Saralasin on plasma aldosterone in hypertensive subjects as in Figure 15, showing that fall in plasma aldosterone induced by Saralasin is inversely related to the pre-Saralasin plasma angiotensin II concentration.

REFERENCES

1. BIRKENHÄGER, W. H., AND SCHALEKAMP, M. A. D. H.: *Control Mechanisms in Essential Hypertension.* Elsevier, Amsterdam, 1976.

2. PAGE I. H., AND BUMPUS, F. M. (EDS.): *Angiotensin.* Springer-Verlag, Berlin, 1974.

3. BROWN, J. J., FRASER, R., LEVER, A. F., ET AL.: *Renin, angiotensin, aldosterone in hypertension,* in Peters, D. K. (ED.): *Twelfth Symposium on Advanced Medicine.* Pitman Medical, London, 1976, pp. 407–424.

4. LARAGH, J. H. (ED.): *Hypertension Manual.* Yorke Medical Books, New York, 1973.

5. ROSS, E. J.: *Aldosterone and Aldosteronism.* Lloyd-Luke, London, 1975.

6. KAPLAN, N. M.: *Clinical Hypertension.* Medcom Press, New York, 1973.

7. FISHER, J. W. (ED.): *Kidney Hormones.* Academic Press, New York, 1971.

8. MORTON, J. J., SEMPLE, P. F., WAITE, M. A., ET AL.: *Estimation of angiotensin I and II in the human circulation by radioimmunoassay,* in ANTONIADES, H. N. (ED.): *Hormones in Human Plasma.* Harvard University Press, Cambridge, Mass., pp. 607–642.

9. BEEVERS, D. G., BROWN, J. J., FRASER, R., ET AL.: *The clinical value of renin and angiotensin estimations.* Kidney Int. 8:S-181, 1975.

10. BEEVERS, D. G., BROWN, J. J., FRASER, R., ET AL.: *Recent developments in the biochemical investigation of hypertension.* Essays Biochem. 1:1975.

11. BROWN, J. J., FRASER, R., LEVER, A. F., ET AL.: *Aldosterone: physiological and pathophysiological variations in man,* in MASON, A. S. (ED.): *Clinics in Endocrinology and Metabolism,* Vol. 1, No. 2 W. B. Saunders, Philadelphia, 1972, pp. 397–449.

12. GENEST, J., KOIW, E., AND KUCHEL, O. (ED.): *An International Textbook on Hypertension.* McGraw-Hill/Blakiston, New York, 1977.

13. OPARIL, S., AND HABER, E.: *The renin-angiotensin system.* N. Engl. J. Med. 291:389, 1974.

14. VANE, J. R.: *The release and fate of vasoactive hormones in the circulation.* Br. J. Pharm. 35:209, 1969.

15. VANE, J. R.: *Sites of conversion of angiotensin I,* in GENEST, J., AND KOIW, E. (EDS.): *Hypertension '72.* Springer-Verlag, Berlin, 1972, pp. 523–532.

16. OPARIL, S., TREGEAR, G. W., KOERNER, T., ET AL.: *Mechanisms of pulmonary conversion of angiotensin I to II in the dog.* Circ. Res. 29:682, 1971.

17. SEMPLE, P. F.: *The concentration of angiotensin I and II in blood from the pulmonary artery and left ventricle of man.* J. Clin. Endocrin. Metab. 44:915, 1977.

18. SEMPLE, P. F., BOYD, A. S., DAWES, P. M., ET AL.: *Angiotensin II and its heptapeptide (2-8), hexapeptide (3-8) and pentapeptide (4-8) metabolites in arterial and venous blood of man.* Circ. Res. 39:671, 1976.

19. SEMPLE, P. F., AND MORTON, J. J.: *Angiotensin II and angiotensin III in rat blood.* Circ. Res. 38 (Suppl. 2): 122, 1976.

20. SEMPLE, P. F., BROWN, J. J., LEVER, A. F., ET AL.: *Renin, angiotensin II and III in acute renal failure: note on the measurement of angiotensin II and III in rat blood.* Kidney Int. 10:S-169, 1976.

21. GOODFRIEND, T. L., AND PEACH, M. J.: *Angiotensin III: (des-aspartic acid¹)- angiotensin II. Evidence and speculation for its role as an important agonist in the renin-angiotensin system.* Circ. Res. 36 and 37 (Suppl. 1):38, 1975.

22. PEACH, M. J., AND CHIU, A. T.: *Stimulation and inhibition of aldosterone biosynthesis in vitro by angiotensin II and analogs.* Circ. Res. 34 (Suppl. 1):7, 1974.

23. BLAIR-WEST, J. R., COGHLAN, J. P., DENTON, D. A., ET AL.: *The effect of the heptapeptide (2-8) and hexapeptide (3-8) fragments of angiotensin II on aldosterone secretion.* J. Clin. Endocrin. Metab. 32:575, 1971.

24. CAMPBELL, W. B., BROOKS, S. N., AND PETTINGER, W. A.: *Angiotensin II- and angiotensin III-induced aldosterone release in vivo in the rat.* Science 184:994, 1974.

25. BANGHAM, D. R., ROBERTSON, I., ROBERTSON, J. I. S., ET AL.: *An international collaborative study of renin assay: establishment of the international reference preparation of human renin.* Clin. Sci. Mol. Med. 48 (Suppl. 2):135, 1975.

26. BROWN, J. J., DAVIES, D. L., LEVER, A. F., ET AL.: *Estimation of renin in human plasma.* Biochem. J. 93:594, 1964.

27. GOULD, A. B., SKEGGS, L. T., AND KAHN, J. R.: *Measurement of renin and substrate concentrations in human serum.* Lab. Invest. 15:1802, 1966.

28. GIESE, J., JORGENSEN, M., NIELSEN, M. D., ET AL.: *Plasma renin concentration measured by use of a radioimmunoassay for angiotensin I.* Scand. J. Clin. Lab. Invest. 26:355, 1970.

29. POULSEN, K., AND JORGENSEN.: *An easy radioimmunological micro-assay of renin activity, concentration and substrate in human and animal plasma, based on angiotensin I trapping by antibody.* J. Clin. End. Metab. 39:816, 1974.

30. BOUCHER, R., VEYRAT, R., DE CHAMPLAIN, J., ET AL.: *New procedures for measurement of human plasma angiotensin and renin activity levels.* Can. Med. Assoc. J. 90:194, 1964.

31. GOULD, A. B., AND GREEN, D.: *Kinetics of the human renin and human substrate reaction.* Cardiovasc. Res. 5:86, 1971.

32. PICKERING, G. W.: "Concluding remarks." In: *International Symposium on Angiotensin, Sodium and Hypertension.* Can. Med. Assoc. J. 90:340, 1964.

33. PICKERING, G. W.: *High Blood Pressure,* ed. 2 Churchill, London, 1968, p. 139.

34. PICKERING, G. W.: *Concluding remarks,* in GENEST, J., AND KOIW E. (EDS.): *Hypertension '72.* Springer-Verlag, Berlin, 1972, pp. 606–607.

35. W. H. O. TECHNICAL REPORT SERIES No. 565: *26th Report of Expert Committee on Biological Standardization,* 1975.

36. LECKIE, B.: *The activation of a possible zymogen in rabbit kidney.* Clin. Sci. 44:301, 1973.

37. LECKIE, B., AND MCCONNELL, A.: *A renin inhibitor from rabbit kidney: conversion of a large inactive renin to a smaller active enzyme.* Circ. Res. 36:513, 1975.

38. BOYD, G. W.: *A protein-bound form of porcine renal renin.* Circ. Res. 35:426, 1974.

39. DERKX, F. H. M., VAN GOOL, J. M. G., WENTING, G. J., ET AL.: *Inactive renin in human plasma.* Lancet 2:496, 1976.

40. LECKIE, B., BROWN, J. J., LEVER, A. F., ET AL.: *Inactive renin in human plasma.* Lancet 2:748, 1976.

41. SKINNER, S. L., CRAN, E. J., GIBSON, R., ET AL.: *Angiotensin I and II, active and inactive renin, renin*

substrate, renin activity and angiotensinase in human liquor amnii and plasma. Am. J. Obstet. Gynecol. 121:626, 1975.

42. LUMBERS, E. R.: *Activation of renin in human amniotic fluid by low pH.* Enzymologia 40:329, 1971.

43. OSMOND, D., SCAIFF, K. O., COOPER, R. M., ET AL.: *Trypsin-induced increase in human plasma renin activity.* Proc. Canad. Fed. Biol. Soc. 17:27, 1974.

44. LECKIE, B., McCONNELL, A., GRANT, K., ET AL.: *An inactive renin in human plasma.* Circ. Res. 40(Suppl. 1):46, 1977.

45. TREE, M.: *Measurement of plasma renin-substrate in man.* J. Endocrin. 56:159, 1973.

46. WAITE, M. A., TREE, M., AND McDERMOTT, E. A.: *The estimation of human renin-substrate concentration by radioimmunoassay.* J. Endocrin. 57:329, 1973.

47. WEIR, R. J., BROWN, J. J., FRASER, R., ET AL.: *Relationship between plasma renin, renin-substrate, angiotensin II, aldosterone and electrolytes in normal pregnancy.* J. Clin. Endocrin. Metab. 40:108, 1975.

48. SKINNER, S. L., LUMBERS, E. R., AND SYMONDS, E. M.: *Analysis of changes in the renin-angiotensin system during pregnancy.* Clin. Sci. 42:479, 1972.

49. SKINNER, S. L., LUMBERS, E. R., AND SYMONDS, E. M.: *Alteration by oral contraceptives of normal menstrual changes of plasma renin activity, concentration, and substrate.* Clin. Sci. 36: 67, 1969.

50. LARAGH, J. H., SEALEY, J. E., LEDINGHAM, J. G. G., ET AL.: *Oral contraceptives: renin, aldosterone and high blood pressure.* JAMA 201:918, 1967.

51. MEDINA, A., DAVIES, D. L., BROWN, J. J., ET AL.: *A study of the renin-angiotensin system in the nephrotic syndrome.* Nephron 12:233, 1974.

52. KHAYYALL, M., MACGREGOR, J., BROWN, J. J., ET AL.: *Increase of plasma renin-substrate after infusion of angiotensin in the rat.* Clin. Sci. 44:87, 1973.

53. BLAIR-WEST, J. R., REID, I. A., AND GANONG, W. F.: *Stimulation of angiotensinogen release by raised blood angiotensin in the dog.* Clin. Sci. Mol. Med. 46:665, 1974.

54. BOYD, G. W., ADAMSON, A. R., FITZ, A. E., ET AL.: *Radioimmunoassay determination of plasma renin activity.* Lancet 1:213, 1969.

55. VALLOTON, M. B.: *Determining plasma-renin activity.* Lancet 1:840, 1969.

56. HABER, E., KOERNER, T., PAGE, L. B., ET AL.: *Application of a radioimmunoassay for angiotensin I to the physiologic measurement of plasma renin activity in normal human subjects.* J. Clin. End. Metab. 29:1349, 1969.

57. WAITE, M. A.: *Measurement of concentrations of angiotensin I in human blood by radioimmunoassay.* Clin. Sci. Mol. Med. 45:51, 1973.

58. BROWN, J. J., FRASER, R., LEVER, A. F., ET AL.: *Further observations on the relationship between plasma angiotensin II and aldosterone during sodium deprivation,* in SAMBHI, M. P. (ED.): *Mechanisms of Hypertension.* Excerpta Medica Amsterdam/New York, 1973, pp. 148–154.

59. OELKERS, W., BROWN, J. J., FRASER, R., ET AL.: *Sensitization of the adrenal cortex to angiotensin II in sodium-depleted man.* Circ. Res. 34:69, 1974.

60. HOLLENBERG, N. K., CHENITZ, W. R., ADAMS, D. F., ET AL.: *Reciprocal influence of salt intake on adrenal glomerulosa and renal vascular responses to angiotensin II in normal man.* J. Clin. Invest. 54: 34, 1974.

61. DEHENEFFE, J., CUESTA, V., BRIGGS, J. D., ET AL.: *Response of aldosterone and blood pressure to angiotensin infusion in anephric man; effect of sodium deprivation.* Circ. Res. 39:183, 1976.

62. CHINN, R. H., AND DÜSTERDIECK, G. O.: *The response of blood pressure to infusion of angiotensin II: relation to plasma concentrations of renin and angiotensin II.* Clin. Sci. 42:489, 1972.

63. BEEVERS, D. G., BROWN, J. J., CUESTA, V., ET AL.: *Inter-relationships between plasma angiotensin II, arterial pressure, aldosterone and exchangeable sodium in normotensive and hypertensive man.* J. Steroid Biochem. 6:779, 1975.

64. PALS, D. T., MASUCCI, F. D., DENNING. G. S., ET AL.: *Role of the pressor action of angiotensin II in experimental hypertension.* Circ. Res. 29:673, 1971.

65. DAVIS, J. O.: *The use of blocking agents to define the functions of the renin-angiotensin system.* Clin. Sci. Mol. Med. 38 (Suppl. 2): 3, 1975.

66. BROWN, J. J., BROWN, W. C. B., FRASER, R., ET AL.: *Effects of the angiotensin II antagonist Saralasin on blood pressure and plasma aldosterone in man in relation to the prevailing plasma angiotensin II concentration.* Prog. Biochem. Pharmacol. 12:230, 1976.

67. BROWN, J. J., BROWN, W. C. B., FRASER, R., ET AL.: *The effects of Saralasin, an angiotensin II antagonist, on blood pressure and the renin-angiotensin-aldosterone system in normal and hypertensive subjects.* Aust. N. Z. J. Med. 6:48, 1976.

68. BROWN, J. J., BROWN, W. C. B., FRASER, R., ET AL.: *Effects of infusing the angiotensin II antagonist, Saralasin on arterial blood pressure and on plasma concentrations of renin and angiotensin II in normal subjects and selected hypertensive patients,* in SAMBHI, M. P. (ED.): *Systemic Effects of Anti-Hypertensive Agents.* Symposia Specialists, Miami, 1976, pp. 499–512.

69. MACGREGOR, J., BRIGGS, J. D., BROWN, J. J., ET AL.: *Renin and renal function,* in LANT, A. F., AND WILSON, G. M.: *Modern Diuretic Therapy in the Treatment of Cardiovascular and Renal Disease.* Excerpta Medica, Amsterdam, 1973, pp. 71–83.

70. DAVIES, D. L., BEEVERS, D. G., BROWN, J. J., ET AL.: *Sodium and the renin-angiotensin system in patients with hypertension.* Proc. IV Int. Congr. Endocrinol., Washington D. C., 1972. Excerpta Medica, Int. Congr. Series No. 273:693, 1973.

71. PATON, A. M., LEVER, A. F., OLIVER, N. W. J., ET AL.: *Plasma angiotensin II, renin, renin-substrate and aldosterone concentrations in acute renal failure in man.* Clin. Nephrol. 3:18, 1975.

72. CUESTA, V., BIANCHI, G., BROWN, J. J., ET AL.: *Arterial pressure and plasma angiotensin II concentration in renal hypertension,* in GIOVANNETTI, S., BONOMINI, V., AND D'AMICO, G. (EDS.): *Proc. VI Int. Congr. Nephrol., Florence, 1975.* Karger, Basel, 1976, pp. 243–254.

73. CARAVAGGI, A. M., BIANCHI, G., BROWN, J. J., ET AL.: *Blood pressure and plasma angiotensin II concentration after renal artery constriction and angiotensin infusion in the dog: (5-ileu) angiotensin II and its breakdown fragments in dog blood.* Circ. Res. 38:315, 1976.

74. MEDINA, A., BELL, P. R. F., BRIGGS, J. D., ET AL.: *Changes of blood pressure, renin and angiotensin I and II after bilateral nephrectomy in patients with chronic renal failure.* Br. Med. J. 4, 694, 1972.

75. LECKIE, B., BROWN, J. J., LEVER, A. F., ET AL.: *Inactive renin in human plasma.* Lancet 2:1412, 1976.

76. BROWN, J. J., DAVIES, D. L., LEVER, A. F., ET AL.: *Influence of sodium loading and sodium depletion on plasma renin in man.* Lancet 2:278, 1963.

77. BROWN, J. J., DAVIES, D. L., LEVER, A. F., ET AL.: *Renin and angiotensin: a survey of some aspects.* Postgrad. Med. J. 42:153, 1966.

78. BRUNNER, H. R., BAER, L., SEALEY, J. E., ET AL.: *Influence of potassium administration and of potassium deprivation on plasma renin in normal and hypertensive subjects.* J. Clin. Invest. 49:2128, 1970.

79. BROWN, J. J., DAVIES, D. L., LEVER, A. F., ET AL.: *Effect of acute haemorrhage in dog and man on plasma renin concentration.* J. Physiol. (Lond.) 182:649, 1966.

80. GROSS, F., BRUNNER, H., AND ZIEGLER, M.: *Renin-angiotensin system, aldosterone and sodium balance.* Recent Prog. Horm. Res. 21:119, 1965.

81. CATT, K. J., CAIN, M. D., ZIMMET, P. Z., ET AL.: *Blood angiotensin II levels of normal and hypertensive subjects.* Br. Med. J. 1:819, 1969.

82. SUNDSFJORD, J. A., AND AAKVAAG, A.: *Plasma angiotensin II and aldosterone excretion during the menstrual cycle.* Acta Endocrinol. 64:452, 1970.

83. KREMER, D., BROWN, J. J., DAVIES, D. L., ET AL.: *Prolonged amiloride therapy in a case of primary hyperaldosteronism with chronic peptic ulceration.* Br. Med. J. 2:216, 1973.

84. KEIM, H. J., DRAYER, J. I. M., THURSTON, H., ET AL.: *Triamterene-induced changes in aldosterone and renin values in essential hypertension.* Arch. Intern. Med. 136:645, 1976.

85. BROWN, J. J., DAVIES, D. L., LEVER, A. F., ET AL.: *Plasma renin in a case of Conn's syndrome with fibrinoid lesions: use of spironolactone in treatment.* Br. Med. J. 2:1636, 1964.

86. BROWN, J. J., DAVIES, D. L., FERRISS, J. B., ET AL.: *Comparison of surgery and prolonged spironolactone therapy in patients with hypertension, aldosterone excess and low plasma renin.* Br. Med. J. 1:729, 1972.

87. KUCHEL, O., FISHMAN, L. M., LIDDLE, G. W., ET AL.: *Effect of diazoxide on plasma renin activity in hypertensive patients.* Ann. Intern. Med. 67:791, 1967.

88. VANDONGEN, R., PEART, W. S., AND BOYD, G. W.: *Adrenergic stimulation of renin secretion in the isolated perfused rat kidney.* Circ. Res. 32:290, 1973.

89. DAVIS, J. O., AND FREEMAN, R. H.: *Mechanisms regulating renin release.* Physiol. Rev. 56:1, 1976.

90. HOLMES, A. M., HESLING, C. M., AND WILSON, T. M.: *Drug-induced secondary hyperaldosteronism in patients with pulmonary tuberculosis.* Q. J. Med. 39:299, 1970.

91. HOLMES, A. M., MARROTT, P. K., YOUNG, J., ET AL.: *Pseudohyperaldosteronism induced by habitual ingestion of liquorice.* Postgrad. Med. J. 46:625, 1970.

92. CONN, J. W., ROVNER, D. R., AND COHEN, E. L.: *Licorice-induced pseudoaldosteronism.* JAMA 205:80, 1968.

93. TRUST, P. M., ROSEI, E. A., BROWN, J. J., ET AL.: *Effect on blood pressure, angiotensin II and aldosterone concentrations during treatment of severe hypertension with intravenous labetalol: comparison with propranolol.* Br. J. Clin. Pharm. 3:799, 1976.

94. MORGAN, T. O.: *In Discussion*. Clin. Sci. Mol. Med. 48 (Suppl. 2): 123, 1975.

95. DOYLE, A. E.: *In Discussion*. Clin. Sci. Mol. Med. 48 (Suppl. 2): 120, 1975.

96. MAXWELL, M. H.: *In Discussion*. Clin. Sci. Mol. Med. 48 (Suppl. 2): 121, 1975.

97. WOODS, J. W., PITTMAN, A. W., PULLIAM, C., ET AL.: *Renin profiling in hypertension and its use in treatment with propranolol and chlorthalidone*. N. Engl. J. Med. 294:1137, 1976.

98. DAVIES, D. L., SCHALEKAMP, M. A., BEEVERS, D. G., ET AL.:*Abnormal relation between exchangeable sodium and the renin-angiotensin system in malignant hypertension and in hypertension with chronic renal failure*. Lancet 1:683, 1973.

99. SCHALEKAMP, M. A., BEEVERS, D. G., BRIGGS, J. D., ET AL.: *Hypertension in chronic renal failure*. Am. J. Med. 55:379, 1973.

100. BEEVERS, D. G., BROWN, J. J., DAVIES, D. L., ET AL.: *The inter-relation of plasma and exchangeable sodium with the components of the renin-angiotensin system in the pathogenesis of hypertension,* in SAMBHI, M. P. (ED.): *Mechanisms of Hypertension*. Excerpta Medica, Amsterdam, 1973, pp. 133 – 139.

101. BROWN, J. J., FRASER, R., LEVER, A. F., ET AL.: *Renin-angiotensin system in the regulation of aldosterone in humans*. in GENEST, J., KOIW, E., AND KUCHEL, O. (ED.): *An International Textbook on Hypertension*. McGraw-Hill/Blakiston, New York, 1977, pp. 529 – 548.

102. ROBERTSON, P. W., KLIDJIAN, A., HARDING, L. K., ET AL.: *Hypertension due to a renin-secreting tumour*. Am. J. Med. 43:963, 1967.

103. KIHARA, I., KITAMURA, S., HOSHINO, T., ET AL.: *A hitherto unreported vascular tumour of the kidney: a proposal of "juxtaglomerular-cell tumour"*. Acta Path. Jap. 18:197, 1968.

104. BROWN, J. J., FRASER, R., LEVER, A. F., ET AL.: *Hypertension and secondary hyperaldosteronism associated with a renin-secreting renal juxtaglomerular-cell tumour*. Lancet 2:1228, 1973.

105. BARRACLOUGH, M. A., BACCHUS, B., BROWN, J. J., ET AL.: *Plasma renin and aldosterone secretion in patients with renal or renal artery lesions*. Lancet 2:1310, 1965.

106. BARRACLOUGH, M. A.: *Sodium and water depletion with acute malignant hypertension*. Am. J. Med. 40:265, 1966.

107. BROWN, J. J., LEVER, A. F., AND ROBERTSON, J. I. S: *Renal hypertension: aetiology, diagnosis and treatment,* in BLACK, D. A. K., AND JONES, N. F. (EDS.): *Renal Disease*, ed. 4. Blackwell, Oxford, 1977.

108. PEART, W. S.: *Hypertension and the kidney,* in BLACK, D. A. K. (ED.): *Renal Disease*, ed. 3. Blackwell, Oxford, 1972, pp. 705 – 737.

109. DAY, R. P., AND LEUTSCHER, J. A.: *Big renin: a possible pro-hormone in the plasma of a patient with Wilms' tumour*. J. Clin. Endocrinol. Metab. 38:923, 1974.

110. HOSIE, K. F., BROWN, J. J., HARPER, A. M., ET AL.: *The release of renin into the renal circulation of the anaesthetised dog*. Clin. Sci. 38:157, 1970.

111. BROWN, J. J., CURTIS, J. R., LEVER, A. F., ET AL.: *Plasma renin concentration and the control of blood pressure in patients on maintenance haemodialysis*. Nephron 6:329, 1969.

112. BROWN, J. J., DUSTERDIECK, G. O., FRASER, R., ET AL.: *Hypertension and chronic renal failure*. Br. Med. Bull. 27:128, 1971.

113. MAGGIORE, Q., BIAGINI, M., ZOCCALI, C., ET AL.: *Long-term propranolol treatment of resistant arterial hypertension in haemodialysed patients*. Clin. Sci. Mol. Med. 48 (Suppl. 2): 73, 1975.

114. MOORE, S. B., AND GOODWIN, F. J.: *Effect of beta-adrenergic blockade on plasma-renin activity and intractable hypertension in patients receiving regular dialysis treatment*. Lancet 2:67, 1976.

115. PETTINGER, W., PARKER, T., HULL, A., ET AL.: *Propranolol in refractory high-renin dialysis*. Lancet 2: 1361, 1976.

116. GILL, J. R., GEORGE, J. M., SOLOMON, A., ET AL.: *Hyperaldosteronism and renal sodium loss reversed by drug treatment for malignant hypertension*. N. Engl. J. Med. 270:1088, 1964.

117. MCALLISTER, R. G., VAN WAY, S. W., DAYANI, K., ET AL.: *Malignant hypertension: effect of therapy on renin and aldosterone*. Circ. Res. 28 and 29 (Suppl. 2): 160, 1971.

118. BROWN, J. J., DAVIES, D. L., LEVER, A. F., ET AL.: *Plasma renin concentration in human hypertension: III-renin in relation to complications of hypertension*. Br. Med. J. 1:505, 1966.

119. DAUDA, G., MOHRING, J., HOFBAUER, K., ET AL.: *The vicious circle in acute malignant hypertension of rats*. Clin. Sci. Mol. Med. 45 (Suppl. 1): 251, 1973.

120. BEEVERS, D. G., BROWN, J. J., CUESTA, V., ET AL.: *The role of angiotensin II in the control of aldosterone and blood pressure in normal and hypertensive man,* in: *Proc. Sixth Meeting of Internat. Study Group for Steroid Hormones, Rome, 1973*. Pergamon Press, Oxford, 1974, pp. 291 – 300.

121. BROWN, J. J., CUESTA, V., DAVIES, D. L., ET AL.: *Mechanism of renal hypertension*. Lancet 1:1219, 1976.

122. BIANCHI, G., TENCONI, L. T., AND LUCCA, R.: *Effect in the conscious dog of constriction of the renal artery to a sole remaining kidney on haemodynamics, sodium balance, body fluid volumes, plasma renin concentration and pressor responsiveness to angiotensin.* Clin. Sci. 38:741, 1970.

123. BIANCHI, G., BALDOLI, E., LUCCA, R., ET AL.: *Pathogenesis of arterial hypertension after the constriction of the renal artery leaving the opposite kidney intact both in the anaesthetised and in the conscious dog.* Clin. Sci. 42:651, 1972.

124. WEIR, R. J., BROWN, J. J., FRASER, R., ET AL.: *Plasma renin, renin-substrate, angiotensin II and aldosterone in hypertensive disease of pregnancy.* Lancet 2:291, 1973.

125. WEIR, R. J., BRIGGS, E., MACK, A., ET AL.: *Blood pressure in woman after 1 year of oral contraception.* Lancet 1:467, 1971.

126. WEIR, R. J., BRIGGS, E., MACK, A., ET AL.: *Blood pressure in women taking oral contraceptives.* Br. Med. J. 1:533, 1974.

127. WEIR, R. J., DAVIES, D. L., FRASER, R., ET AL.: *Contraceptive steroids and hypertension.* J. Steroid Biochem. 6:961, 1975.

128. BROWN, J. J., DAVIES, D. L., LEVER, A. F., ET AL.: *Plasma concentrations of renin in a patient with Conn's syndrome and fibrinoid lesions of the renal arterioles: effect of spironolactone treatment.* J. Endocrinol. 33:279, 1965.

129. KIRKENDALL, W. M., FITZ, A. E., AND ARMSTRONG, M. L.: *Hypokalaemia and the diagnosis of hypertension.* Dis. Chest. 45:337, 1964.

130. CONN, J. W., COHEN, E. L., AND ROVNER, D. R.: *Suppression of plasma renin activity in primary aldosteronism.* JAMA 190:213, 1964.

131. DISTLER, A., BARTH, C., ROSCHER, S., ET AL.: *Hochdruck und Aldosteronismus bei solitaren Adenomen und bei Nodularer Hyperplasie der Nebeunierenrinde.* Klin. Wschr. 47:688, 1969.

132. BAER, L., SOMMERS, S. C., KRAKOFF, L. R., ET AL.: *Pseudo-primary aldosteronism: an entity distinct from true aldosteronism.* Circ. Res. 26 and 27 (Suppl. 1):203, 1970.

133. BIGLIERI, E. G., SCHAMBELAN, M., SLATON, P. E., ET AL.: *The intercurrent hypertension of primary aldosteronism.* Circ. Res. 26 and 27 (Suppl. 1):195, 1970.

134. NICHOLLS, M. G., ESPINER, E. A., HUGHES, H., ET AL.: *Primary aldosteronism: a study in contrasts.* Am. J. Med. 59:334, 1975.

135. FERRISS, J. B., BROWN, J. J., FRASER, R., ET AL.: *Results of adrenal surgery in patients with hypertension, aldosterone excess and low plasma renin concentration.* Br. Med. J. 1:135, 1975.

136. FERRISS, J. B., BROWN, J. J., FRASER, R., ET AL.: *Hypertension with aldosterone excess and low plasma renin: preoperative distinction between patients with and without adrenocortical tumour.* Lancet 2:995, 1970.

137. AITCHISON, J., BROWN, J. J., FERRISS, J. B., ET AL.: *Quadric analysis in the distinction between patients with and without adrenocortical tumours in hypertension with aldosterone excess and low plasma renin.* Am. Heart J. 82:660, 1971.

138. STOCKIGT, J. R., COLLINS, R. D., AND BIGLIERI, E. G.: *Determination of plasma renin concentration by radioimmunoassay: diagnostic import of precise measurement of subnormal renin in hyperaldosteronism.* Circ. Res. 28 and 29 (Suppl. 2): 175, 1971.

139. LUETSCHER, J. A., GANGULY, A., MELADA, G. A., ET AL.: *Pre-operative differentiation of adrenal adenoma from idiopathic adrenal hyperplasia in primary aldosteronism.* Circ. Res. 34 (Suppl. 1): 175, 1974.

140. BROWN, J. J., FERRISS, J. B., FRASER, R., ET AL.: *Apparently isolated excess of deoxycorticosterone in hypertension: a variant of the mineralocorticoid excess syndrome.* Lancet 2:243, 1972.

141. GENEST, J., AND NOWACZYNSKI, W.: *Aldosterone and electrolyte balance in hypertension.* J. R. Coll. Physicians Lond., 5:77, 1970.

142. MELBY, J. C., DALE, S. L., AND WILSON, T. E.: *18-hydroxydeoxycorticosterone in hypertension.* Circ. Res. 28 and 29 (Suppl. 2): 143, 1971.

143. GENEST, J., NOWACZYNSKI, W., KUCHEL, O., ET AL.: *The adrenal cortex and essential hypertension.* Recent Progr. Horm. Res. 32:377, 1976.

144. BIGLIERI, E. G., HERRON, M. A., AND BRUST, W.: *17-hydroxylation deficiency in man.* J. Clin. Invest. 45:1946, 1966.

145. BROWN, J. J., FRASER, R., MASON, P. A., ET AL.: *Severe hypertension with lack of secondary sex characteristics due to partial 17-alpha-hydroxylase deficiency.* Scott. Med. J. 21:288, 1976.

146. CAREY, R. M., DOUGLAS, J. G., SCHWEIKERT, J. R., ET AL.: *The syndrome of essential hypertension and suppressed plasma renin activity.* Arch. Intern. Med. 130:849, 1972.

147. DUNN, M. J., AND TANNEN, R. L.: *Low-renin hypertension.* Kidney Int. 5:317, 1974.

148. LEBEL, M., SCHALEKAMP, M. A., BEEVERS, D. G., ET AL.: *Sodium and the renin-angiotensin system in essential hypertension and mineralocorticoid excess.* Lancet 2:308, 1974.

149. SCHALEKAMP, M. A., LEBEL, M., BEEVERS, D. G., ET AL.: *Body-fluid volume in low-renin hypertension.* Lancet 2:310, 1974.

150. BROWN, J. J., LEVER, A. F., ROBERTSON, J. I. S., ET AL.: *Renal abnormality of essential hypertension.* Lancet 2:320, 1974.

151. PADFIELD, P. L., BEEVERS, D. G., BROWN, J. J., ET AL.: *Is low-renin hypertension a stage in the development of essential hypertension or a diagnostic entity?* Lancet 1:548, 1975.

152. BROWN, J. J., LEVER, A. F., ROBERTSON, J. I. S., ET AL.: *Pathogenesis of essential hypertension.* Lancet 1:1217, 1976.

153. SPARK, R. F., AND MELBY, J. C.: *Hypertension and low plasma renin activity: presumptive evidence of mineralocorticoid excess.* Ann. Intern. Med. 75:831, 1971.

154. CRANE, M. G., HARRIS, J. J., AND JOHNS, V. J.: *Hyporeninemic hypertension.* Am. J. Med. 52:457, 1972.

155. PADFIELD, P. L., ALLISON, M. E. M., BROWN, J. J., ET AL.: *Effect of intravenous furosemide on plasma renin concentration: suppression of response in hypertension.* Clin. Sci. Mol. Med. 49:353, 1975.

156. DOYLE, A. E., AND JERUMS, G.: *Sodium balance, plasma renin and aldosterone in hypertension.* Circ. Res. 27 (Suppl. 2):267, 1970.

157. OELKERS, W., MAGNUS, R., AND SAMWER, K. F.: *Das Verhalten der Plasmareninkonzentration nach akuter Natriurese und nach Orthostase bei Gesunden und Hypertonikern.* Klin. Wschr. 48:598, 1970.

158. BRUNNER, H. R., SEALEY, J. E., AND LARAGH, J. H.: *Renin subgroups in essential hypertension.* Circ. Res. 33 (Suppl. 1): 99, 1973.

159. THOMAS, G. W., LEDINGHAM, J. G. G., BEILIN, L. J., ET AL.: *Renin unresponsiveness in essential hypertension: a community study.* Clin. Sci. Mol. Med. 51 (Suppl. 3): 185, 1976.

160. BÜHLER, F. R., LARAGH, J. H., BAER, L., ET AL.: *Propranolol inhibition of renin secretion: a specific approach to diagnosis and treatment of renin-dependent renal disease.* N. Eng. J. Med. 287:1209, 1972.

161. BÜHLER, F. R., BURKART, F., LUTOLD, B. E., ET AL.: *Antihypertensive beta-blocking action as related to renin and age: a pharmacologic tool to identify pathogenic mechanisms in hypertension.* Am. J. Cardiol. 36:653, 1975.

162. ROBERTSON, J. I. S., BÜHLER, F. R., GEORGE, G. F., ET AL.: *Round table on renin suppression and the hypotensive action of beta-adrenergic blocking drugs.* Clin. Sci. Mol. Med. 48 (Suppl. 2):109, 1975.

163. HAMER, N. J.: *Renin and beta-adrenoreceptor blockade — the mechanism of the hypotensive effect?* Br. J. Clin. Pharm. 3:425, 1976.

164. BRUNNER, H. R., LARAGH, J. H., BAER, L., ET AL.: *Essential hypertension: renin and aldosterone, heart attack and stroke.* N. Engl. J. Med. 286:441, 1972.

165. BRUNNER, H. R., SEALEY, J. E., AND LARAGH, J. H.: *Renin as a risk factor in essential hypertension: more evidence.* Am. J. Med. 55:295, 1973.

166. GOODWIN, F. J.: *Why measure renin?,* in LEDINGHAM, J. G. G. (ED.): *Tenth Symposium on Advanced Medicine* Pitman Medical, London, 1974, pp. 188–200.

167. GOLDBY, F. S., AND BEILIN, L.: *New thoughts on essential hypertension.* Br. Med. J. 2:594, 1972.

168. Leading Article: *Angiotensin, myocardial infarction and strokes.* Lancet 1:1273, 1972.

169. SCHALEKAMP, M. A. D. M., AND BIRKENHÄGER, W. H.: *Renin levels in hypertension.* N. Engl. J. Med. 286:1319, 1972.

170. STROOBANDT, R., FAGARD, R., AND AMERY, A. K. P. C.: *Are patients with essential hypertension and low renin protected against heart attack and stroke?* Am. Heart J. 86:781, 1973.

171. DOYLE, A. E., JERUMS, G., JOHNSTON, C. I., ET AL.: *Plasma renin levels and vascular complications in hypertension.* Br. Med. J. 2:206, 1973.

172. GENEST, J., BOUCHER, R., KUCHEL, O., ET AL.: *Renin in hypertension: how important as a risk factor?,* in SAMBHI, M. P. (ED.): *Mechanisms of Hypertension.* Excerpta Medica, Amsterdam/New York, 1973, p. 317.

173. MROCZEK, W. J., FINNERTY, F. A., AND CATT, K. J.: *Lack of association between plasma-renin and history of heart attack and stroke in patients with essential hypertension.* Lancet 2:464, 1973.

174. PEART, W. S., LARAGH, J. H., HICKLER, R. B., ET AL.: *Round table on renin as a risk factor in hypertension.* Clin. Sci. Mol. Med. 48 (Suppl. 2): 117, 1975.

175. CHRISTLIEB, A. R., GLEASON, R. E., HICKLER, R. B., ET AL.: *Renin: a risk factor for cardiovascular disease.* Ann. Intern. Med. 81:7, 1974.

176. BEEVERS, D. G., BROWN, J. J., FERRISS, J. B., ET AL.: *Renal abnormalities and vascular complications in primary hyperaldosteronism: evidence on tertiary hyperaldosteronism.* Q. J. Med. 45:401, 1976.

177. BRUNNER, H. R., GAVRAS, H., LARAGH, J. H., ET AL.: *The risk of low-renin hypertension: an updated analysis.* Abstracts, 9th Annual Meeting of European Society for Clinical Investigation. Rotterdam, April, 1975, p. 53.

178. TIGERSTEDT, R., AND BERGMAN, P. G.: *Niere und Kreislauf.* Skand. Arch. Physiol. 8:223, 1898.

179. OELKERS, W., SCHÖNESHÖFER, M., SCHULTZE, G., ET AL.: *Effect of prolonged low-dose angiotensin II infusion on the sensitivity of adrenal cortex in man.* Circ. Res. 36 and 37 (Suppl. 1):49, 1975.

180. LEDINGHAM, J. M., AND COHEN, R. D.: *The role of the heart in the pathogenesis of renal hypertension.* Lancet 2:979, 1963.

181. GUYTON, A. C., AND COLEMAN, T. G.: *Quantitative analysis of the pathophysiology of hypertension.* Circ. Res. 24 (Suppl. 1):1, 1969.

182. TOBIAN, L., AND BINION, J. I.: *Artery wall electrolytes in renal and DOCA hypertension.* J. Clin. Invest. 33:1407, 1954.

183. DICKINSON, C. J., AND YU, R.: *Mechanisms involved in the progressive pressor response to very small amounts of angiotensin in conscious rabbits.* Circ. Res. 21 (Suppl. 2):157, 1967.

184. FOLKOW, B.: *The haemodynamic consequences of adaptive structural changes of the resistance vessels in hypertension.* Clin. Sci. 41:1, 1971.

185. GUTHRIE, G. P., GENEST, J., AND KUCHEL, O.: *Renin and the therapy of hypertension.* Ann. Rev. Pharm. Tox. 16:287, 1976.

186. THOMAS, G. W., LEDINGHAM, J. G. G., AND BEILIN, L.: *Renin responses to intravenous frusemide in essential hypertension.* Clin. Sci. Mol. Med. 50:19P, 1976.

187. KREMER, D., BODDY, K., BROWN, J. J., ET AL.: *Amiloride in the treatment of primary hyperaldosteronism and essential hypertension.* Clin. End. (Oxford) 7:151, 1977.

188. DEVINE, B. L., FIFE, R., AND TRUST, P. M.: *Minoxidil for severe hypertension after failure of other hypotensive drugs.* Brit. Med. J. 2:667, 1977.

An Approach to Mineralocorticoid Hormone Hypertension*

Edward G. Biglieri, M.D.

The recognition of mineralocorticoid hypertension becomes increasingly more important, and the availability of specific hormone measurements and diagnostic techniques can identify mineralocorticoid hormones (MCH) as the cause or modifier of some hypertensive states. The principal MCH secreted by the adrenal zona glomerulosa is aldosterone. The amount of aldosterone bound to corticosteroid-binding globulin is small and metabolism of this MCH is rapid. Its production is regulated primarily by the renin-angiotensin system except in some disease states. Deoxycorticosterone (DOC) is an MCH also secreted by the adrenal cortex but by the zona fasciculata. Under certain conditions and in certain disease states, DOC can be secreted in increased amounts and can also effect all the electrolyte abnormalities attributed to syndromes of aldosterone excess. Such hypertensive syndromes are unusual, and they can be identified and treated. In addition, DOC can also serve as a marker of certain types of MCH excess syndromes. Even cortisol, when produced in excessive quantities, has MCH-like properties in promoting sodium retention, accelerating potassium depletion, and producing hypertension. In determining the diagnosis of a hypertensive patient, the possibility of an MCH excess syndrome must be entertained. The best indicator of MCH excess is a reduced serum potassium concentration or evidence of urinary potassium wasting. The presence of unprovoked hypokalemia or hypokalemia provoked by sodium loading warrants careful scrutiny for an adrenal MCH cause of hypertension.[1]

ADRENOCORTICAL CAUSES OF HYPERTENSION WITH HYPOKALEMIA (Table 1)

Syndrome of Primary Aldosteronism

The most common cause of adrenocortical hypertension is aldosterone excess produced either by an adrenocortical adenoma or micro- or macronodular hyperplasia of the adrenal gland. Patients with this disorder have a reduced serum potassium concentration and mild to severe elevation of blood pressure. Despite prolonged and sustained hypertension, it has little effect clinically on target organs such as the heart and kidney.

*This study was supported in part by U.S. Public Health Service Research Grants HE-11046 from the National Heart Institute and AM-06415 from the National Institute of Arthritis and Metabolic Diseases. The studies were carried out in the General Clinical Research Center (RR-00083) at San Francisco General Hospital Medical Center, with support by the Division of Research Resources, National Institutes of Health.

91

Table 1. Adrenocortical causes of hypertension*

| | Syndrome of Primary Hyperaldosteronism | 11β- and 17α-Hydroxylation Deficiency (Low-Aldosterone Hypertension) | Cushing's Syndrome | | |
			Adrenal Adenoma	Adrenal (Pituitary Adenoma)	Hyperplastic Ectopic ACTH
Potassium (serum)	↓	N to ↓	N to ↓	N to ↓	↓
PRA	↓	↓	N to ↑	N to ↑	N
Aldosterone production	↑	↓	N	N	N to ↓
Cortisol production	N	N to ↓	↑	↑	↑

* ↓ = decreased, ↑ = increased, and N = normal.

Major retinopathy is rarely present. Under these circumstances, some assessment of the renin-angiotensin system is indicated, and the most frequently used technique is measurement of plasma renin activity (PRA). The principal actions of aldosterone are sodium retention and facilitation of potassium excretion. With continued sodium retention and expansion of the extracellular fluid and plasma volume, the renin-angiotensin system becomes suppressed.[2, 3] Thus, a situation exists in which renin and aldosterone are not parallel, but instead aldosterone production is high and PRA is suppressed owing to the excessive production of aldosterone. It is important when considering this diagnosis to make sure that cortisol metabolism is normal by measuring urinary 17-hydroxycorticosteroid or plasma cortisol levels.

Syndromes of Low Aldosterone Hypertension

The best examples of this type of MCH hypertension are those forms of congenital adrenal hyperplasia associated with either 11β-hydroxylation deficiency or 17α-hydroxylation deficiency.[4, 5] In both of these disorders, the nature of the defect is such that in response to a falling plasma cortisol level, ACTH production increases and DOC is the principal mineralocorticoid secreted. This can eventually produce a hypertensive and hypokalemic syndrome clinically similar to that of primary aldosteronism. However, aldosterone production is reduced in these patients because the enzymatic defects preclude normal aldosterone production. Consequently, PRA eventually becomes suppressed. Thus, a situation exists in which in the presence of hypertension and hypokalemia there is no evidence of aldosterone excess but instead DOC excess. Clinically, the two types of congenital adrenal hyperplasia are readily distinguishable because, in the 11β-hydroxylation deficiency type, the formation of adrenal androgens is accelerated and results in virilization. In contrast, in patients with 17 α-hydroxylation deficiency, the formation of both glucocorticoid hormones and androgenic steroids is impaired, resulting in primary amenorrhea and absence of puberty in the female and pseudohermaphroditism in the male. In these conditions, normal or low cortisol production and its failure to respond to ACTH further identify the nature of the enzymatic lesion.[6]

Other observations suggest that possibly other MCHs exist that produce a symptom complex and biochemical profile of low aldosterone hypertension with low PRA. 18-Hydroxy-DOC, although a weak MCH, could play a role in suppressing renin and subsequently aldosterone production.[7] The importance of this MCH in clinical disorders remains to be firmly established. Liddle described a familial renal disorder with hypertension and hypokalemia that were resistant to treatment with both spironolactone and salt restriction. Aldosterone excretion was negligible and renin was reduced. Triamterene, however, reduced blood pressure and increased potassium concentration.[8] Other cases have been described in which hypertension was associated with extremely low production of both glucocorticoid hormones and MCHs in the presence of reduced PRA.[9] These should be good cases in which to look for additional MCHs. Recently, a patient was described with apparently ACTH-induced hypertension and mild hyperaldosteronism with strong evidence that another ACTH-controlled MCH was responsible for the electrolyte and hypertensive changes.[10] In these types of hypertension, the search for MCHs continues. In contrast, patients with low renin hypertension but normal aldosterone production should prove to be a fruitful area in which to search for combinations of normal regulatory factors that sustain normal aldosterone production or an additional aldosterone regulatory substance.

Cushing's Syndrome

CUSHING'S SYNDROME DUE TO AN ADRENOCORTICAL ADENOMA. Cushing's syndrome can be recognized clinically and should be considered in all hypertensive patients. Over two thirds of the patients with Cushing's syndrome have hypertension and mild degrees of hypokalemia. Both PRA and aldosterone are usually within normal limits owing to the influence of cortisol. However, PRA may be increased because of the primary increase in renin substrate.[11] Increased levels of urinary cortisol metabolites, 17-hydroxy-steroids, and plasma cortisol establish an adrenocortical adenoma as the cause of this syndrome.

CUSHING'S DISEASE (PITUITARY ADENOMA). Because the drive to the adrenal gland in this form of Cushing's syndrome is ACTH produced by the adenoma, MCHs can also participate in the hypertensive process and the potassium wasting. Several mineralocorticoid hormones, especially DOC and corticosterone, are increased by ACTH. There is no reason to suspect that DOC and corticosterone alone increase the frequency of hypertension and hypokalemia in this form of Cushing's syndrome, but they may contribute.[12]

CUSHING'S SYNDROME DUE TO "ECTOPIC" PRODUCTION OF ACTH. This increasingly common malignant form of Cushing's syndrome is almost invariably associated with hypertension and hypokalemia. The major increases in cortisol production are almost always associated with increased secretion of DOC and corticosterone.[12] The high levels of DOC and corticosterone contribute to the profound hypokalemia that occurs. Plasma renin activity in this disorder tends to be normal and not suppressed.

Mineralocorticoid Abnormalities Produced by Antihypertensive Therapy

The treatment of hypertension almost invariably involves the use of a diuretic or volume-depleting agent. Unless adequate precautions are taken, such medications can effect potassium wasting and mild to moderate hypokalemia in the hypertensive patient. 17-Hydroxy-steroid or plasma cortisol levels are within normal limits in these patients, but both PRA and aldosterone can be elevated during the maintenance of chronic hypovolemia with diuretic therapy. This becomes an important differential consideration in patients with suspected primary MCH disorders. The presence of elevated PRA strongly suggests secondary hyperaldosteronism. Adequate assessment of the renin-angiotensin system and aldosterone level can only be made after diuretic therapy has been stopped for 2 to 3 weeks, the amount of time required to replete adequately the potassium depletion that may have occurred.

SALIENT DIAGNOSTIC AND THERAPEUTIC FEATURES
OF HYPERMINERALOCORTICOID CONDITIONS (Table 2)

Syndrome of Primary Hyperaldosteronism

Primary hyperaldosteronism can be caused by a distinct adrenocortical adenoma or by a hyperplastic abnormality. A carcinoma of the adrenal gland that solely produces an excess of aldosterone is exceedingly rare. Once excessive aldosterone production is documented, determination of changes in plasma aldosterone concentration (PAC) is useful in establishing the precise diagnosis. If PAC after overnight recumbency (i.e., recumbency for at least 6 hours[13]) is greater than 20 ng./dl. (our normal range is 4 to 14 ng./dl.) during sodium intake of 120 mEq./day[13] and falls after 4 hours of upright posture,[13, 14] an adrenocortical adenoma is the probable cause of the hyperaldosteronism. This fall in PAC is presumably due to the modulating influence of ACTH when the renin-angiotensin system is virtually suppressed so as to be inoperative. In addition, an elevated level of DOC after overnight recumbency has only been observed in patients with an adenoma or adrenocortical malignancy, which are rare. Plasma renin concentration or PRA is considerably suppressed.[15] The DOCA test, i.e., administration of deoxycorticosterone acetate (10 mg. every 12 hours) for 3 days, fails to alter aldosterone production: neither urinary excretion of aldosterone nor PAC decreases into the normal range.[1] Administration of spironolactone in doses of 200 to 600 mg./day for a period of 4 to 6 weeks usually normalizes blood pressure in these patients.[16] An adenoma is the cause of primary hyperaldosteronism in more than 85 percent of patients presenting with the syndrome. An adenoma can be located by scintiscan utilizing [131]I-19-iodocholesterol[17, 18] in over 80 percent of the cases. Surgical removal of the adenoma and affected gland results in normalization of all abnormalities. If the medical condition of the patient precludes any major operative procedure, long term management can be accomplished with spironolactone at diminishing dose levels, with the ultimate maintenance dose usually between 100 and 150 mg./day.

The course and management of patients with adrenal hyperplasia are different. Plasma aldosterone concentration is the key to diagnosis: the level is invariably less than 20 ng./dl. after overnight recumbency and increases promptly during 4 hours in the upright posture.[13, 14] Plasma DOC levels are within normal limits. Plasma renin concentration or PRA is suppressed and shows limited and subnormal responses to upright posture. Administration of DOCA to patients with this form of hyperaldosteronism evokes two types of responses and thus differentiates forms of hyperplasia: suppression of aldosterone production into the normal range indicates indeterminate hyperaldosteronism and lack of suppression into the normal range identifies idiopathic hyperaldosteronism (IHA). This separation is important from a therapeutic point of view. The IHA group shows minimal to no response to large doses of spironolactone, whereas 100 to 200 mg./day of spironolactone is an effective management program for those with indeterminate hyperaldosteronism. At this time, surgery for adrenal hyperplasia remains at best controversial. The bulk of evidence supports limited, if any, improvement with subtotal or total adrenalectomy in patients with all forms of adrenal hyperplasia. The diagnosis of cases of indeterminate hyperaldosteronism appears to be increasing; these cases could represent an extremely important pivotal group between low renin hypertension and a more established form of primary hyperaldosteronism such as IHA or APA. Continued followup of these patients is important because it may very well represent a significant transitional phase. A rare form of primary hyperaldosteronism exists that is called glucocorticoid-remediable hyperaldosteronism. This disorder, most frequently seen in young adults, has all the clinical and biochemical features of primary aldosteronism. It is presumably due to adrenal hyperplasia, and replacement doses of

Table 2. Salient diagnostic and therapeutic features of hypermineralocorticoid conditions*

| | Syndrome of Primary Hyperaldosteronism | | | Low Aldosterone Hypertension | | |
| | Aldosterone-producing Adenoma | Adrenal Hyperplasia | | 11β-Hydroxylation Deficiency | 17α-Hydroxylation Deficiency | Other Types |
		Idiopathic	Indeterminate			
1) PAC after overnight recumbency	>20 ng./dl.	<20 ng./dl.	<20 ng./dl.	↓	↓	↓
2) PAC after 4 hour upright after (1)	↓ (occasionally ↑)	↑	↑	±	±	±
3) Plasma DOC	N	N	N	↑	↑	N
4) PRA	↓↓	↓	↓	↓	↓↓	↓
5) DOCA test	0	0	↑	±	±	±
6) Blood pressure response to spironolactone	+	0	+	±	±	±
7) Blood pressure response to dexamethasone	0	0	0	+	+	0

*PAC = plasma aldosterone, DOC = deoxycorticosterone, PRA = plasma renin activity, ± = not established, N = normal, ↑ = increased, ↓↓ = markedly suppressed, ↓ = suppressed, 0 = no change, and + = favorable.

glucocorticoids normalize blood pressure, the suppressed renin system, and the elevated aldosterone levels. The mechanism for this unusual action of glucocorticoids is unknown. In all forms of adrenal hyperplasia, the [131]I-19-iodocholesterol scintiscan may provide important corroborative information to support the biochemical findings.

Syndromes of Low Aldosterone Hypertension

Low-aldosterone hypertension is found in a small but distinct group of patients in whom an MCH excess syndrome is suspected. In the presence of suppressed renin activity and low-aldosterone production, the implication of another MCH can be postulated. It was through this type of reasoning that MCH excess was suspected in the first diagnosed cases of the 17α-hydroxylation deficiency syndrome of congenital adrenal hyperplasia. Thus, in the presence of reduced renin activity and aldosterone production with hypertension and hypokalemia, the measurement of plasma DOC or DOC production is an important diagnostic maneuver. The finding of a high plasma DOC level or elevated DOC production in such a patient immediately identifies the type of congenital adrenal hyperplasia or possibly the presence of a DOC excess syndrome. The levels of DOC that must be achieved in order to produce hypertension are great indeed, and the reported levels in both the 17α- and 11β-hydroxylation deficiency syndromes are far in excess of 200 ng./dl. Values that are within or slightly above the normal range would have little influence on blood pressure or potassium balance because most of the DOC that circulates is bound, and in the presence of normal amounts of aldosterone its ability to react with the MCH receptors is considerably reduced. Of course, there are other clinical features and measurements that clearly identify the presence of an enzymatic defect of the adrenal gland. In both types of congenital adrenal hyperplasia, replacement doses of glucocorticoid hormones are more than adequate to reduce the elevated ACTH levels, to normalize the levels of DOC production, and to correct the hypertension and potassium depletion. A normal circadian pattern of ACTH secretion is retained in patients with these diseases so that small doses of glucocorticoid hormones administered between 8 p.m. and 10 p.m. can effectively block the early morning ACTH surge and control the symptoms. Thus the dose of glucocorticoid hormone can be extremely small indeed. This is of particular importance in those patients in whom the defect is complete to the point that little or no cortisol is produced. Such patients are exquisitely sensitive to even small doses of MCHs.

Within the low-renin, low-aldosterone group, one is left with a number of intriguing patients that continue to appear in the literature, suggesting another MCH.[9]

SUMMARY

The MCHs that are produced in excess and cause a hypermineralocorticoid state are aldosterone and DOC. The recognition of associated syndromes has been clarified both clinically and biochemically. The possibility that other MCHs exist is suggested by interesting cases that purport to have the metabolic effects of MCHs with no excess of any known steroid. The role MCHs play in essential hypertension or essential hypertension with low PRA still remains speculative. The increased extracellular fluid and exchangeable sodium and the improvement with aminoglutethamide initially described in patients with low-renin hypertension have not been confirmed consistently and must at best remain controversial. There is no convincing evidence that increased MCH activity exists in both blood and urine of these low-renin hypertensive patients. Functionally, however, all hypertensive patients do in some way manifest some of the features of subjects undergoing partial MCH escape. This has been suggested by studies using DOCA in hypertensive patients. All hypertensive patients, regardless of the cause, retain far less salt before sodium escape occurs, implying that, at least functionally, the extracellular fluid volume seems to be expanded. Whether this is due to MCH activity or to some other interplay between MCHs and other factors, e.g., the autonomic nervous system or blood pressure itself, is not clear. Another MCH may indeed be an essential ingredient in explaining these phenomena.

REFERENCES

1. BIGLIERI, E. G., STOCKIGT, J. R., AND SCHAMBELAN, M.: *Adrenal mineralocorticoids causing hypertension.* Am. J. Med. 52:623, 1972.

2. BIGLIERI, E. G., AND FORSHAM, P. H.: *Studies on expanded extracellular fluid and responses to various stimuli in primary aldosteronism.* Am. J. Med. 30:564, 1961.

3. CONN, J. W., COHEN, E. L., AND ROVNER, D. R.: *Suppression of plasma renin activity in primary aldosteronism.* JAMA 190:213, 1964.

4. BIGLIERI, E. G., AND MANTERO, F.: *The characteristics, course and implications of the 17-hydroxylation deficiency in man,* in FINKELSTEIN, M., ET AL. (eds.) *Research on Steroids,* vol. 5. Società Editrice Universo, Rome, 1973, 385–399.

5. BIGLIERI, E. G.: *A perspective on aldosterone abnormalities.* Clin. Endocrinol. 5:399, 1976.

6. BONGIOVANNI, A. M., AND ROOT, A. W.: *The adrenogenital syndrome.* N. Engl. J. Med. 268:1283, 1342, 1391, 1963.

7. MELBY, J. C., DALE, S. L., AND WILSON, T. E.: *18-Hydroxy-deoxycorticosterone in human hypertension.* Circ. Res. 28,29(Suppl. II):II-143, 1971.

8. LIDDLE, G. W., BLEDSOE, T., AND COPPAGE, W. S., JR.: *A familial renal disorder simulating primary aldosteronism but with negligible aldosterone secretion.* Trans. Am. Assoc. Phys. 89:199, 1963.

9. SANN, L., REVOL, A., ZACHMAN, M., ET AL.: *Unusual low plasma renin hypertension in a child.* J. Clin. Endocrinol. Metab. 43:265, 1976.

10. NEW, M. I., PETERSON, R. E., AND SAENGER, P.: *Evidence for an unidentified ACTH-induced steroid hormone causing hypertension.* J. Clin. Endocrinol. Metab. 43:1283, 1976.

11. KARKOFF, L., NICHOLIS, G., AND AMSEL, B.: *Pathogenesis of hypertension of Cushing's syndrome.* Am. J. Med. 58:216, 1975.

12. SCHAMBELAN, M., SLATON, P. E., JR., AND BIGLIERI, E. G.: *Mineralocorticoid production in hyperadrenocorticism: role in pathogenesis of hypokalemic alkalosis.* Am. J. Med. 51:299, 1971.

13. BIGLIERI, E. G., SCHAMBELAN, M., BRUST, N., ET AL.: *Plasma aldosterone concentration: further characterization of aldosterone-producing adneomas.* Circ. Res. 34,35(Suppl. I): I-183, 1974.

14. GANGULY, A., MELADA, G. A., LUETSCHER, J. A., ET AL.: *Control of plasma aldosterone in primary aldosteronism: distinction between adenoma and hyperplasia.* J. Clin. Endocrinol. Metab. 37:765, 1973.

15. SCHAMBELAN, M., BRUST, N. L., CHANG, B. C. F., ET AL.: *Circadian rhythm and effect of posture on plasma aldosterone concentration in primary aldosteronism.* Clin. Endocrinol. Metab. 43:115, 1976.

16. BIGLIERI, E. G., AND SCHAMBELAN, M.: *Management of primary hyperaldosteronism,* in ONESTI, G., KIM, K. E., AND MOYER, J. H. (eds.): *Hypertension: Mechanisms and Management.* Grune & Stratton, New York, 1973, 493–498.

17. SEABOLD, J. E., COHEN, E. L., AND BEIERWALTES, W. H.: *Adrenal imaging with ^{131}I-19-iodocholesterol in the diagnostic evaluation of patients with aldosteronism.* J. Clin. Endocrinol. Metab. 42:41, 1976.

18. HOGAN, M. J., MCRAE, J., SCHAMBELAN, M., ET AL.: *Location of aldosterone-producing adenomas with ^{131}I-19-iodocholesterol.* N. Engl. J. Med. 294:410, 1976.

Glucocorticoid Hypertension

Peter G. Pletka, M.D., and Roger B. Hickler, M.D.

In the classic description of the syndrome that now bears his name, Cushing in 1932 described 12 patients with obesity, moon facies and plethora, 9 of whom had hypertension.[1] He attributed this syndrome to the effect of basophil adenomata in the pituitary but did not discount the adrenal as contributing to some of the features observed. Ten years later Albright showed the features of this syndrome to be due to the increased secretion of adrenal hormones.[2] Since then systemic hypertension has been a well recognized feature of this syndrome, ranging in incidence from 80 to 90 percent of patients in all reported series.[3-6]

Over the last 20 years, additional disorders of cortisol metabolism have been described in which hypertension plays a prominent part. In 1956 Eberlein and Bongiovanni described a hypertensive form of virilizing adrenal hyperplasia to be due to 11β-hydroxylase deficiency resulting in decreased cortisol production,[7] and in 1966 Biglieri and coworkers described hypertension in women with absence of sexual characteristics associated with a 17α-hydroxylation defect.[8]

Although many of the clinical features in the various syndromes can be explained on the basis of an abnormality in cortisol synthesis or metabolism, the presence of hypertension can be explained with any degree of certainty in only a small minority of cases.

It is the purpose of this presentation to review the various hypertensive conditions in which abnormalities of cortisol metabolism have been described and to examine those mechanisms which may be responsible for its pathogenesis.

BIOSYNTHESIS AND METABOLISM OF CORTICOSTEROIDS

An understanding of the various conditions resulting from abnormalities of corticosteroid production is impossible without a brief review of the biosynthetic pathway (Fig. 1). The main glucocorticoids in man, the steroids that have a predominant effect on carbohydrate and protein metabolism, are cortisol and corticosterone. Both of these hormones have in addition distinct mineralocorticoid effects and may influence salt and water homeostasis under both basal and pathologic conditions, an important point to remember when considering conditions in which they are produced to excess.

Cortisol, together with the androgenic steroids, is produced in the zona fasciculata and zona reticularis of the adrenal gland, while aldosterone is generated in the zona glomerulosa.

The synthesis of cortisol and androgens is dependent on adequate secretion of ACTH from the pituitary gland. This secretion follows a diurnal pattern reaching peaks in the morning and low levels by late afternoon, and is reflected by a similar cortisol secretory pattern. The total secretory rate of cortisol is between 15 and 30 mg./24 hrs. Cortisol has a half-life of approximately 80 minutes, is metabolized mostly in the liver, and secreted in the urine where it is measured as 17-ketogenic steroids and 17-hydroxy-corticosteroids (Porter-Silber chromogens).

In Cushing's syndrome the primary defect is one of excess cortisol production, which may be the result of an autonomous dysfunction of the adrenal gland such as an adrenal carcinoma or adenoma or secondary to excess ACTH production either from the pituitary or a nonadrenal tumor.

In 11β-hydroxylation defects, which may be either congenital such as in the adreno-genital syndrome, or acquired as in some cases of carcinoma of the adrenal, production of cortisol is impaired. Hypertension results because of an accumulation of desoxycor-ticosterone, a cortisol precursor with marked mineralocorticoid activity. Since the suppressive influence of cortisol on ACTH is absent and desoxycorticosterone does not influence ACTH secretion, the overall effect will be an increase in production of desoxycorticosterone and its metabolites, as well as a shunting of cortisol precursors into the androgen pathway, resulting in virilization.

In 17α-hydroxylase deficiency, both the production of androgen and cortisol is impaired and desoxycorticosterone again is formed in excess which results in hypertension, accompanied by hypogonadism due to decreased production of the sex hormones.

Although corticosterone has 50 percent of the glucocorticoid activity of cortisol, its production rate is only one fifteenth to one tenth that of cortisol and it may play only a minor role under basal conditions. However, its mineralocorticoid effect is greater than that of cortisol and when secreted to excess it may have profound salt and water retaining activities.

CUSHING'S SYNDROME

Cushing's syndrome is the prototype of glucocorticoid hypertension. The clinical features of this syndrome have been well documented and are the result of chronic overproduction of cortisol.

The clinical spectrum ranges from the patient with florid features consisting of truncal obesity, moon facies with plethora, muscular weakness and bruising, which are readily recognizable, to patients with subtle cushingoid features such as moderate obesity, striae, and often diabetes mellitus, in whom the diagnosis cannot be made except by laboratory investigations. Another group that may present a diagnostic problem is one consisting mostly of women who are middle-aged, moderately obese, with hirsutism, in whom hypertension is detected. Many of these will turn out to have essential hypertension and normal plasma cortisol levels.

Ross and coworkers[6] reviewed the clinical features of Cushing's syndrome in 601 patients and found that truncal obesity occurred in 88 percent, moon facies and plethora in 75 percent, menstrual irregularities in 60 percent, muscular weakness in 61 percent and bruising in 41 percent. Other features commonly associated with Cushing's syndrome but having a low diagnostic value because they occur in many patients without Cushing's syndrome are acne, striae, edema, hirsutism, and abnormal glucose tolerance tests.

The diagnosis of Cushing's syndrome, although often made clinically, always requires laboratory confirmation. The laboratory investigations should address themselves to two issues:

1. To firmly establish the diagnosis and,
2. Once the diagnosis is made, to differentiate the various causes of this syndrome

which include (a) pituitary induced adrenal hyperplasia, (b) ectopic ACTH syndrome and (c) adrenal tumors.

The diagnosis is established by tests that determine the basal secretory rates of the various hormones that may be secreted in this conditon and measured in the urine and plasma.

24-Hour Urinary 17-Hydroxycorticosteroid, 17-Ketogenic Steroid and Ketosteroid Excretion. Urinary hydroxycorticosteroids reflect most accurately the cortisol secretory rates and are nearly always elevated in all cases of Cushing's syndrome. However, in view of the secretory variability that may occur even in proven cases of Cushing's syndrome, these measurements require repetition on several occasions before a definite diagnosis can be made.

Measurement of 17-ketogenic steroid excretion, although useful as an index of cortisol production, is relatively nonspecific since in addition to measuring cortisol and its metabolites it also measures pregnentriol, which may be increased in certain cases of congenital adrenal hyperplasia. It also has to be taken into account that both 17-hydroxycorticosteroid and 17-ketogenic steroid excretions are often increased in simple obesity, hyperthyroidism, and pregnancy and are affected by many medications.

Urinary ketosteroid excretion analyses, although in many ways having outlived their usefulness, are still being used. Traditionally, it is a test of adrenal androgen production. However, it is a poor test of cortisol production or excretion since only 5 to 10 percent of cortisol secreted by the adrenal is metabolized into ketosteroids.

Plasma Cortisol Levels. These are among the most useful and commonly used laboratory tests for diagnosing Cushing's syndrome. In view of the diurnal variation of cortisol secretion, plasma cortisol levels are best measured in the evening when concentrations are usually less than 8 μg./100 ml. Patients with Cushing's syndrome lack the normal diurnal rhythm and it is unusual to find levels below 8 μg./100 ml. Plasma and cortisol levels in the morning range between 12 and 25 μg./100 ml. and may overlap with values found in the early stages of the disease. During the later stages, levels of 15 or 35 μg./100 ml. (two- to fivefold normal) are recorded at any time of day.

Low-dose Dexamethasone Suppression Test. If 24-hour urinary 17-hydroxycorticosteroid or 17-ketogenic steroid excretion is increased and evening cortisol levels exceed 8 μg./100 ml., it is best to proceed with the suppression test. If the patient is not hospitalized, the "overnight" suppression test may be used where 1 mg. of dexamethasone is given before midnight and plasma cortisol levels are measured in the morning. In patients with Cushing's syndrome this dose will not suppress ACTH secretion and cortisol levels in excess of 12 μg./100 ml. are usually found. If the patient is hospitalized, the 2-day test should be used. A dosage of 0.5 mg. of dexamethasone is given every 6 hours for 2 days and if on the second day plasma cortisol levels do not decrease below 5 μg./100 ml. and 24-hour urinary 17-hydroxycorticosteroid below 2.5 mg./24 hr., a diagnosis of hypercortisolism can be made.

Once the presence of hypercortisolism is established, the different causes of this condition have to be identified.

Four tests are commonly used to differentiate hyperplasia, adenomas and carcinomas of the adrenal cortex, namely ACTH stimulation, high-dose dexamethasone suppression, metyrapone inhibition and plasma ACTH levels.

Each test should be used according to the suspicions of the clinician as to the probable cause of Cushing's syndrome, and more than one test is necessary to confirm the diagnosis.

ACTH stimulation results in increased plasma cortisol and urinary 17-hydroxycorticosteroid in patients with pituitary induced hyperplasia, commonly in adrenal adenomas, but NOT in carcinomas.

High-dose dexamethasone, 2 mg. every 6 hours for 2 days, will NOT suppress adrenal carcinomas and adenomas, usually not ectopic ACTH-induced hyperplasia, but will suppress pituitary-induced hyperplasia.

Metyrapone inhibition (an adrenal inhibitor blocking 11β-hydroxylation) results in an increased excretion of 17-hydroxycorticosteroids and 17-ketogenic steroids in normal subjects. A similar but more pronounced response will occur in pituitary-induced hyperplasia, but NOT in adrenal adenomas and carcinomas. With ectopic ACTH production the response is variable.

Plasma ACTH levels are high in pituitary Cushing's syndrome, high in ectopic ACTH syndrome, and low in adrenal carcinomas and adenomas.

Intravenous pyelography, tomography and adrenal venography are used to localize the adrenal abnormality, and roentgenograms of the sella turcica may disclose sellar erosions characteristic of pituitary tumors.

The frequency with which Cushing's syndrome occurs among the hypertensive population is not entirely known. On the basis of autopsies the incidence of Cushing's syndrome has been estimated at 0.1 percent of the population, and if one considers that 15 to 20 percent of the population has hypertension and that hypertension occurs in 80 percent of patients with Cushing's syndrome, then the incidence can be calculated as being 1:300 of the hypertensive population. This is consistent with the observation at the Peter Bent Brigham Hospital where 1:400 of randomly selected hypertensive patients were found to have Cushing's syndrome.[9] In other studies, however, laboratory evidence of cortisol hypersecretion has been reported in a startling 36 percent of patients simulating essential hypertension, an observation which to our knowledge has not been reproduced.[10]

Hypertension occurs in 80 to 90 percent of all patients with endogenous Cushing's syndrome and increases in frequency after the fifth decade. Ross and coworkers found in their series of 50 patients that 23 of 24 patients aged over 40 had hypertension.[6]

The 80 to 90 percent occurrence of hypertension in the naturally occurring disease, irrespective of its underlying etiology, is in sharp contrast to the 10 to 20 percent incidence of hypertension in iatrogenic Cushing's syndrome. Although all of these conditions have in common the presence of a state of hypercortisolism, the pathophysiology and clinical features of each of these conditions are somewhat different and it is appropriate to discuss each one separately.

ADRENAL HYPERPLASIA DUE TO PITUITARY DISORDERS

This condition is the most common cause of Cushing's syndrome and represents 60 to 65 percent of patients in all reported series.[4-6] The majority of cases are in women usually in the third and fourth decades, although cases in the extremes of life have also been reported.

The primary disorder is an inappropriately high pituitary secretion of ACTH in the presence of an elevated plasma cortisol level. In 5 to 10 percent of patients a pituitary tumor is present, most commonly a basophil or chromophobe adenoma resulting in an enlarged sella turcica. In the remainder, either small basophil adenomata or more frequently no abnormal pathology is detected at surgery or autopsy.[3]

The elevated ACTH levels are responsible for the increase in plasma cortisol which is usually 2 to 5 times normal levels. These levels suppress only partially with low-dose dexamethasone, while high-dose dexamethasone usually reduces plasma cortisol levels to less than 5 μg./100 ml. and 24-hour urinary 17-hydroxycorticosteroid excretion to less than 5 mg./24 hr.

The clinical picture is characteristically the one described, of which hypertension is a constant feature. Hypertension may be the presenting condition in about 10 percent of

102

cases, some patients having levels in excess of 200/110 mm. Hg, which may progress rapidly to the malignant phase.[11] Hypertensive complications are responsible for a large percentage of deaths recorded in the untreated disorder and still account for some deaths after surgical correction.

In addition to the hypertension, the presence of hypokalemia and metabolic alkalosis in 10 to 15 percent of cases, although less common than in adrenal tumors and ectopic ACTH syndrome, suggests the presence of a hormone with marked mineralocorticoid activity. Plasma aldosterone, deoxycorticosterone and corticosterone levels are usually all within normal limits,[12, 13] although in some cases increased levels have been recorded.[14] The finding of normal aldosterone levels in the presence of increased ACTH secretion is consistent with the observation that continuous ACTH infusion only transiently increases aldosterone production.[15, 16] However, the finding of normal deoxycorticosterone and corticosterone is surprising since experimental intravenous infusion of ACTH results in elevation of both these two steroids.[15, 17] However, ACTH levels in this condition may only be slightly increased, in contrast to ectopic ACTH syndrome, and not sufficient to sustain production of these two hormones.

In the search for a mineralocorticoid which may be responsible for the hypertension, Melby and coworkers reported an increased excretion of 18-hydroxy-tetrahydro-deoxycorticosterone (18-OH-TH-DOC) and 18-hydroxy-deoxycorticosterone (18-OH-DOC) in patients with pituitary-induced Cushing's syndrome as well as the ectopic ACTH syndrome.[18] They considered that a threefold increase in secretion of these hormones, if accompanied by a corresponding increase in DOC, is sufficient to produce arterial hypertension. In two of nine patients with pituitary-induced Cushing's syndrome in whom 18-OH-DOC was measured, it was increased 2 and 30 times normal, and in all nine patients 18-OH-TH-DOC urinary excretion was increased two- to fourfold.[18] However, despite these elevations, it is too early to tell whether these hormones are responsible for the hypertensive and mineralocorticoid effects observed; and results of further studies have to be awaited.

In considering the possible hormonal causes of hypertension and hypokalemic alkalosis, the question also arises whether cortisol itself may not be responsible. There are several mechanisms that can be considered through which cortisol could cause hypertension:

1. Cortisol has a distinct mineralocorticoid effect which under suitable conditions of very high secretion could result in marked salt and water retention.
2. Cortisol stimulates the renin-angiotensin system.
3. Cortisol has been shown to potentiate the vascular effects of catecholamines.

The mineralocorticoid activity of cortisol is only $\frac{1}{200}$ to $\frac{1}{300}$ the activity of aldosterone (Table 1), but its secretion in normal subjects is 200 to 300 times that of aldosterone so that under basal conditions it may play an equivalent role to aldosterone in sodium homeostasis. In pituitary-induced Cushing's syndrome, the two- to fivefold increase in cortisol secretion may be sufficient to cause hypokalemic alkalosis in a small number of patients. However, it is unlikely to be entirely responsible for the pathogenesis of hypertension, despite the finding of sodium retention and extracellular fluid volume expansion,[6, 19] since the chronic administration of hydrocortisone in equivalent doses does not result in an equal incidence of hypertension.[20]

Both ACTH and cortisol have been shown to increase plasma renin substrate (PRS), the globulin on which renin acts to release angiotensin I.[21, 22] Krakoff and coworkers have recently shown an increased concentration of PRS in patients with Cushing's syndrome,[23] and also in patients receiving synthetic glucocorticoids,[24] and have speculated that this mechanism may play a role in the genesis of hypertension by allowing a

Table 1. Relative glucocorticoid and mineralocorticoid activity

Corticosteroid	Glucocorticoid Activity	Mineralocorticoid Activity
Cortisol	1	1
Cortisone	0.8	0.8
Aldosterone	0.3	300
Corticosterone	0.5	1.5
Deoxycorticosterone	0	20
Prednisone	4	0.3
Prednisolone	5	0.3
Methylprednisolone	5	0
Dexamethasone	30	0
Fludrocortisone	8	250

given amount of renin to generate more angiotensin, similar to the effect seen with oral contraceptive agents.

Corticosteroids have also been shown to potentiate the pressor effects of catecholamines,[25, 26] probably through an effect on arterial smooth muscle contractility. Although the mechanism of action is not clearly understood, several hypotheses have been proposed. The studies of Bohr and associates,[27, 28] and of Raab,[29] have suggested that corticosteroids may increase their reactivity to catecholamines by altering the ionic gradient across the smooth muscle cell. Besse and Bass[30] suggested that cortisol may act by increasing the affinity of the adrenergic receptors to catecholamines. Cortisol also has been shown to potentiate the effects of catecholamines in isolated aortic strips by inhibiting catechol-O-methyltransferase, an enzyme involved in the inactivation of epinephrine.[31] Since patients with Cushing's syndrome as well as normal subjects given pharmacologic doses of glucocorticoid have an increased vascular reactivity to catecholamines,[25, 32] it may be speculated that cortisol may play a role in the genesis of hypertension by potentiating the effects of normal levels of circulating catecholamines on the cardiovascular system.

ECTOPIC ACTH SYNDROME

The ectopic ACTH production from nonadrenal tumors accounts for about 15 to 20 percent of all cases of Cushing's syndrome. It is most commonly the result of tumors of the lung, thymomas, and carcinomas of the pancreas, although it may occur with almost any malignancy. Carcinoma of the lung, however, accounts for more than all the other tumors combined.[33]

Patients with this syndrome differ from those with pituitary-dependent cortisol production in several important ways. Men are represented far more commonly than women. It is a rare disorder in children. The typical adiposity, peripheral muscular atrophy, plethora and striae are often absent. Replacing these features is a clinical picture dominated by wasting, generalized weakness, and weight loss, as well as other features associated with malignancy.

Similar to pituitary-dependent Cushing's syndrome, ACTH and cortisol levels are elevated, but much more so, with secretory rates 10 to 30 times normal. The absence of cushingoid features despite the high levels of cortisol is a reflection of the short duration of the disease with early mortality.

Laboratory diagnosis of this condition is based on the finding of markedly elevated ACTH levels in the absence of pituitary disease, and high plasma cortisol and urinary 17-hydroxycorticosteroid excretion, which usually do not suppress with high-dose dexamethasone. Hypertension is a frequent finding and is commonly of marked severity associated in a majority of cases with hypokalemic metabolic alkalosis.[6, 12]

In contrast to pituitary-dependent Cushing's syndrome, plasma DOC and corticosterone levels are increased, perhaps reflecting the higher production of ACTH. Aldosterone levels are usually within normal limits.[12, 17] The cortisol in this situation clearly can be responsible for the marked mineralocorticoid effects observed and contribute to the development of hypertension. The production of corticosterone, which has no effect on blood pressure, and DOC with both pressor and mineralocorticoid activity, almost certainly contribute to these features. However, it is of interest that only plasma cortisol levels bear an inverse relationship with the reduced plasma potassium levels observed.[34] Further mineralocorticoid activity may be attributed to the presence of an increased 18-OH-DOC and 18-OH-TH-DOC secretion.

ADRENAL NEOPLASMS

Adrenal neoplasms may be benign or malignant. Adrenal corticoadenomas are the least common cause of Cushing's syndrome and are responsible for between 5 and 15 percent of cases in this condition. The striking feature is that nearly all cases reported are in women. The clinical features are identical to those with pituitary-induced adrenal hyperplasia, but are usually more rapid in onset.

Adenomas may be difficult to differentiate from carcinomas pathologically except that they are usually smaller in size, rarely exceeding 5 cm. in diameter. Adrenal carcinomas are the most common cause of Cushing's syndrome in childhood and are responsible for between 10 and 15 percent of all cases seen. They are frequently unilateral but may occasionally be bilateral. They are palpable in 40 to 60 percent of patients, who may present with cushingoid features and evidence of metastases in other parts of the body, most commonly the liver and the lungs. Similar to adrenal adenomas, the clinical course is short and the majority of patients die within months of the diagnosis.[11]

The diagnosis rests with the finding of markedly elevated cortisol levels associated with low or normal ACTH levels, nonsuppressibility with high-dose dexamethasone and no increase in plasma cortisol with metyrapone. Adrenal carcinomas differ markedly from other causes of Cushing's syndrome in the variety of steroids excreted. Excretion of large amounts of 17-ketosteroids is usual. There is often evidence of a partial defect in 11β-hydroxylation resulting in divergence of progesterone and pregnonalone (see Fig. 1) to the androgenic precursors of ketosteroids. Despite this there is a marked increase in cortisol secretion as well as its precursors, 11-deoxycortisol and DOC. The increased secretion of androgenic steroids is responsible for some of the virilizing features noted in 90 percent of females with carcinoma of the adrenal and 30 percent with adrenal adenomas. Hypertension and hypokalemic alkalosis are common in both benign and malignant tumors and may in part be related to the increased secretion of DOC as well as the high level of cortisol. Aldosterone secretion is usually not increased.[12, 13, 17]

IATROGENIC CUSHING'S SYNDROME

The prolonged administration of corticosteroids in pharmacologic doses results in the development of clinical features which are indistinguishable from those of the natural disease. However, in contrast to the frequent occurrence of hypertension in the natural disease, it only occurs in one fifth of patients treated with steroids. It appears that the dose, duration of treatment, and type of corticosteroid used are important in the iatrogenic genesis of hypertension.

The frequent use in the past of cortisone, with its marked mineralocorticoid effects in high doses, resulted in a high incidence of hypertension. In one group of 100 patients given over 525 mg. of cortisol per week, the incidence of hypertension was 25 percent, while in those using less than 525 mg. per week, it was 18 percent.[20] Savage and coworkers[35] reported an overall incidence of hypertension of 16.6 percent in patients treated with cortisone and its analogues for periods of 1 to 11 years. Unfortunately, in this study exact information regarding the corticosteroid used and the duration of treatment before the development of hypertension was not included, but it can be presumed that many received cortisone for a protracted period of time, since prednisone given in single or divided daily doses of 10 mg. for 9 months produced no case of hypertension in another study.[36] The more frequent use in the last decade of steroids with little or no mineralocorticoid activity is associated with a much lower incidence of hypertension. In a series of 170 patients treated with prednisone only 5 developed this complication.[37] The acute use of steroids even in high doses usually does not cause hypertension in normal subjects.[38] Even when continued for periods of 1 to 7 months the development of hypertension is exceptional.[38] However, when underlying renal disease is present, hypertension is an invariable result.[38] In one series, patients with proteinuria and renal disease of different etiologies treated with cortisone all developed hypertension within 3 weeks.[38] It is a common clinical observation that in this group of patients hypertension often develops during periods of improvement of the underlying condition. The recently introduced use of alternate day therapy may be beneficial for patients with renal disease. In a study of 45 renal transplant recipients, 31 patients had their steroid therapy changed from daily to an alternate day regimen, keeping the dose per 24 hours constant. In 18 of these patients, a reduction of blood pressure was observed and in 11 patients blood pressure remained unchanged. In three patients the blood pressure increased, although a rejection episode may have been responsible for the increase in blood pressure in one patient.[39]

CONGENITAL ADRENAL HYPERPLASIA

There are two syndromes of congenital adrenal hyperplasia associated with hypertension, one described by Eberlein and Bongiovanni,[7] and another by Biglieri.[8] In contrast to the hypertension in Cushing's syndrome where excess cortisol is secreted, the hypertension in these cases is paradoxically associated with a deficiency of cortisol.

In 11β-hydroxylase deficiency, as described by Eberlein and Bongiovanni, the production of corticosterone and aldosterone from 11-deoxycorticosterone and cortisol from 11-deoxycortisol is impaired (Fig. 1). The decreased cortisol production results in increased ACTH which stimulates secretion of androgens, which are not dependent on 11β-hydroxylation, and results in precocious puberty and virilism in boys and pseudohermaphroditism in girls (Fig. 2).

In the 17α-hydroxylase deficiency, as described by Biglieri, in addition to the blockage in the synthesis of cortisol, the production of adrenal androgens and estrogens is impaired (Figs. 1 and 2). Therefore, virilism is not seen, and instead a failure of sexual development is observed with hypogonadism and amenorrhea in females, and ambiguous genital development in males. These defects in sexual development are frequently not observed until after puberty, but the biosynthetic abnormalities are present from birth resulting in hypertension and metabolic alkalosis.

Adrenal steroids not dependent on 17 α-hydroxylation are present in excess amounts — blood levels and urinary excretions of progesterone, DOC, corticosterone, 18-hydroxycorticosterone and 17-ketosteroids are increased. However, aldosterone levels

106

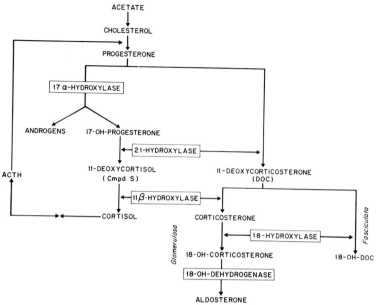

Figure 1. Biosynthesis of corticosteroids.

are subnormal or undetectable. The low aldosterone level may be the result of a DOC-mediated increase in extracellular volume resulting in suppression of plasma renin activity and decreased aldosterone production. Another mechanism may be the decreased intra-adrenal production of aldosterone from 18-hydroxycorticosterone since the reduced plasma renin activity does not always prevent aldosterone secretion. When

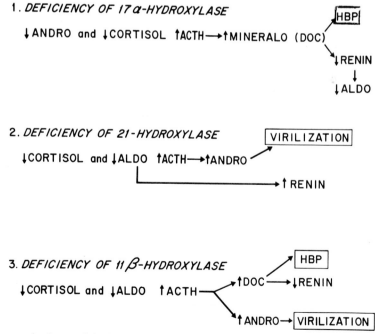

Figure 2. Enzymatic abnormalities in congenital adrenal hyperplasia.

ACTH is administered to patients with aldosterone-producing adenomata in which plasma renin activity is nearly absent, a transient elevation of aldosterone secretion does occur followed by decreased aldosterone production when ACTH is discontinued.[16]

In another syndrome of congenital adrenal hyperplasia associated with 21-hydroxylase deficiency, hypertension does not occur (Fig. 2). The effect of the 21-hydroxylase deficiency is to inhibit both the glucocorticoid and mineralocorticoid pathways. The ACTH excess due to cortisol deficiency results in increased secretion of androgens and thereby virilization of the external genitalia frequently observed at birth. The lack of mineralocorticoid activity due to low aldosterone production may occasionally result in salt wasting and dehydration leading to death if not treated. Plasma renin activity may be increased in this condition, but plasma aldosterone concentration is decreased.

ESSENTIAL HYPERTENSION

The voluminous literature in the last two or three decades attempting to link the adrenal cortex with essential hypertension is clear evidence of the increasing importance that investigators attach to this gland in the causation of hypertension.[40]

There is now considerable evidence that disturbances in regulation of mineralocorticoids may play an active role in the etiology of essential hypertension, especially in the group of patients with low plasma renin activity. Increased aldosterone levels with diminished clearance rates[41] and increased elevated 18-OH-DOC have been reported.[18] However, changes in DOC or corticosterone secretion have not been demonstrated.[41] Other adrenal corticosteroids with variable mineralocorticoid activity have been found to be increased in essential hypertension.[40]

The role played by cortisol, if any, is not entirely clear. Genest and coworkers reported low cortisol levels in some patients with essential hypertension,[41] and Kornel and colleagues[42, 43] found that cortisol excretion was impaired and that certain conjugates of 17-hydroxycorticosteroids were present in the blood and in the urine in reduced concentrations, suggesting an abnormality in cortisol metabolism in essential hypertension.

The importance of cortisol in the maintenance of normal blood pressure and hypertension is well known, and the effects of cortisol on vascular reactivity, especially in response to pressor agents, has been described. However, none of these observations is sufficient to implicate this hormone in the etiology of essential hypertension.

TREATMENT OF GLUCOCORTICOID-INDUCED HYPERTENSION

The treatment of patients with Cushing's syndrome is dependent in large part on the underlying etiology, and is influenced by the duration of the disease and the severity of the clinical features. Hypertension has been recognized as a common feature in all cases of naturally occurring Cushing's syndrome and has been responsible for a significant degree of the morbidity and mortality of this condition. Plotz and coworkers described a 50 percent mortality within 5 years in untreated patients, many of whom died of hypertensive complications.[3] Since the introduction of definitive methods of treatment the mortality has markedly decreased. The best results have been obtained in patients with adrenal adenomas in whom surgical removal has been followed by a cure in nearly 100 percent of cases.[5]

In patients with pituitary-induced adrenal hyperplasia, three modalities of treatment have been advocated:

1. Irradiation to the pituitary.
2. Bilateral adrenalectomy.
3. Ortho,-para,-dichlorodiphenyl dichloroethane (o,p'-DDD) administration.

The use of pituitary irradiation has been recommended by some because of the absence of complications, in contrast to the morbidity associated with adrenal surgery followed by lifelong steroid replacement. Unfortunately, pituitary irradiation is only successful in 20 percent of cases, the remainder having to undergo adrenal surgery later.[5]

Total bilateral adrenalectomy is the only dependable curative procedure in this condition, but hypertension is relieved in only about 75 percent of cases.[4, 11] The blood pressure response to adrenalectomy is inversely proportional to the duration of the disease. This may relate to the observation that the hypertensive disease has been found to be more severe and frequent when the disease was present over 5 years compared to when it was present less than 2 years.[4] The blood pressure under some circumstances may not be reversible. O'Neal and coworkers[4] reported that 3 of 7 patients who remained hypertensive after adrenalectomy had marked arteriolar changes on renal biopsy, including the presence of fibrinoid necrosis.[4]

The use of o,p'-DDD in pituitary-induced Cushing's syndrome has a striking degree of success. In one series, a cure was experienced by all 8 patients in whom this medication was used.[5] The advantage of o,p'-DDD is that it selectively destroys the zona fasciculata and zona reticularis while sparing the zona glomerulosa, but its disadvantage lies in the time it takes to attain the desired effect (usually 4 to 6 months), and this precludes its use in cases where there may be a degree of urgency, as in the presence of severe hypertension.

Cushing's syndrome due to ectopic ACTH production by adrenal tumors has been treated by radiation therapy, surgery and chemotherapy with very poor results. In a series of 18 patients with this syndrome, all died within 1 to 18 months.[5] However, in a larger series, 10 of 105 patients were cured by surgical resection of the tumor. In those patients in whom the tumor was nonresectable and who continued to manifest signs of hypercortisolism, the use of adrenal inhibitors (such as aminoglutethimide and metyrapone) or bilateral adrenalectomy has had a temporary beneficial effect.

In patients with adrenal carcinoma, resectability of the tumor has been associated with survival for up to 9 years in some series, although the majority of patients die within a period of months or at the most 1 to 2 years. O,p'-DDD has been utilized with some success in cases where the tumor is nonresectable with survival up to 2 years.[5]

In contrast to patients with Cushing's syndrome in whom improvement in hypertension is dependent on adequate surgical removal of the adrenals, the treatment of patients with hypertension due to congenital adrenal hyperplasia is much more satisfactory. In both 11β- and 17α-hydroxylase deficiency, the increased ACTH production resulting from low cortisol levels can be suppressed by the use of dexamethasone which corrects both the hypertension and the associated electrolyte disturbances.

REFERENCES

1. CUSHING, H.: *The basophil adenomas of the pituitary body and their clinical manifestations (pituitary basophilism)*. Bull. Johns Hopkins Hosp. 50:137, 1932.
2. ALBRIGHT, F.: *Cushing's syndrome*, Harvey Lect. 38:123, 1942–1943.
3. PLOTZ, C. M., KNOWLTON, A. T., AND RAGAN, C.: *The natural history of Cushing's syndrome*. Am. J. Med. 13:597, 1952.
4. O'NEAL, L. W., KISSANE, J. M., AND HARTROFT, P. M.: *The kidney in endocrine hypertension*. Arch. Surg. 100:498, 1970.
5. ORTH, D. N., AND LIDDLE, G. W.: *Results of treatment in 108 patients with Cushing's syndrome*. N. Engl. J. Med. 285:243, 1971.

6. Ross, E. J., Marshall-Jones, P., and Friedman, M.: *Cushing's syndrome: diagnostic criteria.* Q. J. Med. 35:149, 1966.

7. Eberlein, W. R., and Bongiovanni, A. M.: *Plasma and urinary corticosteroids in hypertension from a congenital adrenal hyperplasia.* J. Biol. Chem. 223:85, 1956.

8. Biglieri, E. G., Herron, M. A., and Brust, N.: *17-Hydroxylation deficiency in man.* J. Clin. Invest. 45:1946, 1966.

9. Hickler, R. B., Amsterdam, G. A., and Christlieb, A. R.: *Hypertension secondary to disorders of the adrenal cortex,* in A. N. Brest and J. H. Moyer, (eds.): *Cardiovascular Disorders.* F. A. Davis, Philadelphia, 1968, p. 965.

10. Glaz, E., Fudor, E., Debreczeni, L., et al.: *Dynamic changes in plasma aldosterone and cortisol levels and renin activity in patients with oligosymptomatic adreno-cortical hypertension simulating essential hypertension,* in J. Genest and E. Koiw, (eds.): *Hypertension '72.* Springer-Verlag, New York, 1972, p. 227.

11. Raker, J. W., Cope, O., and Ackerman, I. P.: *Surgical experience with the treatment of hypertension of Cushing's syndrome.* Am. J. Surg. 107:153, 1964.

12. Biglieri, E. G., Slaton, P. E., Schambelan, M., et al.: *Hypermineralocorticoidism.* Am. J. Med. 45:170, 1968.

13. Oddie, C. J., Coghlan, J. P., and Scoggins, B. A.: *Plasma deoxycorticosterone levels in man with simultaneous measurement of aldosterone, corticosterone, cortisol and 11-deoxycortisol.* J. Clin. Endocrinol. Metab. 34:1039, 1972.

14. Schambelan, M., Slaton, P. E., Jr., and Biglieri, E. G.: *Mineralocorticoid production in hyperadrenocorticism.* Am. J. Med. 51:299, 1971.

15. Biglieri, E. G., Schambelan, M., and Slaton, P. E., Jr.: *Effect of adrenocorticotropin on desoxycorticosterone, corticosterone and aldosterone excretion.* J. Clin. Endocrinol. Metab. 29:10090, 1969.

16. Newton, M. A., and Laragh, J. H.: *Effect of corticotropin on aldosterone excretion and plasma renin in normal subjects, in essential hypertension, and in primary aldosteronism.* J. Clin. Endocrinol. Metab. 28:1006, 1968.

17. Brown, R. D., and Strott, C. A.: *Plasma deoxycorticosterone in man.* J. Clin. Endocrinol. Metab. 32:744, 1971.

18. Melby, J. C., Dale, S. L., Grekin, R. J., et al.: *(18-OH-DOC) secretion in experimental and human hypertension.* Recent Prog. Horm. Res. 28:287, 1972.

19. Prunty, F. T. G., Brooks, R. V., Dupre, J., et al.: *Adrenocortical hyperfunction and potassium metabolism in patients with "nonendocrine" tumors and Cushing's syndrome.* J. Clin. Endocrinol. Metab. 23:737, 1963.

20. Ragan, C.: *Corticotropin, cortisone, and related steroids in clinical medicine. Practical considerations.* Bull. N.Y. Acad. Sci. 29:355, 1953.

21. Helmer, O. M., and Griffith, R. S.: *Biological activity of steroids as determined by assay of renin-substrate (hypertensinogen).* Endocrinology 49:154, 1951.

22. Lazar, J., and Hoobler, S. W.: *Studies on the role of the adrenal in renin kinetics.* Proc. Soc. Exp. Biol. Med. 138:164, 1971.

23. Krakoff, L., Nicolis, G., and Amsel, B.: *Pathogenesis of hypertension in Cushing's syndrome.* Am. J. Med. 58:216, 1975.

24. Krakoff, L. R.: *Measurement of plasma renin substrate by radioimmunoassay of angiotensin I: concentration in syndromes associated with steroid excess.* J. Clin. Endocrinol. Metab. 37:110, 1973.

25. Mendlowitz, M., Naftchi, N., Weinreb, H. L., et al.: *Effect of prednisolone on digital vascular reactivity in normotensive and hypertensive subjects.* J. Appl. Physiol. 16:89, 1961.

26. Schmid, P. G., Eckstein, J. W., and Abboud, F. M.: *Effect of a 9-α-fluorohydrocortisone on forearm vascular responses of norepinephrine.* Circ. Res. 24:383, 1969.

27. Bohr, D. F., and Cummings, G.: *Comparative potentiating action of various steroids on the contraction of vascular smooth muscle.* Fed. Proc. 17:17, 1958.

28. Bohr, D. F.: *Contraction of vascular smooth muscle.* Can. Med. Assoc. J. 90:174, 1964.

29. Raab, W.: *Transmembrane cationic gradient and blood pressure regulation: interaction of corticoids, catecholamines and electrolytes on vascular cells.* Am. J. Cardiol. 4:752, 1959.

30. Besse, J. C., and Bass, A. D.: *Potentiation by hydrocortisone of responses to catecholamines in vascular smooth muscle.* J. Pharmacol. Exp. Ther. 154:224, 1966.

31. Kalsner, S.: *Mechanism of hydrocortisone potentiation of responses to epinephrine and norepinephrine in rabbit aorta.* Circ. Res. 24:383, 1969.

32. MENDLOWITZ, M., GITLOW, S., AND NAFTCHI, N.: *Work of digital vasoconstriction produced by infused norepinephrine in Cushing's syndrome.* J. Appl. Physiol. 13:252, 1958.

33. LIDDLE, G. W., ISLAND, D. P., NEY, R. L., ET AL.: *Nonpituitary neoplasms and Cushing's syndrome.* Arch. Intern. Med. 111:471, 1963.

34. CHRISTY, N. P., AND LARAGH, J. H.: *Pathogenesis of hypokalemic alkalosis in Cushing's syndrome.* N. Engl. J. Med. 265:1083, 1961.

35. SAVAGE, V., COPEMAN, W. S. C., CHAPMAN, L., ET AL.: *Pituitary and adrenal hormones in rheumatoid arthritis.* Lancet 1:232, 1962.

36. NUGENT, C. A., WARD, S., MacDIAMOND, W. D., ET AL.: *Glucocorticoid toxicity. Single contrasted with divided daily doses of prednisone.* J. Chronic Dis. 18:323, 1965.

37. MOUNSELL, K., PEARSON, R. S. B., AND LIVINGSTONE, J. C.: *Long term corticosteroid treatment of asthma.* Br. Med. J. 1:661, 1968.

38. PERERA, G. A.: *Cortisone and blood pressure.* Proc. Soc. Exp. Biol. Med. 76:583, 1951.

39. DIETHELM, A. G., STERLING, W. A., HARTLEY, M. W., ET AL.: *Alternate day prednisone therapy in recipients of renal allografts. Risks and benefits.* Arch. Surg. 111:867, 1976.

40. GENEST, J., NOWACZYNSKI, W., KUCHEL, O., ET AL.: *The adrenal cortex and essential hypertension.* Recent Prog. Horm. Res. 32:377, 1976.

41. NOWACYZNSKI, W., KUCHEL, O., AND GENEST, O.: *Aldosterone, deoxycorticosterone and corticosterone metabolism in benign essential hypertension,* in J. GENEST AND W. KOIW, (EDS.): *Hypertension '72.* Springer-Verlag, New York, 1972, p. 245.

42. KORNEL, L., AND MOTOMASHI, K.: *Corticosteroids in human blood. II. Free and conjugated hydroxycorticosteroids in essential hypertension.* J. Clin. Endocrinol. Metab. 25:904, 1965.

43. KORNEL, L., MIYABO, S., SAITO, Z., ET AL.: *Corticosteroids in human blood. VIII. Cortisol metabolites in plasma of normotensive subjects and patients with essential hypertension.* J. Clin. Endocrinol. Metab. 40:949, 1975.

Stress and Hypertension: Interrelations and Management*

Herbert Benson, M.D., Jamie B. Kotch, A.B., and Karen D. Crassweller, A.B.

Essential hypertension is by definition of unknown etiology. Many believe its pathogenesis to be multifactorial.[1] This chapter is written to support the hypothesis that a major causative factor of hypertension is "stress." Evidence will be presented in this chapter which strongly suggests that stressful situations requiring behavioral adjustment lead to hypertension. Since behavioral events theoretically contribute to hypertension, it is not unreasonable to assume that behavioral interventions can be used in the therapy of hypertension. The evidence establishing the effectiveness of such behavioral interventions will also be presented.

EPIDEMIOLOGIC CONSIDERATIONS

Epidemiologic investigations have shown a consistent relation between elevated systemic arterial blood pressure (hypertension) and a number of environmental variables. Epidemiologic factors that have been associated with the prevalence of hypertension include urban vs. rural living, race, socioeconomic status and its accompanying standard of living, occupation and education. A consistent theme underlying the study of such demographic variables in elevated blood pressure has been the concept of environmental stress.[2, 3] Terms such as "stress," "social stress," and "occupational stress" have been vague and difficult to quantify. This lack of firm definition has seriously impeded research. However, when stress is defined in terms of environmental situations that require continuous behavioral adjustment on the part of the individual, a consistent relation between stress and hypertension is found.[4]

Comparison of blood pressure patterns of two population groups is most commonly made in terms of difference in the prevalence of hypertension or in the proportion of the population showing relatively elevated blood pressure. Urban populations in both the United States[5-7] and other countries[8-15] have higher blood pressure levels or hypertensive mortality rates[6] than their neighboring rural populations. Exceptions are found in studies of blacks in Jamaica[16, 17] and in Mississippi[18] where females from rural areas have higher mean systolic and diastolic pressures than urban females. The concept of increased blood pressures in urban areas is logical. Since the complexities of urban life far exceed those of rural living, the city poses many more situations which require behavioral adjustment.

*Supported in part by grants from the U. S. Public Health Service (RR 01032 from the General Clinical Research Centers Program of the Division of Research Resources, MH 25101, and HL 10539).

113

Variations in blood pressure have also been correlated with indices of socioeconomic status, although data on the distribution of blood pressure by social class have been contradictory.[19-21] Relatively high standards of living, higher incomes, more extensive education, and professional or skilled occupations are associated with a greater prevalence of elevated blood pressure.[10, 22] However, others have reported that hypertension prevalence rates decrease as measures of socioeconomic status improve.[6, 15, 23-27] Yet other investigations reveal that the relation between social class and elevated arterial blood pressure is confounded by sociocultural variables. For example, the Health Examination Survey conducted between October 1959 and December 1962 did not offer a clear association between yearly income and blood pressure in the Caucasian population investigated.[28] A more distinct relation between salary and blood pressure is noted, however, in the black population. Greater prevalence of elevated blood pressure is witnessed in blacks with incomes less than $2,000 per year or with less than five years of schooling than in those with higher incomes and more education.[28]

Arterial pressures of adult American blacks are higher than those of the white adult population.[6, 7, 14, 15, 18, 25, 26, 28-33] This racial difference exists for both sexes and for all age groups. However, this racial factor is much less significant in the northwest United States and in large metropolitan areas.[28] Black populations in "high stress" neighborhoods of Detroit (those areas marked by low socioeconomic status) have a greater prevalence of hypertension than do blacks in middle class neighborhoods.[24, 26, 34] However, when white and black women are matched for social class and its corresponding stressor conditions, no blood pressure differences are present.[18, 25] Investigations outside the United States also reveal that blacks do not always have higher blood pressures than whites.[35] These data suggest that the stresses inherent in a lower class position may transcend any racial influences. Again, the need for continuous behavioral adjustment may be the common denominator of such demographic variables as socioeconomic class and race. High occupational or financial status, with its attendant responsiblities are indeed stressful and demand specific behavioral adjustments. Similarly, the life situations faced daily by the ghetto inhabitant or the racial pressures endured by the black person are also stressful.

Life-threatening events are the most obvious environmental circumstances which cause stress and require behavioral adjustment. In 1947, when an explosion equalling the force of an atomic bomb shook the town of Texas City, marked increases in arterial blood pressure were witnessed in the inhabitants that persisted for days after the explosion.[36] During World War II, elevated blood pressures were observed among the besieged Russian population of Leningrad[37, 38] and were also noted among the soldiers going to battle.[37]

Elevated systemic arterial blood pressure has been associated with rapid cultural change resulting from industrialization, by adoption of cultural traits of another group, and by migration to different environments.[39] For example, the prevalence of hypertension has been directly related to the degree of "westernization" in several Pacific island populations.[10, 40-42] Furthermore, the migration of rural inhabitants to more urban environments within the same country resulted in elevated blood pressure.[43] Higher mean blood pressures have been noted in Zulu adults who recently moved to an urban community, as compared to urban residents of longer standing. Such data suggest that behavioral adaptation to urban life indeed may be stressful and a significant factor contributing to hypertension.[9, 13]

Involved in the process of cultural change is the breakdown of traditional mores and the adoption of new value systems and behaviors. Previously sanctioned patterns of behavior which can no longer be expressed may lead to repeated autonomic nervous system arousal.[44] This occurred in the Zulus where the extended family, a social tradition in the rural Zulu community, is associated with elevated blood pressure in the ur-

114

ban community.[11] The view that increases in blood pressure represent a failure of adaptation to a new environment is held by some researchers.[13]

Striking examples of the inherent problems in adaptation may be seen in migrant groups, where specific attitudes contribute to a difficult adjustment.[6] Black migrants living in a Chicago slum who viewed their neighbors as undesirable had higher blood pressures than those with neutral or positive attitudes. The greatest prevalence of hypertension is recorded for those who wished to move from their housing locations, but were uncertain of their chances of moving. These results do not necessarily indicate a causal relation between environment or negative attitudes and elevated blood pressures. However, the conflict and uncertainty resulting from environmental change can be stressful and may lead to an increase in systemic arterial blood pressure.[45]

Educational status appears to be an intervening variable in occupational stress. A greater prevalence of elevated blood pressure was noted in white-collar workers with less education than their colleagues.[6] Similarly, a comparison of high school and college graduates in managerial positions in the same company revealed more illness and more signs prognostic of cardiovascular disease and hypertension in the high school graduates.[46] Indeed, such a discrepancy between occupational status and education may be quite stressful, and lead to negative health effects for the "self-made man".[47]

In summary, epidemiologic studies have shown a direct relation between the prevalence of hypertension and a wide variety of demographic variables. A common denominator of these many variables appears to be the presence of situations which require behavioral adjustment.

PHYSIOLOGY OF STRESSFUL EVENTS LEADING TO HYPERTENSION

Stressful situations requiring behavioral adjustment appear to elevate blood pressure by means of a physiologic response, the emergency reaction, first described by Dr. Walter B. Cannon.[48] Cannon reasoned that this innate, integrated hypothalamic response prepared an animal for behavioral action such as running or fighting when faced with threatening environmental situations. The emergency reaction termed the defense-alarm reaction by others[49, 50] and popularly called the fight-or-flight response, is characterized by coordinated increases in catecholamine production, blood pressure, heart and respiratory rates, and markedly increased skeletal muscle blood flow.[48, 50] Direct electrical stimulation of specific areas of the hypothalamus, mesencephalic tegmentum, and central gray matter in laboratory animals induces the fight-or-flight response.[51] In the conscious animal, direct stimulation of hypothalamic regions produced behaviors ranging from mild alerting to fully developed emergency reactions culminating in fight or flight.[52] In anesthetized cats, topical stimulation of such areas led to an integrated response consisting of increases in arterial blood pressure, splanchnic and skin vasoconstriction, muscle vasodilatation, pupil dilatation, retraction of the nictitating membrane and pilo-erection.[50] The muscle vasodilatation in response to "emotional stress" in humans,[53] or to direct hypothalamic stimulation in the cat was found to be mediated in part by sympathetic cholinergic fibers[50, 51, 54] and represented only one aspect of a complex cardiovascular response which prepared the animal for strenuous muscular exercise.[55] This hypothalamic response with its autonomic and behavioral components most probably had profound evolutionary significance, since animals with the most highly developed fight-or-flight response may have had an increased probability of surviving and reproducing. Natural selection thus favored the perpetuation of the response and it has probably persisted for eons.

Situations requiring behavioral adjustment (stressful events) lead to elicitation of the fight-or-flight response.[4] Today's complex society presents man with many stressful situations which have led to the excessive elicitation of the response. In addition, its behavioral features of running and fighting are socially unacceptable or inappropriate.

Continuous arousal of the fight-or-flight response may result in hemodynamic changes which lead to hypertension. The changes in essential hypertension are analogous to those occurring in acute pressor responses to "stressful" stimuli, and in preparation for severe muscular exercise.[56-58] During acute pressor responses to emotional "stress" induced by mental arithmetic under time pressure, there was an increased cardiac output and an increased vascular resistance in the kidneys, splanchnic and skin areas associated with skeletal muscle vasodilatation.[59] Normotensive and essential hypertensive subjects both showed the same qualitative vascular response to "stressful" stimuli, but the response was of longer duration in hypertensive patients, and there was an exaggeration of visceral and skin vasoconstriction which was not balanced by a corresponding skeletal muscle vasodilatation.[57, 59] The persistence of these vascular resistance patterns in essential hypertension suggested that essential hypertension did not necessarily result from unusual or newly acquired patterns of hemodynamic response, but rather represented a fixation of a vascular resistance response found normally in acute pressor reactions and during strenuous muscular exercise.[56-58] The existence of a normal cardiac output in essential hypertension[60] is, however, discrepant with the hemodynamic patterns found in acute pressor reactions.

Chronic or repeated hypothalamic stimulation (elicitation of the fight-or-flight response) may lead to a "fixation" of the hemodynamic pattern of selective visceral vasoconstriction and muscle vasodilatation, and may possibly contribute to sustained elevations in arterial blood pressure.[56] Indeed, chronic stimulation of the hypothalamic defense area in the rat resulted in a significant increase of the "resting" mean blood pressure level.[61] Hypothalamic mediation of cardiovascular response to chronic mentally "stressful" environmental stimuli may thus play a significant role in the gradual development of essential hypertension, when environmental conditions are conducive to repeated or chronic arousal of the hypothalamic defense area.[51, 56, 62]

THE RELAXATION RESPONSE: A BEHAVIORAL-PHYSIOLOGIC APPROACH TO HYPERTENSION

If repeated elicitation of the fight-or-flight response and its accompanying sympathetic nervous system arousal contributes to the development of hypertension, then an opposite hypothalamic response, characterized by decreased sympathetic nervous system activity theoretically should counteract such pathophysiologic effects and be useful in the prevention and therapy of hypertension. Such a reaction, which directly counters the fight-or-flight response, indeed exists and was first termed by Hess the trophotropic response.[52] Electrical stimulation of an area of the anterior hypothalamus of a cat's brain produced

> hypo- or adynamia of the skeletal musculature, accompanied by lowering of the blood pressure. . . We are evidently dealing here with an antagonist of dynamogenic zone! We are actually dealing with a protective mechanism against overstress belonging to the trophotropic-endophylactic system and promoting restorative processes. We emphasize that these adynamic effects are opposed to ergotropic reactions which are oriented toward increased oxidative metabolism and utilization of energy.[52]

This hypothalamic-mediated trophotropic response defined in the cat by Hess has subsequently been more extensively investigated in man, and has been termed the relaxation response.[63, 64] The relaxation response, consisting of human physiologic changes opposite to those of the fight-or-flight response,[64-67] is characterized by decreased O_2 consumption, heart and respiratory rates, arterial blood lactate and markedly increased skin resistance. The EEG demonstrated an increase in the intensity of slow alpha waves and occasional theta wave activity.[65] There is a slight increase in resting forearm muscle blood flow probably secondary to decreased sympathetic adrenergic activity.[67] The physiologic changes, when viewed in their totality, are different from those of sleep or of sitting quietly with closed eyes.[65] These physiologic changes which occur concomitantly are most consistent with a generalized decrease in sympathetic nervous system activity.

Techniques have existed for centuries, usually within a religious context, which enable an individual to bring forth the relaxation response and its associated physiologic changes.[63, 64] Practices eliciting the relaxation response may be found in practically every culture of man: in Christian and Jewish meditative prayers, in Eastern religions such as in Zen, Hinduism, Shintoism and Taoism,[63, 64] and in cultic Eastern practices such as Transcendental Meditation and Yoga. Despite the apparent diversity of these widespread techniques, four elements appear to be integral and are necessary for elicitation of the relaxation response:

A Mental Device: There should be a constant mental stimulus, e.g., a sound, word or phrase repeated silently or audibly. The purpose of this procedure is to free one's self from logical, externally oriented thought.

A Passive Attitude: This element is perhaps the most important. If distracting thoughts do occur during the repetition, they should be disregarded and one's attention should be passively redirected to the repetition. One should not worry about how well he is performing the technique.

Decreased Muscle Tonus: The subject should be in a comfortable posture so that minimal muscular work is required.

A Quiet Environment: A quiet environment with minimal environmental stimuli should be chosen. During the practice of the technique, the practitioner is instructed to close his eyes. A place of worship is often suitable as is a quiet room.

For example, these four elements are found in "The Prayer of the Heart" or "The Prayer of Jesus," a repetitive prayer which dates back to the beginning of Christianity and was used in meditation and mystical practices.[68] It was described in the fourteenth century at Mt. Athos in Greece by Gregory of Sinai:

> Sit down alone and in silence. Lower your head, shut your eyes, breathe out gently, and imagine yourself looking into your own heart. Carry your mind, i.e., your thoughts, from your head to your heart. As you breathe out, say 'Lord Jesus Christ, have mercy on me.' Say it moving your lips gently, or simply say it in your mind. Try to put all other thoughts aside. Be calm, be patient and repeat the process very frequently.[68]

In Judaism, similar practices date back to the second century B.C. and are found in one of the earliest forms of Jewish mysticism, Merkabolism.[69] In this practice of meditation, the subject sat with his head between his knees and whispered hymns, songs and repeated a name of a magic seal.

In the East, meditation which elicited the relaxation response was developed much earlier and became a major element not only in religion but also in everyday life. Age-old practices of Yoga strive for "union" of the self with a supreme being or principle. Yogic meditation is concentration upon a single point to cancel out all distractions that are associated with everyday life.[63] Writings from Indian scriptures, the Upanishads, dated sixth century B.C., note that individuals might attain "a unified state with the Brahman [the Deity] by means of restraint of breath, withdrawal of senses, meditation, concentration, contemplation and absorption."[70]

Secular techniques have also been known to produce physiologic effects characteristic of the relaxation response. Some of these include Autogenic Training,[71] Progressive Relaxation,[72] hypnosis,[73-76] and Sentic Cycles.[77] It is important to note that the relaxation response is not unique to any specific technique or religious practice. In fact, investigations have demonstrated that the physiologic responses associated with the relaxation response can be elicited equally well by many techniques.[78]

A SIMPLE NONCULTIC TECHNIQUE WHICH ELICITS THE RELAXATION RESPONSE

A simple technique which elicits the relaxation response has been developed in our laboratory and may be easily learned by following a simple set of instructions.[64, 79] This technique is but one of scores of techniques which incorporate the four basic elements which elicit the relaxation response. The instructions are:

1. Sit quietly in a comfortable position.
2. Close your eyes.
3. Deeply relax all your muscles, beginning at your feet and progressing up to your face. Keep them deeply relaxed.
4. Breathe through your nose. Become aware of your breathing. As you breathe out, say the word "ONE" silently to yourself. For example, breathe IN . . . OUT, "ONE"; IN . . . OUT, "ONE"; etc. Breathe easily and naturally.
5. Continue for 10 to 20 minutes. You may open your eyes to check the time, but do not use an alarm. When you finish, sit quietly for several' minutes at first with your eyes closed and later with your eyes opened. Do not stand up for a few minutes.
6. Do not worry about whether you are successful in achieving a deep level of relaxation. Maintain a passive attitude and permit relaxation to occur at its own pace. When distracting thoughts occur, try to ignore them by not dwelling upon them and return to repeating "ONE." With practice, the response should come with little effort. Practice the technique once or twice daily, but not within two hours after any meal, since the digestive processes seem to interfere with the elicitation of the relaxation response.[64]

THE USEFULNESS OF THE RELAXATION RESPONSE IN THE THERAPY OF HYPERTENSION

Prospective investigations have demonstrated that the regular elicitation of the relaxation response lowers blood pressure in both medicated and nonmedicated hypertensive subjects.[80-86] For example, in one investigation done by our laboratory,[80, 81] 86 hypertensive subjects who were attending introductory lectures of Transcendental Meditation agreed to delay their learning of the technique in order to participate in the study. Prior to their acceptance in the investigation, blood pressures were measured three to four times over a period of 15 to 20 minutes and had to exceed either 140 mm. Hg systolic or 90 mm. Hg diastolic or both, on the last blood pressure recording. These arbitrary levels are higher than those considered to be normotensive.[87] Weekly control measurements of blood pressure were made for approximately six weeks before the subjects were taught to elicit the relaxation response through this practice of meditation. Subjects meditated twice daily for at least two weeks; each subject's blood pressure was then measured approximately every two weeks for an average of 20 to 25 weeks. Measurements were taken at random times of the days, but never during meditation. Measurements were repeated every five minutes until both systolic and diastolic pressures were within 5 mm. Hg of the preceding measurement. On each day of blood pressure measurement for the control and experimental periods the subjects completed a questionnaire which assessed the amount and type of medication they were taking, their dietary habits, and their frequency of meditation.

Each subject was instructed to adhere to the medication schedule prescribed by his physician. During the study, 50 of the original 86 volunteers had altered either their antihypertensive medications or their diets and were thus excluded. Of the remaining 36 patients, 22 received no antihypertensive medications during the study and 14 remained on constant drug therapy during both the premeditation-control and postmeditation-experimental periods. In the 22 unmedicated subjects, blood pressures averaged 146.5 mm. Hg systolic and 94.6 mm. Hg diastolic during the control period. During the experimental period, when the subjects were regularly eliciting the relaxation response through the practice of Transcendental Meditation, blood pressures decreased significantly to 139.5 mm. Hg systolic (p < 0.001) and 90.8 mm. Hg diastolic (p < 0.002) (Fig. 1). In the 14 subjects who remained on constant antihypertensive medications, control blood pressures averaged 145.6 mm. Hg systolic and 91.9 mm. Hg diastolic. During the experimental period, systolic blood pressure decreased significantly to 135.0 mm. Hg (p < 0.01) and diastolic blood pressures decreased to 87.0 mm. Hg (p < 0.05) (Fig. 2). In subjects who chose to stop the regular practice of meditation, both systolic and diastolic pressures returned to their initial hypertensive levels within four weeks after termination of the meditational practice.[88]

Datey and coworkers witnessed decreases in systolic and diastolic blood pressure in hypertensive patients who elicited the relaxation response through the practice of another Yogic technique called Shavasan.[82] In this investigation, 47 subjects were grouped according to both severity of hypertension and the extent of drug therapy. In the patients who were not taking any antihypertensive medication, an average mean

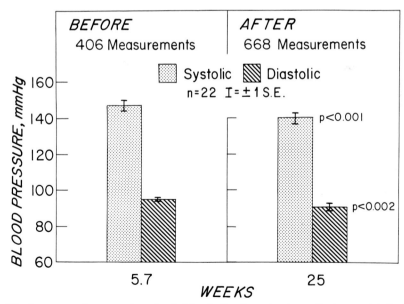

Figure 1. Blood pressure decreases in untreated borderline hypertensive patients associated with regular elicitation of the relaxation response. The blood pressure measurements were made at periods of the day unrelated to the elicitation of the relaxation response.

119

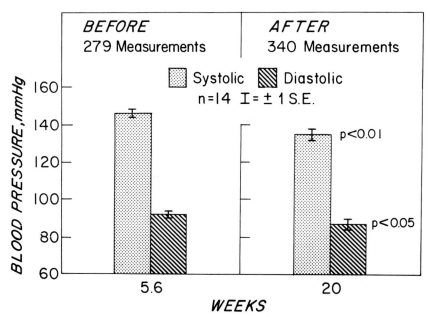

Figure 2. Blood pressure decreases in treated hypertensive patients associated with regular elicitation of the relaxation response. The blood pressure measurements were made at periods of the day unrelated to the elicitation of the relaxation response.

blood pressure of 134 mm. Hg was significantly reduced ($p < 0.05$) to 107 mm. Hg post-intervention. In those whose hypertension was well controlled with the use of antihypertensive drugs, no attempt was made to reduce it further. However, for the majority of patients, the drug requirement was gradually reduced ($p < 0.05$) with no change in mean blood pressure. Lastly, patients whose blood pressure was inadequately controlled despite pharmacologic therapy experienced a decrease of 10 mm. Hg in mean blood pressure after practicing Shavasan. Results of this study, however, are difficult to evaluate, since the method and circumstances of blood pressure recording were not described.

In two well-controlled longitudinal investigations, Patel[83, 84] combined Yogic relaxation with biofeedback techniques in the treatment of 20 medicated hypertensive patients. Results showed that the average systolic blood pressure in these subjects was reduced by 20.4 ± 11.4 mm. Hg while mean diastolic pressure was reduced by 14.2 ± 7.5 mm. Hg ($p < 0.001$). The total drug requirement in 12 patients decreased by an average of 41.9 percent. In this study, a control group matched for age and sex was employed. Length of testing sessions, number of attendances and the procedure for blood pressure measurements were kept the same in the control as in the treatment group. However, instead of receiving instruction in the relaxation technique, control patients were asked to rest on a couch. Results showed that systolic blood pressure in the control group was reduced by 0.5 ± 14.5 mm. Hg and diastolic blood pressure by 2.1 ± 6.2 mm. Hg. Control subjects experienced no significant change in medication requirement.

Further substantiation of the usefulness of the relaxation response in the treatment of hypertension has come from Blackwell and coworkers.[85] Although their investigation was limited due to a small sample size, results indicate there were significant reductions in blood pressure after 12 weeks of the practice of Transcendental Meditation.

Stone and DeLeo[86] produced significant decreases in systolic and diastolic blood pressure using a Buddhist meditation exercise to elicit the relaxation response. After six months of practicing the technique twice daily, the treatment group exhibited significant decreases ($p < 0.05$) in systolic and diastolic pressures from their pretreatment measurements. Average systolic blood pressure dropped from 146 ± 2 mm. Hg to 131 ± 4 mm. Hg; average diastolic blood pressure decreased from 95 ± 3 mm. Hg to 85 ± 2 mm. Hg. These blood pressure decreases in the meditators were also significantly different ($p < 0.05$) than those of the age-and-race-matched control subjects who received no psychotherapeutic instruction. Changes in peripheral sympathetic nervous system activity, as reflected by levels of dopamine-beta-hydroxylase (DBH) in plasma, were also evaluated, and plasma volume and plasma renin activity were measured. Plasma DBH levels decreased markedly ($p < 0.05$) in the treated patients post-intervention, and were also significantly less ($p < 0.05$) than the DBH levels of the control group. Pretreatment measurements of plasma renin activity were similar in the control and treatment groups. However, after six months of meditation, furosemide-stimulated plasma renin activity values in the upright posture were significantly lower ($p < 0.05$) than pretreatment values in the treated hypertensive subjects.

SIDE EFFECTS OF THE RELAXATION RESPONSE

The side effects of the relaxation response appear to be minimal. They are essentially those of prayer. No adverse side effects have been observed when the response is regularly elicited for two daily periods of 20 to 30 minutes. However, we have noted some of the subjective feelings experienced by a small percentage of people who elicit the relaxation response. These include feeling of warmth in the hands, feelings of weightlessness and sensations of floating, mild sexual arousal, lacrimation, and various visual phenomena (personal observations, Herbert Benson). When the relaxation response is elicited much more frequently, such as for many hours daily over a period of several months, some individuals have experienced feelings of withdrawal from life and symptoms ranging from mild disorientation to hallucinatory behavior (personal observations, Herbert Benson). Some patients already taking propranolol have been noted to develop marked bradycardias necessitating the lowering of the dose of propranolol. Several patients suffering from diabetes mellitus have reported that it was necessary for them to decrease their daily amount of insulin because of hypoglycemic reactions after they had regularly started eliciting the relaxation response. These side effects are at the present time of anecdotal nature. Systematic investigation is necessary to establish their validity.

CONCLUSION

Epidemiologic and physiologic evidence strongly suggests that stressful circumstances which require behavioral adjustment may lead to hypertension. The fact that hypertension can be treated by a behavioral intervention, the relaxation response, strongly supports this concept. The relaxation response, which is essentially without side effects, should therefore be strongly considered in the therapy of hypertension. It costs nothing other than sitting quietly twice daily for 10 to 20 minutes. Not only may it be used in the therapy of established hypertension and thereby perhaps lower the required dose of antihypertensive medications, but it may also be a valuable therapeutic modality in the treatment of borderline and labile hypertension. In these frequently encountered clinical states, it is often difficult to decide whether or not to start pharmacologic antihypertensive therapy. In these cases the relaxation response may have particular efficacy. Furthermore, the relaxation response does not commit a patient to lifelong therapy and may, indeed, be alleviating the primary factors which are leading to the development of more profound, fixed essential hypertension.

ACKNOWLEDGMENT

We wish to thank Nancy E. MacKinnon for her excellent secretarial assistance.

REFERENCES

1. PAGE, I. H., AND McCUBBIN, J. W.: *Renal Hypertension.* Year Book Medical Publishers, Chicago, 1968.
2. GLOCK, C. Y., AND LENNARD, H. L.: *Studies in hypertension. V. Psychologic factors in hypertension: an interpretative review.* J. Chronic Dis. 5:174, 1957.
3. SCOTCH, N. A., AND GEIGER, H. J.: *The epidemiology of essential hypertension. A review with special attention to psychologic and socio-cultural factors. (II) Psychologic and socio-cultural factors in etiology.* J. Chronic Dis. 16:1183, 1963.
4. GUTMANN, M. C., AND BENSON, H.: *Interaction of environmental factors and systemic arterial blood pressure: a review.* Medicine 50:543, 1971.
5. BERKSON, D. M., STAMLER, J., LINDBERG, H. A., ET AL.: *Socioeconomic correlates of atherosclerotic and hypertensive heart disease.* Ann. N. Y. Acad. Sci. 84:835, 1960.
6. STAMLER, J., BERKSON, D. M., LINDBERG, H. A., ET AL.: *Socioeconomic factors in the epidemiology of hypertensive disease,* in STAMLER, J., ET AL. (ED.): *The Epidemiology of Hypertension.* Grune & Stratton, New York, 1967, p. 289.
7. NATIONAL CENTER FOR HEALTH STATISTICS: *Blood pressure of adults by race and area.* Vital and Health Statistics, PHS Pub. No. 1000, Series 11, No. 5, 1964.
8. BENSON, H., COSTAS, R., GARCIA-PALMIERI, M. R., ET AL.: *Coronary heart disease risk factors: a comparison of two Puerto Rican populations.* Am. J. Public Health 56:1057, 1966.
9. GAMPEL, M. B., SLOME, C., SCOTCH, N., ET AL.: *Urbanization and hypertension among Zulu adults.* J. Chronic Dis. 15:67, 1962.
10. MADDOCKS, I.: *The influence of standard of living on blood pressure in Fiji.* Circulation 24:1220, 1961.
11. SCOTCH, N. A.: *Sociocultural factors in the epidemiology of Zulu hypertension.* Am. J. Public Health 53:1205, 1963.
12. MADDOCKS, I.: *Blood pressures in Melanesians.* Med. J. Aust. 1:1123, 1967.
13. SCOTCH, N.: *A preliminary report on the relation of sociocultural factors to hypertension among the Zulu.* Ann. N. Y. Acad. Sci. 84:1,000, 1960.
14. RÉE, G. H.: *Arterial pressures in a West African (Gambian) rural population.* J. Trop. Med. Hyg. 76:65, 1973.
15. KOTCHEN, J. M., KOTCHEN, T. A., SCHWERTMAN, N. C., ET AL.: *Blood pressure distributions of urban adolescents.* Am. J. Epidemiol. 99:315, 1974.
16. MIALL, W. E., KASS, E. H., LING, J., ET AL.: *Factors influencing arterial pressure in the general population in Jamaica.* Br. Med. J. 2:497, 1962.
17. MIALL, W. E., DEL CAMPO, E., FODOR, J., ET AL.: *Longitudinal study of heart disease in a Jamaican rural population.* Bull. WHO 46:685, 1972.
18. LANGFORD, H. G., WATSON, R. L., AND DOUGLAS, B. H.: *Factors affecting blood pressure in population groups.* Trans. Assoc. Am. Physicians 81:135, 1968.
19. HENDERSON, M., APOSTOLIDES, A., ENTWISLE, G., ET AL.: *A study of hypertension in a black urban community: preliminary epidemiologic findings.* Prev. Med. 3:334, 1974.
20. BORHANI, N. O., AND BORKMAN, T. S.: *Alameda County blood pressure study.* California State Department of Public Health, 1968.
21. ANTONOVSKY, A.: *Social class and the major cardiovascular diseases.* J. Chronic Dis. 21:65, 1968.
22. MIALL, W. E., AND OLDHAM, P. D.: *Factors influencing arterial blood pressure in the general population.* Clin. Sci. 17:409, 1958.
23. APOSTOLIDES, A., HEBEL, J. R., McDILL, M. S., ET AL.: *High blood pressure: its care and consequences in urban centers.* Int. J. Epidemiol. 3:105, 1974.
24. HARBURG, E., SMEDES, T., STRAUCH, P., ET AL.: *Progress report: stress and heredity in negro-white*

blood pressure differences. United States Public Health Service and Michigan Heart Association (HS 00164-05), 1970.

25. SYME, S. L., OAKES, T. W., FRIEDMAN, G. D., ET AL.: *Social class and racial differences in blood pressure.* Am. J. Public Health 64:619, 1974.

26. HARBURG, E., ERFURT, J. C., CHAPE, C., ET AL.: *Socioecological stressor areas and black/white blood pressure: Detroit.* J. Chronic Dis. 26:595, 1973.

27. YODFAT, Y.: *The prevalence of cardiovascular disease in different ethnic and socioeconomic groups in Beit Shemesh, Israel.* Isr. J. Med. Sci. 8:1685, 1972.

28. GORDON, T., AND DEVINE, B.: *Hypertension and hypertensive heart disease in adults.* Vital and Health Statistics, Government Printing Office, Washington, D. C., 1966. (PHS Publication No. 1000), p. 1.

29. LENNARD, H. L., AND GLOCK, C. Y.: *Studies in hypertension. VI. Differences in the distribution of hypertension in negroes and whites: an appraisal.* J. Chronic Dis. 5:186, 1957.

30. MCMAHON, F. G., COLE, P. A., AND RYAN, J. R.: *A study of hypertension in the inner city. A student hypertension survey.* Am. Heart J. 85:70, 1973.

31. SOLBERG, L. A., AND MCGARRY, P. A.: *Cerebral atherosclerosis in negroes and caucasians.* Atherosclerosis 16:141, 1972.

32. STAMLER, J.: *Lectures in Preventive Cardiology.* Grune & Stratton, New York, 1967.

33. STAMLER, J., STAMLER, R., AND PULLMAN, T. N.: *The Epidemiology of Hypertension.* Grune & Stratton, New York, 1967.

34. HARBURG, E., ERFURT, J. C., HAUENSTEIN, L. S., ET AL.: *Socio-ecological stress, suppressed hostility, skin color, and black-white male blood pressure: Detroit.* Psychosom. Med. 35:276, 1973.

35. BECKER, B. J. P.: *Cardiovascular disease in the Bantu and coloured races of South Africa.* S. Afr. J. Med. Sci. 11:107, 1946.

36. RUSKIN, A., BEARD, O. W., AND SCHAFFER, R. L.: *"Blast hypertension." Elevated arterial pressures in the victims of the Texas City Disaster.* Am. J. Med. 4:228, 1948.

37. GRAHAM, J. D. P.: *High blood pressure after battle.* Lancet 11:239, 1945.

38. WRIGHT, I. S.: *Cardiovascular diseases. Role of psychogenic and behavior patterns in development and aggravation.* N. Y. State J. Med. 75:2128, 1975.

39. SYME, S. L., HYMAN, M. M., AND ENTERLINE, P. E.: *Some social and cultural factors associated with the occurrence of coronary heart disease.* J. Chronic Dis. 17:277, 1964.

40. PRIOR, I. A. M.: *A health survey in a rural Maori community.* N.Z. Med. J. 61:333, 1962.

41. PRIOR, I. A. M.: *Population studies in New Zealand and the South Pacific,* in FEJFAR, Z. (ED.): *WHO Report on Cardiovascular Epidemiology in the Pacific,* 1970, p. 28.

42. LABARTHE, D., REED, D., BRODY, J., ET AL.: *Health effects of modernization in Palau.* Am. J. Epidemiol. 98:161, 1973.

43. CRUZ-COKE, R.: *Environmental influences and arterial blood pressure.* Lancet 11:885, 1960.

44. CASSEL, J.: *Hypertension and cardiovascular disease in migrants: a potential source of clues?* Int. J. Epidemiol. 3:204, 1974.

45. OSTFELD, A. M., AND SHEKELLE, R. B.: *Psychological variables and blood pressure,* in STAMLER, J., ET AL. (ED.): *The Epidemiology of Hypertension.* Grune & Stratton, New York, 1967, p. 321.

46. CHRISTENSON, W. N., AND HINKEL, L. E.: *Differences in illness and prognostic signs in two groups of young men.* JAMA 177:247, 1961.

47. THEORELL, T., AND LIND, E.: *Systolic blood pressure, serum cholesterol and smoking in relation to sociological factors and myocardial infarction.* J. Psychosom. Res. 17:327, 1973.

48. CANNON, W. B.: *The emergency function of the adrenal medulla in pain and the major emotions.* Am. J. Physiol. 33:356, 1914.

49. HESS, W. R., AND BRUGGER, M.: *Das subkortikale Zentrum der affektiven Abwehrreaktion.* Helv. Physiol. Acta 1:33, 1943.

50. ABRAHAMS, V. C., HILTON, S. M., AND ZBROZYNA, A. W.: *Active muscle vasodilatation produced by stimulation of the brain stem: Its significance in the defense reaction.* J. Physiol. 154:491, 1960.

51. ABRAHAMS, V. C., HILTON, S. M., AND ZBROZYNA, A. W.: *The role of active muscle vasodilatation in the alerting stage of the defense reaction.* J. Physiol. 171:189, 1964.

52. HESS, W. R.: *The Functional Organization of the Diencephalon.* Grune & Stratton, New York, 1957.

53. BLAIR, D. A., GLOVER, W. E., GREENFIELD, A. D., ET AL.: *The activation of cholinergic vasodilator nerves in the human forearm during emotional stress.* J. Physiol. 148:633, 1959.

54. UVNÄS, B.: *Cholinergic vasodilator nerves.* Fed. Proc. 25:1618, 1966.

55. HILTON, S. M.: *Hypothalamus regulation of the cardiovascular system.* Br. Med. Bull. 22:243, 1966.

56. BROD, J.: *Circulation in muscle during acute pressor responses to emotional stress and during chronic sustained elevation of blood pressure.* Am. Heart J. 68:424, 1964.

57. BROD, J.: *Essential hypertension: haemodynamic observations with a bearing on its pathogenesis.* Lancet II:773, 1960.

58. BROD, J.: *Haemodynamic response to stress and its bearing on the haemodynamic basis of essential hypertension,* in CORT, J. H. (ED.): *The Pathogenesis of Essential Hypertension.* Proceedings of the Prague Symposium, State Medical Publishing House, Prague, 1961, p. 256.

59. BROD, J., FENCL, V., HEJL, Z., ET AL.: *Circulatory changes underlying blood pressure elevation during acute emotional stress (mental arithmetic) in normotensive and hypertensive subjects.* Clin. Sci. 18:269, 1959.

60. EICH, R. H., CUDDY, R. P., SMULYAN, H., ET AL.: *Haemodynamics in labile hypertension.* Circulation 34:299, 1966.

61. FOLKOW, B., AND RUBINSTEIN, E. H.: *Cardiovascular effects of acute and chronic stimulation of the hypothalamic defense area in the rat.* Acta Physiol. Scand. 68:48, 1966.

62. HENRY, J. P., AND CASSEL, J. C.: *Psychosocial factors in essential hypertension. Recent epidemiologic and animal experimental evidence.* Am. J. Epidemiol. 90:171, 1969.

63. BENSON, H., BEARY, J. F., AND CAROL, M. P.: *The relaxation response.* Psychiatry 37:37, 1974.

64. BENSON, H.: *The Relaxation Response.* William Morrow, New York, 1975.

65. WALLACE, R. K., BENSON, H., AND WILSON, A. F.: *A wakeful hypometabolic physiologic state.* Am. J. Physiol. 221:795, 1971.

66. WALLACE, R. K., AND BENSON, H.: *The physiology of meditation.* Sci. Am. 226:84, 1972.

67. LEVANDER, V. L., BENSON, H., WHEELER, R. C., ET AL.: *Increased forearm blood flow during a wakeful hypometabolic state.* Fed. Proc. 31:405, 1972.

68. FRENCH, R. M. (TRANS.): *The Way of a Pilgrim.* Seabury Press, New York, 1968.

69. SCHOLEM, G. G.: *Jewish Mysticism.* Schocken Books, New York, 1967.

70. ORGAN, T. W.: *The Hindu Quest for the Perfection of Man.* Ohio University Press, Athens, Ohio, 1970.

71. LUTHE, W., (ED.): *Autogenic Therapy.* Vols. 1–5. Grune & Stratton, New York, 1969.

72. JACOBSON, E.: *Progressive Relaxation.* University of Chicago Press, Chicago, 1938.

73. BARBER, T. X.: *Physiological effects of hypnosis.* Psychol. Bull. 58:390, 1961.

74. BARBER, T. X.: *Physiological effects of hypnosis and suggestion,* in *Biofeedback and Self-Control.* Aldine-Atherton, Chicago, 1971.

75. GORTON, B. E.: *Physiology of hypnosis.* Psychiatr. Q. 23:317, 457, 1949.

76. CRASILNECK, H. B., AND HALL, J. A.: *Physiological changes associated with hypnosis: a review of the literature since 1948.* Int. J. Clin. Exp. Hypn. 7:9, 1959.

77. CLYNES, M.: *Toward a view of man,* in CLYNES, M., AND MILSUM, J. (EDS.): *Biomedical Engineering Systems.* McGraw-Hill, New York, 1970.

78. BENSON, H.: *Your innate asset for combatting stress.* Harvard Business Review 52:9, 1974.

79. BEARY, J. F., AND BENSON, H.: *A simple psychophysiologic technique which elicits the hypometabolic changes of the relaxation response.* Psychosom. Med. 36:115, 1974.

80. BENSON, H., ROSNER, B. A., MARZETTA, B. R., ET AL.: *Decreased blood pressure in pharmacologically treated hypertensive patients who regularly elicited the relaxation response.* Lancet I:289, 1974.

81. BENSON, H., ROSNER, B. A., MARZETTA, B. R., ET AL.: *Decreased blood pressure in borderline hypertensive subjects who practiced meditation.* J. Chronic Dis. 27:163, 1974.

82. DATEY, K. K., DESHMUKH, S. N., DALVI, C. P., ET AL.: *'Shavasan': A yogic exercise in the management of hypertension.* Angiology 20:325, 1969.

83. PATEL, C. H.: *Yoga and biofeedback in the management of hypertension.* Lancet II:1053, 1973.

84. PATEL, C. H.: *Twelve-month follow-up of yoga and biofeedback in the management of hypertension.* Lancet I:62, 1975.

85. BLACKWELL, B., HANENSON, I., BLOOMFIELD, S., ET AL.: *Transcendental meditation in hypertension.* Lancet I:223, 1976.

86. STONE, R. A., AND DELEO, J.: *Psychotherapeutic control of hypertension.* N. Engl. J. Med. 294:80, 1976.

87. KANNEL, W. B., SCHWARTZ, M. J., AND MCNAMARA, P. M.: *Blood pressure and risk of coronary heart disease: the Framingham study.* Dis. Chest 56:43, 1969.

88. BENSON, H., MARZETTA, B. R., AND ROSNER, B. A.: *Decreased blood pressure associated with the regular elicitation of the relaxation response: a study of hypertensive subjects,* in ELIOT, R. S. (ED.): *Contemporary Problems in Cardiology,* Vol. 1, Stress and the Heart, Futura, Mt. Kisco (New York), 1974.

124

Rational Approach to the Hypertensive Workup

Sheldon G. Sheps, M.D., Cameron G. Strong, M.D., and Robert C. Northcutt, M.D.

ESTABLISHING THE DIAGNOSIS OF HYPERTENSION

The exact definition of high blood pressure (hypertension) remains a thorny problem. Systemic arterial pressure is the driving force for tissue perfusion. The level of this pressure varies in different parts of the body and in different positions in relation to gravity; there are great variations throughout the day in response to bodily functions and external stress. Such variability makes it difficult to characterize the blood pressure in an individual based on a single, casual, indirect blood pressure reading. Pickering[1] has reviewed his long-standing opinion decrying an arbitrary dividing line between normal and high blood pressure: "The relationship between arterial pressure and mortality is quantitative; the higher the pressure, the worse the prognosis." Utilizing a truly portable continuous intra-arterial recording of blood pressure, he obtained data showing great variations during daily activities in both normotensive and hypertensive individuals. In spite of this, office blood pressure determinations taken with the usual precautions, that is, with the patient comfortable, resting, and quiet, and with proper technique, are reasonably replicable. The everyday management of patients with hypertension relies heavily on such casual measurements of blood pressure. Blood pressure measured in this way correlates with mortality and morbidity.

A common problem, particularly at a time when there is great publicity regarding the consequences of undiscovered and untreated hypertension, is the anxiety induced by the very taking of the blood pressure measurement. Such a defense reflex or alarm reaction may be allayed by multiple readings on separate occasions. The issue of how many blood pressure readings to obtain at a single office visit has been approached by Mathieu and associates.[2] They obtained four blood pressure readings in the supine position, 10 minutes apart. The first reading was generally highest, and there was very little change from the second to the fourth reading. Through mathematical analysis it was possible to predict (with 95 percent confidence intervals of less than 5 mm. Hg diastolic and 10 mm. Hg systolic) the fourth blood pressure value from the first two of four readings. Our own experience with an automatic indirect blood pressure machine (Arteriosonde, Roche) indicates that there is very little difference in the mean of the first three of six blood pressure measurements obtained in the sitting position at 5-minute intervals from the mean of the next three. Such attempts at attaining "office basal blood pressure" have considerable value in reducing the defense or alarm reaction.

Overt evidence of anxiety in the office as indicated by tachycardia may not be helpful in predicting which subjects would continue to be hypertensive.[3] Sokolow and colleagues[4] have developed a semiautomatic portable blood pressure recorder and have demonstrated that the severity of vascular complications varies with the level of blood

125

pressure but that the correlation was better with the recorder than with casual blood pressure determinations. Home blood pressure recordings have been used to great benefit for many years, both in the initial evaluation and in the management of hypertensive patients.

A blood pressure recording should be made with attention to the technical details necessary for accuracy. The cuff should be adequate to transmit the pressure evenly to the underlying brachial artery. As a guide, the width should cover about two-thirds of the distance between the shoulder and the elbow, and the length should be sufficient to encircle at least two-thirds of the circumference of the arm. If the cuff completely encircles the arm, the possibility of cuff inadequacy and falsely high readings is greatly lessened.[5] For very obese patients, a much larger cuff (usually called a thigh cuff) may be substituted. One can also take the blood pressure by auscultation over the radial artery with the standard cuff wrapped about the forearm. The problem of the "auscultatory gap" is avoided by palpating for disappearance of the radial pulse with increasing cuff pressure, inflating the cuff to a pressure 30 mm. higher, and then auscultating in the usual manner. If, to avoid the previous step, the cuff is inflated to well above 200 mm. Hg, this may cause discomfort and it may contribute to the alarm reaction and produce false elevations in blood pressure. The patient being screened should be in a comfortable, relaxed sitting position, and the arm should be at the level of the heart. Readings should be obtained from both arms. In addition, at least one recording should be made with the patient standing quietly for 2 minutes to determine whether there is postural hypotension and preparatory to administering drugs. For repeated readings, several minutes should be allowed to elapse between each reading.

There continues to be disagreement over the diastolic reading. Is it best taken as the pressure at which a muffling occurs in the Korotkoff sounds (phase IV) or that at which the sounds disappear (phase V)? Most observers regard the fifth phase, the disappearance of sound, as a more reliable and reproducible end point. Both values should be recorded if there are differences of more than 5 mm. Hg.[5]

Blood pressure is a continuum, and so it is difficult to establish precise criteria for the diagnosis of hypertension. Also, blood pressure is related to age and sex; and in addition to the prevalence of elevated blood pressure in blacks, any degree of hypertension in blacks has a worse prognosis than it would have in a comparable white population. The clinician must consider what level of blood pressure constitutes an increased risk of complications and death from hypertension and, equally important, what the efficacy and risks are of any measures used to reduce elevated blood pressure.

The World Health Organization (WHO) defines hypertension as a casual blood pressure of more than 160/95 mm. Hg. Persons who have a casual blood pressure reading of less than 140/90 mm. Hg are considered normotensive, and those whose blood pressure is in between these values have borderline hypertension. Because men, particularly those who are less than 45 years old, suffer more from hypertensive complications than do women, many authorities lower the value for normal to 130/90 mm. Hg in this group of males. Patients classified as having borderline (labile) hypertension should be followed annually because they are at increased risk for experiencing established hypertension.[6] The more efforts that are made to obtain basal office readings or home blood pressure determinations before the diagnosis of persistent hypertension is made, the fewer false classifications will be assigned.

Another problem concerns systolic hypertension. Systolic hypertension is generally said to be present if the diastolic pressure is within normal limits but systolic pressure is elevated. This is not uncommon in older persons, but it also occurs in adolescents. Actuarial and epidemiologic data indicate that systolic hypertension is important in the development of cardiovascular complications and congestive heart failure.[7] When antihypertensive drugs are used in this condition, they lower diastolic pressure as well as systolic pressure, and it is not clear whether elderly patients with atherosclerotic disease can tolerate the lower diastolic blood pressures without significant impairment of organ perfusion. A controlled prospective study of the efficacy and safety of treatment in purely systolic hypertension, particularly in the elderly, is needed.

EVALUATING TARGET ORGAN DAMAGE AND CAUSE

Clinical Examination

The evaluation of a hypertensive patient is the foundation of rational therapy. It should precede the administration of antihypertensive drugs except in an emergency. If the patient is already receiving therapy, much of the evaluation may be made without discontinuing the treatment; a decision can be made later whether to withhold or alter therapy to permit certain studies.

The initial evaluative effort is directed toward the possible causes of the hypertension, its severity, and the amount of target organ damage that may be present. This information is valuable both in making therapeutic decisions and in determining prognosis. The initial consultations should establish the continuing presence of hypertension and provide a family and personal history of hypertension and its complications. It is also important to determine what drugs, prescribed and over-the-counter varieties, the patient is taking. Of particular interest are birth control pills and other estrogen-containing compounds, corticosteroids, sympathomimetic amines and stimulants, and carbenoxalone; in addition, the ingestion of large amounts of licorice and sodium bicarbonate is significant. Sometimes, having the patient discontinue using a particular agent is the only treatment needed. Table 1 is a patient questionnaire that we have found helpful in focusing attention on information needed in the hypertension evaluation.

Family History

Because hypertension is a familial disorder, the family history is important in determining the approach to treatment. If the parents of a hypertensive patient died before they were 60 years old from cerebrovascular accident, myocardial infarction, or renal failure, or if the patient's siblings have hypertension, the physician may decide to treat the patient more aggressively. Even if treatment is not altered, the family history may assist the physician's efforts in educating and motivating the patient. Particularly important findings are the presence in other members of the family of polycystic kidneys, medullary cancer of the thyroid, pheochromocytoma, renal calculi and hyperparathyroidism, or some hereditary forms of renal parenchymal disease. Recurrent bacterial infection of the urinary tract may contribute to renal parenchymal dysfunction. Hypertension of sudden onset and rapid progression suggests a secondary cause. A positive family history does not exclude the possibility of secondary causes.

Associated Disorders

The presence of hyperlipidemia, gout, diabetes, polycythemia vera, obesity, or other disorders in the patient or his family also plays an important role in the management of the patient. Such a disorder may increase the risk of atherosclerotic complications or complicate the pharmacologic management of the hypertension.

Target Organs

Questions should be directed toward detecting symptoms and signs referable to the target organs of hypertensive disease. The *heart* responds to hypertension by enlargement of the left ventricle, first through hypertrophy and later through dilatation. The

Table 1. Information for the hypertension consultation

	Yes	No		Yes	No
Family history of elevated B.P.:					
Mother	___	___	Brothers	___	___
Father	___	___	Sisters	___	___

Patient history:

First told of elevated B.P.	YEAR
First treated for elevated B.P.	YEAR
Highest level of B.P. known	
Current B.P. medicine:	

Other medications currently or recently taken:

Last day taken:
Bad reactions:

	Yes	No		Yes	No
Elevated B.P. in pregnancy	___	___	Birth control pills	___	___
Hormone pills	___	___			

Have you had any history of the following problems?

	Yes	No		Yes	No
Kidney disease	___	___	Shortness of breath	___	___
Infections	___	___	Asthma or wheezing	___	___
Stones	___	___	Heart failure	___	___
Blood in urine	___	___	Diabetes	___	___
Albumin in urine	___	___	Goiter or thyroid disease	___	___
Frequency of urination	___	___	Elevated cholesterol or		
Urinating after bed	___	___	fats in blood	___	___
Ankle swelling	___	___	Distress in legs with		
Leg or muscle cramps	___	___	walking	___	___
Flushing spells or			Gout	___	___
sweating spells	___	___	Numbness or tingling of		
Recent weight gain	___	___	face, hands, or arms	___	___
Recent weight loss	___	___			
Heart palpitations	___	___	Stroke	___	___
Chest pains	___	___	Blurred vision	___	___
Heart attacks	___	___	Headaches	___	___
Family history of kidney			Impotency	___	___
disease	___	___			

enlargement is asymptomatic until congestive failure supervenes. However, palpation and auscultation may reveal a forceful, somewhat prolonged apical impulse, cardiac enlargement, gallop rhythm, and arrhythmia. Mitral and aortic murmurs of regurgitation may be heard. When hypertensive heart disease is complicated by coronary artery disease, the symptoms of angina pectoris, myocardial infarction, and congestive failure may ensue.

There are usually no *central nervous system* symptoms until a complication such as a stroke, subarachnoid hemorrhage, or hypertensive encephalopathy develops. Dizziness and morning headache are not usually related to hypertension unless malignant or accelerated hypertension is present. Atherosclerotic involvement of carotid arteries may be detected through auscultation for bruits and visualization of microemboli in the retinal circulation. There may be a history of transient ischemic attacks. If such a history is obtained and such findings are present, determining retinal artery pressures will be very helpful in subsequent evaluation.

The *kidney* is involved early in hypertension, primarily through a decrease in the renal blood flow, although this abnormality is not readily detected by routine clinical methods. The relationship of a previous history of toxemia of pregnancy, bacterial infection of the kidneys or bladder, or renal calculi to hypertension is not clear. A history of unusual flank pain or trauma and unexplained gross hematuria may indicate a renal or renovascular cause. Palpation of the abdomen may detect renal masses, and auscultation anteriorly may reveal bruits that suggest renovascular disease.

Examination of the *peripheral vasculature* is very important. An atherosclerotic renovascular disorder may be suggested by the presence of peripheral aneurysms or occlusive arterial disease. Careful palpation of the femoral pulses for a reduction in amplitude *and* a delay in timing relative to the radial pulse is important in considering the presence of *coarctation of the aorta*. This may be confirmed if a reduced blood pressure is found in the thigh (using a thigh cuff). If coarctation is suspected, the patient's back should be inspected for enlarged intercostal arteries, and the heart should be examined for evidence of aortic valve involvement. When coarctation is suspected but the blood pressures in the arm and leg are normal, the blood pressure determination should be repeated after exercise. When the cardiac output is increased, the disparity in blood pressure between the upper and the lower extremities is much more pronounced. Turner's syndrome is also associated with coarctation of the aorta. Acquired causes of coarctation of the aorta include Takayasu's disease (idiopathic medial aortopathy); this disorder is more common in non-Western populations but it is being seen more frequently among Occidentals in our recent experience.

Skin

Inspection of the skin may reveal neurofibromatosis. The hypertension seen in association with this condition is as frequently due to pheochromocytoma as it is to a renal artery dysplasia and stenosis.[8] Orofacial neuromas, a component of multiple endocrine neoplasia, type 2, is a highly significant finding, indicating multiple endocrine disorders of autosomal dominant inheritance: medullary carcinoma of the thyroid, pheochromocytoma, and chief cell hyperplasia of the parathyroid. Evidence of truncal striae and obesity along with atrophy of the skin and other characteristics may suggest hypercortisolism. Urochrome pigmentation indicates renal failure.

Optic Fundus

A window on arteriolar change is available for assessment: the optic fundus can be examined for early changes due to hypertension. About 35 years ago at the Mayo Clinic, Keith, Wagener, and Barker proposed a prognostic classification of essential hypertension based on the changes observed in the optic fundus (Table 2). It should be noted that the presence of retinal hemorrhages alone places the patient in group 2 and that this subgroup of group 2 has a distinctly poorer prognosis than for those in group 2 without retinal hemorrhage(s). The term "angiospastic" is sometimes used in place of group 1 to describe the generalized narrowing and focal constrictions seen in the ocular fundus of patients with acute hypertensive states of recent origin; these are often secondary, such as with renovascular hypertension or pheochromocytoma. We continue to use this classification and consider it helpful in assessing prognosis. Thus, if on the initial examination the patient's diastolic pressure is very high and there are few if any changes in the optic fundus, emotional lability is likely to be playing a major role; but if the pressure is not particularly high, and there are hemorrhages and exudates in the fundus, the prognosis is much worse. The ophthalmoscopic grouping is positively correlated with severity of diastolic hypertension and with the incidence of certain hypertensive complications such as azotemia, proteinuria, inversion of the T wave in

Table 2. Ophthalmoscopic classification
of hypertension*

| | Keith-Wagener-Barker group | | | |
Findings	1	2	3	4
Retinal arterioles				
Sclerosis	<1	1 or more	0–4	0–4
General narrowing	0–4	0–4	0–4	0–4
Focal narrowing	0–4	0–4	0–4	0–4
Hemorrhages	–	±	±	±
Exudates	–	–	+	±
Papilledema	–	–	–	+

*Grading of sclerosis: 1. brightening or increased luster of arterioles, mild depression of veins at points of arteriolar crossing; 2. burnished coppery color of arterioles with definite depression of underlying veins, widening of apparent arteriovenous crossing spaces; 3. polished silver color of arterioles, widening of apparent arteriovenous crossing spaces with change in course of veins ("right angle crossings"), complete invisibility of portions of veins crossing arterioles and distal dilatation of veins; and 4. arterioles visible only as fibrous cords without a bloodstream. Grading of narrowing: 1. reduction of caliber of arterioles to ¾ average caliber (or ½ caliber of veins); 2. reduction of caliber of arterioles to ½ average caliber; 3. reduction of caliber of arterioles to ⅓ average caliber; and 4. arterioles threadlike or invisible. + = present; ± = may or may not be present; – = absent.

the electrocardiogram, myocardial infarction, congestive heart failure, and cerebrovascular accident (Fig. 1).[9]

A classification of hypertension based mainly on the development of complications, such as left ventricular hypertrophy and renal failure, clearly indicates that the prevention of such complications has been missed. In other words, the vast majority of patients who have the most to gain, i.e., those who do not have evidence of organ damage, would have been overlooked. The examination of the optic fundus remains one of the most useful office procedures in evaluation of the hypertensive patient.

The Laboratory Evaluation: Blood Tests

The initial laboratory evaluation of the hypertensive patient should include tests that will help the physician to evaluate vascular disease in the target organs, assess coexisting risk factors for atherosclerotic vascular disease, and determine the likelihood that there is an underlying curable cause of the hypertension. Many of these tests are available as a package (a chemistry profile).

Serum Creatinine Concentration as a Measure of Renal Function

Serum creatinine is superior to blood urea nitrogen as an indicator of glomerular filtration rate. In many instances a more accurate measure of glomerular filtration rate is needed for comparison later in the course of the disease to judge any change in renal function. Twenty-four-hour creatinine clearances have been used extensively for this purpose. We believe that, for a similar cost, much more accurate information can be obtained with measurement of 2-hour clearances begun 30 minutes after subcutaneous injection of radioiodine iothalamate.

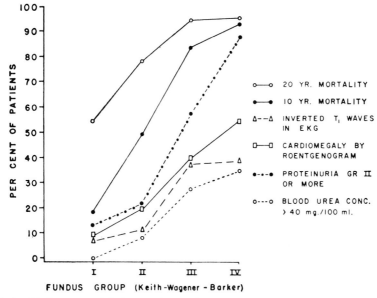

Figure 1. Relationship between ophthalmoscopic grouping and mortality and certain clinical findings or complications of hypertension. (From Breslin, D. J., Gifford, R. W., Jr., Fairbairn, J. F., II, et al.: *Prognostic importance of ophthalmoscopic findings in essential hypertension.* JAMA 195:335, 1966. By permission of the American Medical Association.)

Serum Potassium Concentration

The possibility of hypokalemia due to primary aldosteronism should be sought by measurement of serum potassium concentration. The patient with primary aldosteronism is very unlikely to have a normal concentration of serum potassium, although this may happen rarely in the patient who is on a diet very low in salt. Potassium excretion can be promoted in such patients by placing them for 1 week on a diet containing 150 to 280 mEq. of sodium daily; this will produce hypokalemia and raise the suspicion that primary aldosteronism is causing the hypertension. It is also important to have a baseline determination of serum potassium as a guide for subsequent diuretic therapy.

Serum Triglyceride and Cholesterol

Serum triglyceride and cholesterol should be measured in all patients who are less than 65 years of age in an attempt to evaluate and control these risk factors for atherosclerotic vascular disease.

Serum Uric Acid Concentration

Twenty-five percent of patients with untreated hypertension have elevated serum uric acid concentrations. The use of thiazide diuretics and a low salt diet may double that incidence and produce gouty arthritis or gouty nephropathy.

Serum Calcium Concentration

Primary hyperparathyroidism is approximately five to eight times more common among patients with hypertension than it is in the general population. If patients with this disorder are to be detected and treated appropriately, by surgery, serum calcium measurements should be made before therapy is begun with diuretics, because such treatment may elevate the serum calcium concentration.

Plasma Glucose

The possibility of coexisting diabetes mellitus in the hypertensive patient should be investigated by measuring the 2-hour postprandial plasma glucose. Some clinics have found this timing restriction too cumbersome, and they rely instead on fasting or random plasma glucose determinations as screening methods. The postprandial determination is preferable, however, if scheduling permits.

Hemogram

Information derived from the hemogram is needed for general health assessment and to search for polycythemia, which may complicate management, or anemia, which may reflect renal insufficiency.

The Laboratory Evaluation: Urinalysis

A complete urinalysis should be performed on a fresh first-morning specimen. Examination for cells, bacteria, and formed elements is exceedingly important. The presence of blood casts or red blood cell casts is indicative of active glomerulitis, either primary or secondary to the glomerulonephritis of connective tissue diseases. Proteinuria, nonspecific casts, and microscopic hematuria may be the first clues to the presence of polycystic renal disease. A urine culture should be considered in the presence of pyuria or any history suggestive of urinary tract infection. Asymptomatic bacilluria is more common in patients with hypertension of any cause, and it is especially to be sought in patients with polycystic renal disease or chronic pyelonephritis causing the hypertension.

The Laboratory Evaluation: Other Tests

Electrocardiogram

Electrocardiographic evidence of cardiac hypertrophy may be found in many untreated hypertensives. The electrocardiogram should be evaluated also for evidence of conduction disturbance and ischemic heart disease.

Posteroanterior Chest Roentgenogram

Evidence of cardiac hypertrophy may be found in many untreated patients with hypertension. Age, associated coronary artery disease, and severity of the hypertension will affect the occurrence of this finding. Its presence strengthens the indications for antihypertensive therapy at any blood pressure level and adversely affects prognosis.

Evidence of aortic aneurysm and unfolding of the thoracic aorta should be sought on chest x-ray films. There may be notching and secondary erosion of the ribs from dilatation of the intercostal arteries in patients with coarctation of the aorta.

In addition to chamber enlargement, evidence of pulmonary congestion and interstitial edema should be sought as manifestations of left ventricular failure.

The Excretory Urogram

We regard the excretory urogram performed with carefully timed films at 2 and 3 minutes after injection of the contrast medium as an important component of the diagnostic investigation of hypertensive patients. Decisions on management often hinge on the findings of excretory urography, especially when the results suggest adrenal mass, chronic renal disease, renal obstruction, pyelonephritis, renal cystic disease, renal artery stenosis, renal lithiasis, or renal neoplasm. Three major urographic features (disparity in renal length, delayed appearance time, and hyperconcentration on late films) are commonly found singly or in combination in patients with renovascular hypertension and are uncommonly found in patients with essential hypertension.[10] This procedure should not be carried out in patients who have a history of significant allergic reaction to the contrast medium, in patients with very mild hypertension, or in those in the older age groups (over 60); in those instances it is preferable to obtain a KUB study with tomographic cuts to search for a disparity in renal size and shape. Any hint from the careful history, including especially the factors listed below, or initial laboratory studies of renal or renovascular disease would be very helpful in making that decision.

1. Age less than 30 years
2. Diastolic blood pressure greater than 120 mm. Hg at any age
3. Continuous or systolic-diastolic bruit in the epigastrium, upper abdominal quadrants, or flanks
4. Hypertension of very recent onset
5. Recent acceleration of previously chronic, quiescent course
6. History of acute flank pain, hematuria, urinary tract infection, renal calculi, impaired renal function, or renal trauma
7. Palpable kidney
8. Hypertension resistant to good medical treatment

Urinary Metanephrines

Abnormalities in catecholamine biochemistry are the key to the diagnosis of pheochromocytoma, although certain clinical hints, as listed below, are very helpful, because the majority of patients with pheochromocytoma are symptomatic.

1. Unusual lability of blood pressure
2. Symptomatic paroxysms of hypertension, tachyarrhythmias
3. Spells: 4 "P"s (head pain, palpitation, pallor, perspiration)
4. Accelerated hypertension
5. Hypermetabolism; recent weight loss
6. Abnormal carbohydrate metabolism
7. Pressor response during induction of anesthesia or to antihypertensive drugs
8. Severe hypertension
9. Suprarenal mass (x-ray)

Diagnostic studies involve the measurement of excretion of catecholamines and their major metabolites, total metanephrines, and vanillylmandelic acid (VMA). There is considerable daily variability in the excretion of these substances, but the excretion of metanephrines has given the fewest false-negative results[11] — 4 percent — and has been our choice for a screening test (Table 3). Abnormalities are confirmed by VMA and

Table 3. Screening tests for
pheochromocytoma

Test	False negative, %
Urine	
Metanephrines	4 (2/50)
Catecholamines	22 (13/60)
Vanillylmandelic acid	29 (15/52)
Plasma	
Basal catecholamines	47 (26/55)

catecholamine determinations. For metanephrines, only methylglucamine (an ingredient of many x-ray contrast media) may yield a *falsely normal* value (for 72 hours after its use).

Plasma Renin Activity (PRA)

The test for PRA must be performed under specific, controlled circumstances because many seemingly innocent environmental conditions and drugs may alter the plasma renin levels for a long time. Knowledge of the level of PRA is essential to the diagnosis of renovascular hypertension, renin-producing tumors, and mineralocorticoid hypertension and is important as a research tool in studying essential hypertension. However, the value of a PRA determination in the routine care of patients with essential hypertension remains controversial.

Angiotensin II blockade and converting enzyme inhibitors are under intensive investigation at present and may simplify office screening for angiotensin-dependent hypertension.

WHY SEARCH FOR SECONDARY HYPERTENSION?

The relatively low incidence of secondary hypertension and the relatively high cost of testing necessary to detect and delineate the precise nature of the curable forms of hypertension have been cited as reasons to postpone testing for secondary hypertension in the patient with newly discovered hypertension. For example, Gifford[12] has cited an incidence of less than 6 percent curable hypertension among the 5,000 consecutive hypertensive patients first seen at the Cleveland Clinic from 1966 to 1967. Further, it has been estimated that the cost of testing to find a patient with secondary hypertension is $1,727.[13] McNeil and associates[14] have taken the data from the Cooperative Study on Renovascular Disease and analyzed the costs and benefits of identifying and treating hypertensive patients with renovascular disease. The cost of finding a patient with renovascular disease was calculated as about $2,000 and that of a surgical cure, $20,000. Extensive testing has been called a barrier to adequate compliance.

For the health planner with a global viewpoint, these arguments may seem sensible and even reasonable bases for establishment of criteria of medical care.

This poses a dilemma for the physician who treats patients. With perspective confined to considering the best course of evaluation and management for the individual patient, it is difficult to limit studies and reserve further evaluation for patients who present certain clues in the history, physical examination, or baseline laboratory studies, or for those who fail to respond to medical therapy.

Failure to respond to medical therapy is not unique to the patient with secondary hypertension. Patients with renovascular hypertension usually respond to medical therapy, albeit possibly at the expense of the renal mass and function. Failure to respond is more likely due to poor compliance, a poorly chosen combination of medications, nonadherence to diet, or insufficient medication.

Patients with pheochromocytoma usually have a history of spells or episodes, but for those who do not, failure to detect and remove the pheochromocytoma may lead to stroke or fatal cardiac arrhythmia.

The patient with hypertension caused by polycystic renal disease benefits from early diagnosis because infections can be sought and treated, and sequelae such as renal stone formation and hemorrhage into cysts can be managed more correctly. Knowledge of the prognosis can lead to more timely arrangements for management of end-stage renal disease.

The problem of compliance is, of course, eliminated in the patient whose hypertension has been cured by arterial bypass for a renovascular lesion or by excision of an adrenal tumor.

The physician would not have a problem deciding whom to evaluate for curable hypertension if it had not been shown in a 7- to 14-year followup study that surgical therapy is more effective than medical therapy in prolonging life and decreasing morbidity in patients with renovascular hypertension.[15] Surgery is also indicated for aldosterone-producing adrenal adenoma and carcinoma, pheochromocytoma (benign and malignant), obstructive renal disease, and unilateral chronic atrophic pyelonephritis. Prolongation of life and the decreased incidence of stroke and renal failure undoubtedly accrue from the greater lowering of blood pressure achieved by successful surgical management, compared with medical therapy with its attendant problems of side effects, compliance, and variable blood pressure responses with postural change.

The cost of evaluation and surgical treatment compares favorably with the cost of life-long medication. Our patients with essential hypertension benefit from having secondary causes excluded by study, because they and we know that medical therapy is the proper course of management and that prognosis will be determined more directly by what we do together to control the blood pressure and other detected risk factors.

REFERENCES

1. PICKERING, G.: *Hypertension: definitions, natural histories and consequences.* Am. J. Med. 52:570, 1972.

2. MATHIEU, G., BIRON, P., ROBERGE, F., ET AL.: *Blood pressure determinations during medical examinations: how many?* Can. J. Public Health 65:447, 1974.

3. JULIUS, S., ELLIS, C. N., PASCUAL, A. V., ET AL.: *Home blood pressure determination: value in borderline ("labile") hypertension.* JAMA 229:663, 1974.

4. SOKOLOW, M., WERDEGAR, D., KAIN, H. K., ET AL.: *Relationship between level of blood pressure measured casually and by portable recorders and severity of complications in essential hypertension.* Circulation 34:279, 1966.

5. KING, G. E.: *Taking the blood pressure.* JAMA 209:1902, 1969.

6. FREIS, E. D.: *The clinical spectrum of essential hypertension.* Arch. Intern. Med. 133:982, 1974.

7. KOCH-WESER, J.: *The therapeutic challenge of systolic hypertension.* N. Engl. J. Med. 289:481, 1973.

8. LYNCH, J. D., SHEPS, S. G., BERNATZ, P. E., ET AL.: *Neurofibromatosis and hypertension due to pheochromocytoma or renal-artery stenosis.* Minn. Med. 55:25, 1972.

9. BRESLIN, D. J., GIFFORD, R. W., JR., FAIRBAIRN, J. F., II, ET AL.: *Prognostic importance of ophthalmoscopic findings in essential hypertension.* JAMA 195:335, 1966.

10. BOOKSTEIN, J. J., ABRAMS, H. L., BUENGER, R. E., ET AL.: *Radiologic aspects of renovascular hypertension. Part 2. The role of urography in unilateral renovascular disease.* JAMA 220:1225, 1972.

11. REMINE, W. H., CHONG, G. C., VAN HEERDEN, J. A., ET AL.: *Current management of pheochromocytoma.* Ann. Surg. 179:740, 1974.

12. GIFFORD, R. W., JR.: *Evaluation of the hypertensive patient with emphasis on detecting curable causes.* Milbank Mem. Fund Q. 47:170, 1969.

13. FERGUSON, R. K.: *Cost and yield of the hypertensive evaluation: experience of a community-based referral clinic.* Ann. Intern. Med. 82:761, 1975.

14. McNEIL, B. J., VARADY, P. D., BURROWS, B. A., ET AL.: *Measures of clinical efficacy: cost-effectiveness calculations in the diagnosis and treatment of hypertensive renovascular disease.* N. Engl. J. Med. 293: 216, 1975.

15. HUNT, J. C., SHEPS, S. G., HARRISON, E. G., JR., ET AL.: *Renal and renovascular hypertension: a reasoned approach to diagnosis and management.* Arch. Intern. Med. 133:988, 1974.

Hypertension and Renal Parenchymal Disease: Mechanisms and Management

Jan Brod, M.D., Dr. Sc., F.R.C.P. (Lond.)

With Goldblatt's[1] publication of the famous animal model of experimental hypertension and with the rediscovery of the renal humoral pressor system, i.e., renin-angiotensin,[2-6] hopes were raised that the riddle of the left ventricular hypertrophy found in 48 percent of Bright's autopsied patients with chronic renal disease would be solved at last. The silver clip on the renal artery of the experimental dog was supposed to substitute for two million microclips on the afferent arterioles of the human kidney with vascular nephrosclerosis, presumed since Volhard and Fahr[7] to be the morphological substrate of "essential" hypertension. Also it was not difficult to imagine such "microclips" narrowing the small intrarenal vessels in chronic renal parenchymal disease. In support of this contention were the findings of Harrison, Blalock, and Mason,[8] and Prinzmetal and Friedman[9] that the extract of a clipped kidney or of a kidney whose ureter has been tied raises the blood pressure more than the extract of an intact organ. Moreover, the venous blood of a clipped kidney constricts the vessels in a Läwen-Trendelenburg preparation.[10,11]

As for essential hypertension, the aforementioned hypothesis proved to be inadequate for the following reasons. (1) The renal vessels are anatomically normal during the initial stages of the disease.[12, 13] (2) The increased renal vascular resistance[14] encountered in the initial stages is completely reversible by pyrogens,[15] barbiturates,[16] and sleep.[17] Thus, the increase in renal vascular resistance must come from outside the kidney which, rather than being the "culprit," is the affected organ.[18] (3) Plasma renin or angiotensin levels in uncomplicated cases of essential hypertension are as a rule within the normal range;[19-23] and in these cases the angiotensin antagonist Saralasin is without effect on the raised blood pressure[24, 25] unless the hypertension is malignant. (4) The hemodynamic pattern of early essential hypertension with its raised cardiac output and normal total peripheral vascular resistance[26] differs from that produced by a mildly to moderately pressor infusion of angiotensin.[27]

PLASMA RENIN LEVELS AND CHRONIC RENAL DISEASE

In contrast to essential hypertension, the kidney is the obvious cause of hypertension in chronic renal parenchymal disease which is accompanied in 60 to 96 percent of cases by a raised blood pressure.[28] The intrarenal vessels and the renal blood flow are interfered with to some extent in practically every instance of renal pathology. It is not surprising, therefore, that generalized vasoconstriction produced by increased release of renin and enhanced production of angiotensin is generally accepted as being responsi-

137

ble for the raised blood pressure. This appears to be corroborated by the studies of Neff and associates[29] and Kim and associates[30] who have shown that the hypertension of chronic renal disease with renal failure is sustained by a high peripheral vascular resistance if the associated anemia is corrected by transfusion of packed red cells. In addition, Catt and coworkers[21] found high plasma angiotensin II values in 95 percent of his 27 patients with chronic renal disease and hypertension; unfortunately no data are given on the stage and severity of the hypertension nor on the degree of renal functional impairment.

Several studies by others,[20, 22, 23, 31, 32] however, and also our own data failed to find regularly raised plasma renin activity or plasma angiotensin in cases of chronic non-uremic renal disease with hypertension, unless the hypertension was malignant (Fig. 1). Even most cases of renal artery stenosis, considered to be the clinical counterpart of the Goldblatt model, have normal plasma renin activity and the administration of the angiotensin antagonist Saralasin has been ineffective in these patients. Blood pressure lowering occurred only in those relatively rare cases where the renal artery stenosis led to malignant hypertension with high plasma renin activity (Fig. 2).

In the late stages of chronic renal failure, where the maintenance of extracellular fluid volume homeostasis becomes a problem, the plasma renin activity actually is an expression of the extracellular fluid balance, being high in dehydrated patients and low in cases of overhydration.[33]

It is, however, precisely in the overhydrated patients that the blood pressure may become uncontrollably high, which only demonstrates that the simple explanation of the hypertension of chronic renal failure as a straightforward consequence of hyperangiotensinemia is untenable. Moreover, fluctuations of plasma renin activity with fluid balance may, at this final stage, be caused by a lesion of the juxtaglomerular apparatus produced by the chronic renal disease.

HEMODYNAMICS OF HYPERTENSION IN CHRONIC RENAL DISEASE

In contrast to essential hypertension, few studies have been devoted to the hemodynamic basis of hypertension in chronic renal disease. The data from older studies[34-39] were conflicting, some authors finding the cardiac output increased and others finding the total peripheral vascular resistance raised. This was due, no doubt, to the inaccuracy and stressfulness of the methods used, to the difficulty of differentiating the various forms of hypertension by the techniques then available, and to the heterogeneity of the subjects so far as sex, age, and stage of hypertension were concerned.

In 11 patients with chronic renal parenchymal disease in whom age, sex, and degree of kidney damage were not defined, Frohlich and associates[40] found a cardiac index of 3228 ml./min./m.² while in normotensive subjects this parameter averaged 3048 ml./min./m.² Due to a broad scatter of the individual data the difference was insignificant, and the authors concluded that the elevated blood pressure was due to increased peripheral vascular resistance (0.025 mm. Hg/ml./min. as compared to 0.017 mm. Hg/ml./min. in the normotensives). However, in their preliminary analysis of the same problem with modern techniques Brod and coworkers[41] found a tendency toward an elevated cardiac output. A detailed analysis of their 20 subjects (14 males and 6 females with an average age of 36 years; 11 with chronic glomerulonephritis, 7 with chronic pyelonephritis, and 2 with polycystic kidney disease) whose renal function was still relatively well maintained (mean glomerular filtration rate 66 ml./min., but with a broad scatter), who were not in heart failure and whose hypertension was benign, revealed a high cardiac output as the basis of hypertension in at least 15 of them. Their total peripheral vascular resistance was entirely within the normal range. The calculated renal vascular resistance was, of course, raised, the renal vascular bed (and renal blood flow)

138

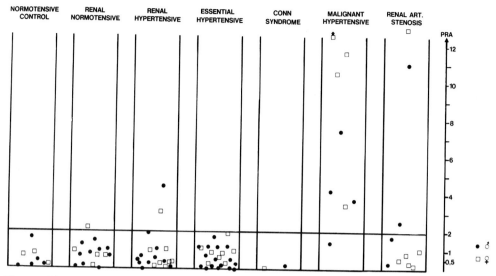

Figure 1. Plasma renin activity (ng./hr.) in our group of normotensive controls and in hypertensive patients of various etiologies. The horizontal line at 2 ng./hr. indicates the upper limit of our normal range. The three renal hypertensive patients whose plasma renin activity was at the upper limit of the normal range or exceeded it did not exhibit any significant differences from the rest of the patients.

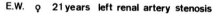

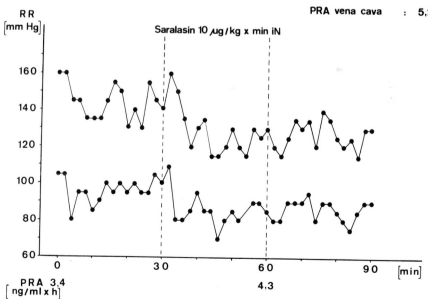

Figure 2. The effect of Saralasin on blood pressure and plasma renin activity in a patient with malignant renovascular hypertension.

having been reduced by the underlying renal disease, and the perfusing pressure being high. It is, however, conceivable that some of the renal vessels may have had a normal or even reduced vascular tone. Of the remaining vascular areas studied, the vascular resistance in skeletal muscle and probably also in the splanchnic area did not differ from that in the normotensive subjects, and only in the skin was the vascular resistance slightly increased (Fig. 3).[42]

That the cardiac output may be raised in nonuremic, nonanemic patients with chronic renal disease and blood pressures repeatedly elevated above 145/95 mm. Hg, was also borne out by our more recent studies in 45 patients whose age varied from 18 to 50 years (mean 33 years), 30 of whom were men and 15 women, and whose glomerular filtration rate averaged 86 ml./min.[43, 44] The cardiac index of the hypertensive renal patients was well above that of the normotensive controls and the normotensive patients with chronic renal disease. In 13 hypertensive patients the cardiac index exceeded the arbitrary value of 3.5 l./min./m.[2], which was reached only by one of the normotensive controls. The cardiac indices in most of the normotensive renal patients were also below this arbitrary level (Fig. 4).

The high cardiac index in the renal hypertensive subjects could not be explained by any difference in age, sex, or the degree of reduction of renal function. When, however, the subjects with chronic renal disease were subdivided according to the World Health Organization criteria for the developmental stages of hypertension, it was apparent that the patients with high cardiac indices were exclusively in stage I-II (stage I being defined as high blood pressure without any clinical evidence of hypertrophy of the heart or changes of the vessels) while the cardiac indices of the patients in stage III were invariably within the normal range (Fig. 5). Thus we may conclude that the high cardiac

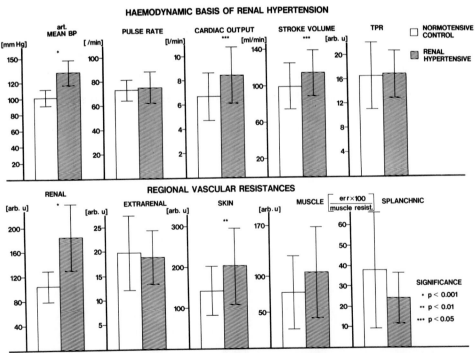

Figure 3. Hemodynamic basis of hypertension in 20 subjects with chronic renal disease and well preserved renal function. The statistical analysis suggests a significantly higher cardiac output, renal and skin vascular resistances in the renal hypertensive subjects. The other parameters did not differ significantly.[42]

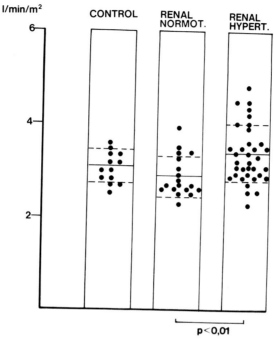

Figure 4. Cardiac index in normotensive control subjects, in normotensives with chronic renal disease, and in subjects with chronic renal disease and hypertension (BP > 145/95).[43, 44]

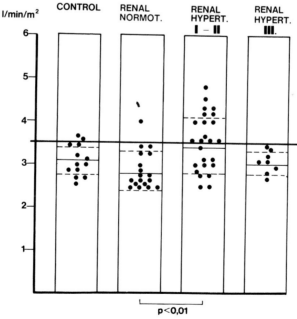

Figure 5. Cardiac index of normotensive controls, renal normotensives, and subjects with chronic renal disease and hypertension. The latter were subdivided according to the WHO criteria into stages I–II, and III. It is obvious that the cardiac output in renal hypertension stage I–II is markedly above that of the other groups.[43, 44]

index is an early event in the development of hypertension of chronic renal disease. This was confirmed by Onesti and coworkers.[45] Accordingly, total peripheral vascular resistance in these patients with chronic renal disease and initial phase of renal hypertension was not strikingly different from that in the normotensive controls or normotensive renal subjects (Fig. 6). Peripheral vascular resistance rose only with the progression of hypertension to stages II and III when signs of hypertrophy and dilatation of the left heart and of vascular damage became apparent. The same applies to the vascular resistance in the forearm muscles (Fig. 7). As previously mentioned, this high peripheral vascular resistance also forms the basis of hypertension in the late stages of renal disease with signs of chronic renal failure.

HEMODYNAMIC EFFECTS OF ANGIOTENSIN

If the hypertension of chronic renal disease is initiated by an increased production of renin, the hemodynamic pattern produced by a mildly or moderately pressor infusion of angiotensin II should simulate that of early renal hypertension. In vitro, the skeletal vessels are most constricted, those of the kidney least.[46] When infused intra-arterially in man, angiotensin produced a massive vasoconstriction in the forearm (Fig. 8). With intravenous infusion in doses raising the mean blood pressure by 30 mm. Hg, angiotensin

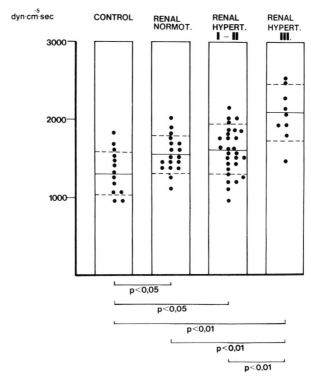

Figure 6. Total peripheral vascular resistance in normotensive controls, in renal normotensives, and in subjects with chronic renal disease and hypertension subdivided as in Figure 5. The total peripheral vascular resistance showed a scatter in the upward direction in the renal patients whose blood pressure was within the normal range, suggesting that the renal disease may affect the arterioles from its earliest phases, but as there was no significant difference between the total peripheral vascular resistance of the patients with the chronic renal disease with normal blood pressure and renal patients with hypertension stage I – II it was obvious that the increase in blood pressure was due to a rise of the cardiac output to which the arterioles did not adjust as they would in normotensive subjects.[43, 44]

142

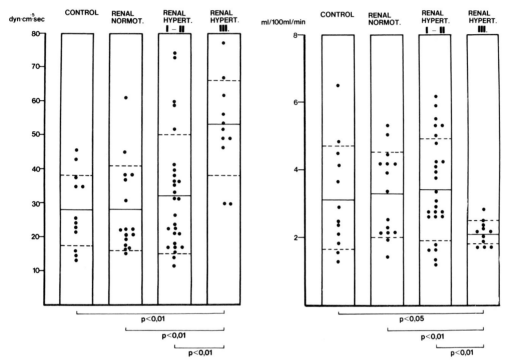

Figure 7. Forearm blood flow and forearm vascular resistance in normotensive controls, in normotensive renal patients, and in patients with chronic renal disease and hypertension subdivided as in Figure 5. It is obvious that these parameters did not differ between the normotensive controls, normotensive renal subjects, and subjects with early renal hypertension. In the late stage of renal hypertension, forearm blood flow was diminished and forearm vascular resistance was significantly higher than in the other subjects.[43, 44]

markedly increased the total peripheral vascular resistance as a result of a strong vasoconstriction in the kidneys and the splanchnic area and of lesser vasoconstriction in the skin, while the constriction of the vessels in the forearm muscles was found to be inconsistent (Fig. 9).[27] In the latter investigation the cardiac output dropped (with one exception) because of a reflex slowing of the heart rate, an effect also reported by others.[47-50] The effect on veins is less certain, McQueen and Morrison[51] and Finnerty[52] reporting a rise of the venous tone whereas De Pasquale and Burch[53] were unable to find any effect of angiotensin on injection into an isolated venous segment. Using a combination of isotopic and plethysmographic methods for the estimation of forearm blood volume and venous distensibility,[54, 55] we found in normotensive subjects that a mildly pressor infusion of angiotensin invariably constricts the peripheral veins, thereby shifting the blood into the central vascular bed with a rise of the central venous pressure (Fig. 10).

There is good evidence at present that apart from its direct constrictor effect on vascular smooth muscle, angiotensin produces part of its hemodynamic effects by stimulating the sympathetic hypothalamic centers[56-59] and the area postrema of the brain stem.[60] This may raise the cardiac output and, along with the visceral vasoconstriction, cause a vasodilation in skeletal muscles. This latter effect and the bradycardia may also be part of the baroreflex counteracting the rise of blood pressure. On the other hand, the afore-

143

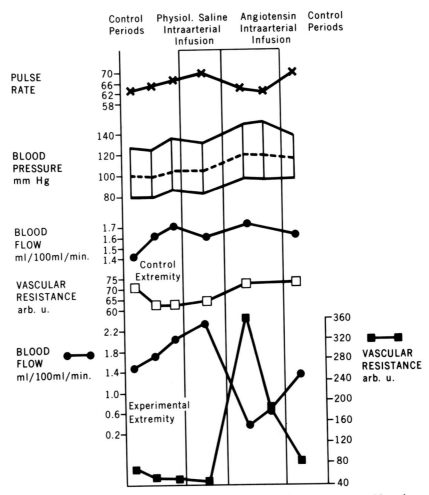

Figure 8. The effect of an intra-arterial injection of angiotensin into the brachial artery. Note the marked fall of blood flow and the striking increase in forearm vascular resistance in the experimental extremity. There is no significant change in the blood flow or vascular resistance in the control extremity. The slight rise of blood pressure and the slowing of the heart rate may be due to the penetration of angiotensin beyond the arterial bed of the extremity.

mentioned increase in central venous pressure may also act to raise the cardiac output.

Thus, the effect of angiotensin is much more complex than previously thought. It will produce a predictable and regular effect only in those areas where the various hemodynamic actions do not conflict. Thus, the vascular resistance will always rise in the kidneys, in the splanchnic area, and to some extent in the skin; and the veins will always constrict. On the other hand, the cardiac output may fall in response to the baroreflex (most frequently) or rise due to central sympathetic stimulation or the Starling effect (rarely); and the vessels in the muscles may dilate (central sympathetic action) or constrict (direct constrictor effect). However, because the powerful vasoconstrictor properties predominate, the total peripheral vascular resistance practically always rises (Fig. 11).

Thus, it is obvious that the hemodynamic pattern produced by a mildly to moderately pressor infusion of angiotensin differs in some important aspects from that of the early

144

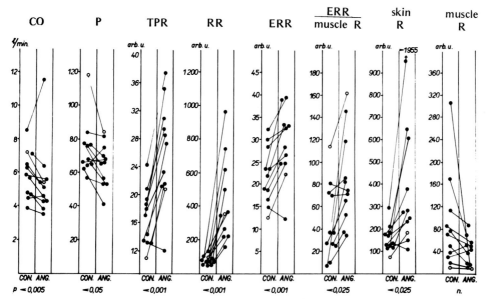

Figure 9. The hemodynamic effect of a moderately pressor intravenous infusion of angiotensin II on the cardiac output (CO), pulse rate (P), total peripheral vascular resistance (TPR), renal vascular resistance (RR), extrarenal vascular resistance (ERR), and the ratio between extrarenal vascular resistance and muscle vascular resistance (ERR/muscle R) which indicates the resistance changes in the splanchnic area, skin vascular resistance (skin R) and muscle vascular resistance (muscle R).[27]

phase of hypertension in chronic renal disease, which, as was mentioned, is manifest by a high cardiac output while the total peripheral vascular resistance remains within the normal range.

MODIFICATIONS OF THE HUMORAL CONCEPT

The inability to find consistently increased plasma levels of renin and angiotensin in renal hypertension led to numerous speculations about altered responsiveness of the vessels in chronic renal disease to normal amounts of angiotensin in the blood. Ames and coworkers[61] found that in the course of a protracted slow infusion of angiotensin in man the blood pressure progressively increases, probably due to a positive sodium balance mediated by the stimulation of aldosterone secretion. This may possibly explain the shift to the left of the regression of mean arterial pressure on plasma angiotensin II in patients with renal hypertension compared to normotensive subjects infused with angiotensin.[62-64] However, such an increased vascular responsiveness to normal plasma angiotensin levels should raise the total peripheral vascular resistance and reflexly diminish the cardiac output, an effect opposite to that found in the initial phase of hypertension in chronic renal disease. In addition, Saralasin should also lower the blood pressure in such a situation, but in our experience does not do so.

The same difficulty applies to several other vasoactive substances recently found in the kidney, all of which have been thought to be possibly connected with the origin of renal hypertension. Grollman and Krishnamurthy[65] separated by dialysis a substance of renal origin which they called nephrotensin and which they claimed could "serve to detect patients with surgically remediable hypertension and elucidate many observations on experimental hypertension". However, the substance is vasoconstrictor and

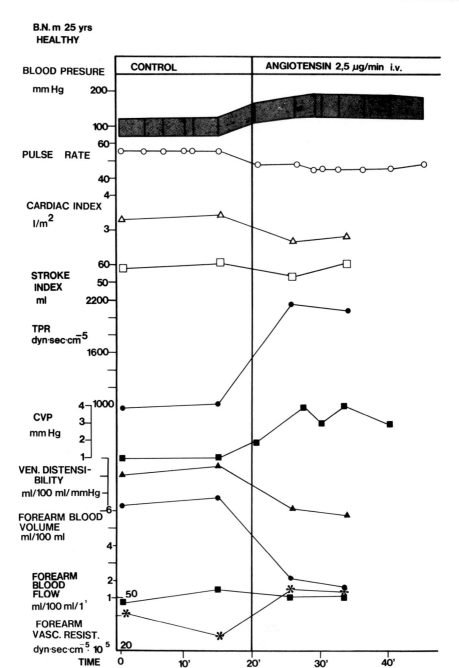

Figure 10. The effect of a mildly pressor intravenous infusion of angiotensin on cardiac index, stroke index, total peripheral vascular resistance (TPR), central venous pressure (CVP), venous distensibility, forearm blood volume, forearm blood flow and forearm vascular resistance. Note the reflex slowing of the heart rate and the drop of the cardiac index as blood pressure rises due to a marked increase in the TPR. The central venous pressure rises while the venous distensibility and forearm blood volume decrease. Due to a rise of the forearm vascular resistance the forearm blood flow does not change during the increase in blood pressure.

146

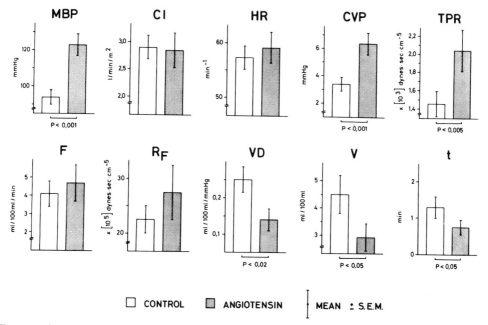

Figure 11. Summary of the effect of a moderately pressor intravenous infusion of angiotensin on the mean blood pressure (MBP), cardiac index (CI), heart rate (HR), central venous pressure (CVP), total peripheral vascular resistance (TPR), forearm blood flow (F), forearm vascular resistance (RF), venous distensibility (VD), volume of blood in the forearm (V), and forearm circulation time (t).[105]

cannot explain the increased cardiac output encountered in early renal hypertensive patients.

The discovery by Grollman[66] that the removal of both kidneys from the body can raise the blood pressure, stimulated the research for possible renal agents with vasodepressor action. This eventually led to the discovery that the renal medulla is the source of material with potent blood pressure lowering properties. This material probably originates in the medullary interstitial cells, lying horizontally between the medullary tubular and vascular structures. These cells contain lipid granules[67] whose number varies inversely with the amount of sodium in the body.[68] It is almost certain that the lipid granules are prostaglandin E_2 which has been extracted from the renal medulla.[69-72] The granules disappear and prostaglandin E_2 is found in increased concentration in the renal venous blood when pressor agents such as norepinephrine or angiotensin are infused intravenously or into the renal artery.[73] The medullary interstitial cells can be cultured in vitro. When these explanted cells are transferred into the peritoneal cavity of a hypertensive animal or their extract is injected, the blood pressure drops to normotensive levels. Muirhead and associates[74] speak of an "antihypertensive renomedullary principle" which has the qualities of a neutral lipid differing from the prostaglandins.

The blood pressure lowering effect of these medullary lipids is due to marked vasodilation, and the cardiac output is raised reflexly. The thought has been expressed by McGiff[75] that inhibition of renal prostaglandin synthesis from their precursor arachidonic acid may be associated with the development of hypertension. Such deficiency, however, should induce generalized vasoconstriction and reflex lowering of the cardiac output, and this differs from the hemodynamic pattern encountered in the initial stages of renal hypertension. In addition, prostaglandin E_2, the only substance whose renal medullary origin is not doubted, does not pass the lung barrier; and therefore its physiological effect on the arterial circulation remains unclear. On the other hand, the site of origin of prostaglandin A, which can pass the lungs, is uncertain. Prostaglandin A is also a potent vasodilator[76] and its deficiency could not explain the hemodynamic pattern of early renal hypertension. In addition, its level in hypertension of renal parenchymal disease is raised and not lowered (Fig. 12).[77]

Prostaglandins are tissue hormones and they may modulate locally the action of angiotensin and norepinephrine.[76] Prostaglandins are also entwined in the action of kinins, the renal release of prostaglandin being dependent upon the activity of the renal kallikrein-kinin system. Nothing is known, so far, about the role of this system in the pathogenesis of hypertension in chronic renal disease.

RENAL VOLUME HOMEOSTASIS AND HYPERTENSION

Apart from producing various vasoactive substances, the kidney is involved in the homeostasis of nitrogenous waste products, of acid-base balance, and of extracellular fluid volume. It has been known for many years, however, that neither an increase in nitrogenous waste products nor an acidosis are linked with any rise in the blood pressure. On the other hand, a positive salt balance has been connected, from the beginning of this century, with high blood pressure. French authors pointed out that a rigorous salt-free diet may reduce high blood pressure,[78] and this observation has been repeatedly confirmed. Epidemiological studies have related the prevalence of hypertension to the magnitude of dietary salt intake.[79] Also, by feeding salt to rats Dahl[80] and Meneely[81] succeeded in elevating their blood pressures without any other experimental interventions.

Balance of the body fluids requires that the kidneys excrete as much salt and water as has been introduced into the body. Long ago, Starling[82] recognized the connection be-

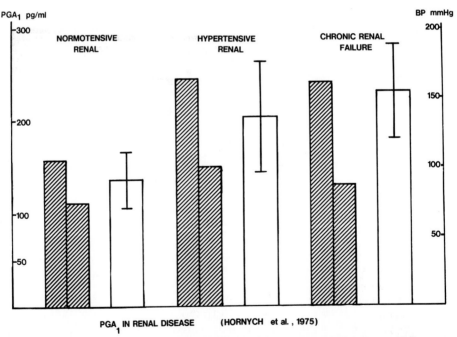

Figure 12. Levels of prostaglandin A_1 in subjects with renal hypertension and chronic renal failure compared with normotensive patients with renal disease. The shaded columns indicate systolic and diastolic blood pressures, the white columns indicate the level of PGA_1 (after Hornych[77] et al., 1975).

tween the body fluid volume, the central venous pressure, the performance of the heart and the renal excretion of fluid. As is shown schematically in Figure 13, a positive salt and water balance normally raises the mean systemic pressure by the increased filling and tension of the venous (capacitance) system.[83] This is responsible for increased venous return to the heart which, in turn, raises the cardiac output and the blood pressure. The enhanced perfusion pressure in the kidneys increases the urinary output of sodium and water, partly by raising the glomerular filtration rate and partly by reducing the tubular reabsorption of salt and water. This will re-establish the balance and may even lead to a slight overshoot in the negative direction, i.e., a drop of the tension in the capacitance bed, a reduced venous return to the heart, and a fall of the cardiac output and the arterial pressure. A decreased renal perfusion pressure, by lowering the urinary water and sodium excretion, will again restore balance.

It is obvious that the arterial blood pressure is the connecting link between the blood volume and the effector organ of extracellular fluid homeostasis, the kidney. From Figure 13 it is clear that with a given sodium intake, there is only one level of blood pressure at which the body neither gains nor loses sodium and water. This is expressed by the renal function curve (Fig. 14) of Guyton and coworkers[84] which also demonstrates how the blood pressure must change when the intake of salt has changed. The system is obviously so effective that a sevenfold increase in the salt intake in dogs raises the blood pressure by less than 10 mm. Hg; the increased salt excretion will quickly restore the balance, so that the authors speak of an "overflow" regulator for arterial pressure.

Such a feedback system requires a perfectly responsive kidney. If the glomerular surface area is reduced by vasoconstriction or destroyed by disease, or if the glomerulotubular balance is disturbed by an enhanced sodium reabsorption due to hyperaldosteronism, a balance between sodium intake and excretion can be achieved only if the renal perfusion pressure rises. The renal function curve shifts to the right but remains parallel to the normal function curve (Fig. 14).

This mechanism was confirmed experimentally in dogs whose kidneys were reduced to one third of their original mass. This maneuver raised the blood pressure insignifi-

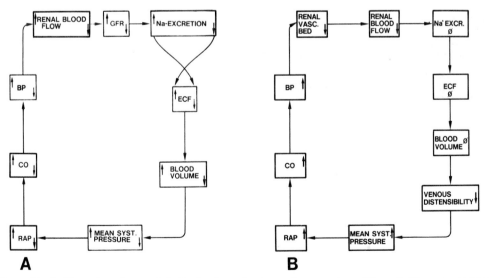

Figure 13. A. The volume homeostatic feedback mechanism under normal conditions. B. The same system when venous distensibility is diminished and renal vascular bed is reduced by disease or vasoconstriction. Under the latter conditions it is obvious that even without a volume change the blood pressure must rise in order to preserve the body fluid and sodium balance.

149

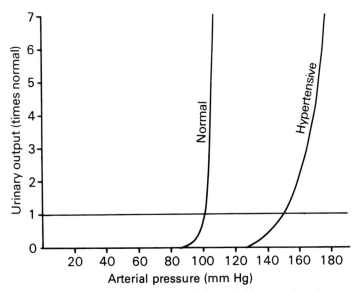

Figure 14. Renal function curve under normal conditions (left) and with reduced renal mass (right). The horizontal line at 1 indicates the usual fluid intake with which the urinary output must be in equilibrium. It is obvious that under normal conditions there is only one level of blood pressure under which the organism neither gains nor loses fluid. It is also clear that with a slight increase or decrease of the fluid intake the blood pressure changes will be only minimal under normal conditions. (By courtesy of Guyton et al.[84])

cantly, but when sodium intake was increased a permanent hypertension was induced, due at first to an increase in the cardiac output while the total peripheral vascular resistance fell slightly. After a few days, however, the cardiac output returned almost to its original level and the elevated blood pressure was sustained by an increased total peripheral vascular resistance.[85, 86] If the hemodynamic basis of the hypertension had been investigated at this slightly later period, the initial rise of the cardiac output would have been overlooked. Similarly, an expansion of blood volume by 20 percent in unanesthetized dogs by repeated transfusions of blood and dextran raised the mean blood pressure from 93.7 to 120 mm. Hg.[87] This was due at first to an increase in the cardiac output, while the total peripheral vascular resistance fell transiently. However, after two hours the cardiac output returned to its original level and hypertension was maintained thereafter by an increased total peripheral vascular resistance.[87]

The mechanism responsible for the subsequent increase in the total peripheral vascular resistance remains unclear. Coleman and Guyton[86] attribute the change to a whole body tissue autoregulation of blood flow. Whether this is due to a flushing out of vasodilating metabolites by an increased blood flow, to local reflexes, or to other factors is unsolved. Another possibility is a rapid increase in the wall/lumen ratio of the vessels subjected to an increased stretch.[88, 89]

The important conclusions to be drawn from the aforementioned experiments are that on reducing the efficiency of the volume homeostatic function of the kidney (1) an increase in the cardiac output is the first mechanism to raise the blood pressure, which is later sustained by an increase in the total peripheral vascular resistance; and (2) once the blood pressure has been raised the fluid balance will be restored, the kidney now being able to excrete the accumulated surplus of salt and water. The entire chain of events with all of the possible secondary influences and implications has actually been reproduced and predicted by a computer system.[90]

Whereas the renal ability to adjust to the requirements of volume homeostasis has

150

been created in the experimental animal within minutes, chronic organic renal disease usually develops over many months or years. It is justified, therefore, to expect that the increased cardiac output will persist longer, and this indeed has been found. The fact that the total peripheral vascular resistance in these early hypertensive patients with chronic renal disease does not fall as it would in normotensive subjects with a similarly elevated cardiac output, suggests, however, that the arterioles at this early stage are already under one of the aforementioned possible influences which eventually rise the total peripheral vascular resistance, or that they are responding to the positive sodium balance or to the physiological levels of angiotensin in the blood.

Borst and Borst-de-Geus demonstrated that the initial increase in weight due to a positive sodium balance produced in a patient by the ingestion of licorice for several weeks will revert to normal when the blood pressure rises.[91] A high cardiac output also has been recorded in patients with oliguric acute renal failure and presumed positive sodium balance,[92, 93] although under these circumstances other factors raising the cardiac output, such as anemia or thiamine deficiency, must be considered. In addition, in 7 patients with acute glomerulonephritis and hypertension, De Fazio and associates[94] found a high cardiac output. The observation by Birkenhäger and associates[95] of 2 severely congested patients with acute glomerulonephritis and hypertension with normal cardiac output and raised total peripheral vascular resistance is not necessarily contradictory. The time interval between the onset of the disease and the evaluation of the hemodynamic parameters is not stated and it is possible that by the time of the study the cardiac output had fallen while the vessels had constricted in response to angiotensin.

In 16 hypertensive patients with chronic renal parenchymal disease whose glomerular filtration rate ranged from 105 to 36 ml./min., Dustan and coworkers[96] found a direct correlation between the weekly average of diastolic pressures measured twice daily and their plasma volume. This differs from our own results (Fig. 15) in which no difference, or a slightly decreasing trend in the circulating blood volume, exchangeable sodium, or extracellular fluid volume, was detected on transition from normotensive renal patients

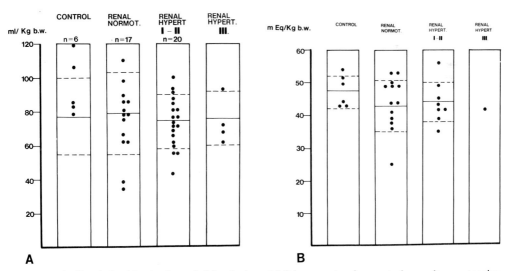

Figure 15. A. Circulating blood volume (ml./kg. body weight) in normotensive controls, renal normotensive subjects, and subjects with chronic renal disease and hypertension (subdivided as in Figure 5). B. Exchangeable Na (mEq./kg. body weight) in normotensive controls, renal normotensive patients, and patients with chronic renal disease and hypertension (subdivided as in Figure 5.)[43, 44]

to patients with chronic renal disease and early and late hypertension. The difference between our own data and those of the previous authors may be due to different laboratory methods or to a difference in the stage and progression of the renal disease. Our findings in renal hypertensive patients, however, are not surprising in view of the foregoing discussion, i.e., once the blood pressure has been raised, the surplus of sodium and water will be excreted from the body and the original balance re-established for as long as the hypertension persists.

There are, however, some renal parenchymal diseases which exhibit a marked tendency to sodium and water retention and eventual formation of edema, i.e., the nephrotic syndrome, in which hypertension either never occurs (lipid nephrosis) or is a late event in the downhill course of the disease (renal amyloidosis, membranous glomerulonephritis). There are other nosological entities in which urinary concentrating power is lost early in their course and which predispose, therefore, to a negative fluid and sodium balance, such as chronic pyelonephritis or other types of interstitial nephropathy, polycystic kidney disease and salt-losing nephritis, but which nonetheless are frequently accompanied by hypertension. Thus, in chronic pyelonephritis, blood pressure elevation may be encountered with equal frequency to that in chronic glomerulonephritis.[28]

The patients with nephrotic syndrome have, in spite of their positive sodium and fluid balance, a normal or low normal circulating blood volume due to hypoalbuminemia and a shift of extracellular fluid out of the vascular compartment; occasionally they may even develop peripheral circulatory failure.[97] The cardiac output of these subjects tends to be low rather than high. The permanent tendency to hypovolemia produces a reflex vasoconstriction and an enhanced production of renin and angiotensin, leading to secondary hyperaldosteronism. Does angiotensin under these conditions contribute to the vascular constriction necessary for the maintenance of a normal blood pressure when the cardiac output is low? Some recent observations with the angiotensin antagonist Saralasin seem to support this idea but further investigation is required. Hypertension probably starts when the glomerular filtration, as a consequence of the progressive scarring of glomeruli, can no longer accommodate at normotensive levels to the body's volume requirements.

The situation is less clear in the group of interstitial nephropathies and polycystic kidney disease. Although their salt-losing tendency becomes manifest only at a relatively advanced stage and explains why some of these patients remain normotensive throughout the whole course of their disease, it is difficult to assume in them a transient positive sodium balance as in the glomerular diseases. A tendency to dehydration will, of course, mobilize the renin-angiotensin-aldosterone system, as already discussed. However, plasma renin activity in this category of hypertensive patients was not different from that encountered in other subjects with chronic renal disease and hypertension or from the normotensive controls. Therefore, additional factors must be considered.

ROLE OF THE CAPACITANCE SYSTEM

It is clear that the pressure in an elastic container depends not only on the volume of the fluid that it contains but also on the capacity of the container. Thus, with a given volume of blood the mean systemic pressure depends on the size, i.e., on the compliance, of the capacitance system. Studies of the pressure-volume relationship in isolated segments of the femoral and jugular veins in dogs with renal hypertension produced by silk perinephritis, suggested a reduced venous compliance.[98] Using a combination of isotopic and plethysmographic methods in our hemodynamic studies on patients with chronic non-uremic renal disease and hypertension, we found that the volume of blood and venous distensibility of the forearm veins have a tendency to decrease even in normotensive patients with chronic renal disease. This is still more marked and attains statistical significance in the hypertensive subjects (Fig. 16).[43] The decreased venous distensibility correlates negatively with the cardiac index in subjects with chronic renal disease and hypertension whose total peripheral vascular resistance is still within normal limits (Fig. 17).

The diminished venous compliance may be due to a greater stiffness of the venous walls of the surrounding tissue gel or to both. Using the wig[99] or capsule technique for measuring tissue compliance, Lucas and Floyer[100] found it to be decreased in reneprival rats and also in animals with a clipped renal artery, the compliance increasing within a short time after removal of the clip. Due to the increased resistance of the tissue to accepting surplus fluid from the blood, the infused saline persisted for a longer period of time in the blood of these animals and, by raising the venous pressure, increased the cardiac output and the arterial pressure (Fig. 18).

Thus, it appears that a narrowed and more rigid capacitance system may be another factor initiating or contributing to the pathogenetic chain of events (even without the necessity of a transient rise of the circulating blood volume) which, in view of the restricted renal adjustability to the requirements of volume homeostasis, will eventually lead to a permanent hypertension (Fig. 13).

What the factor (or factors) adversely affecting the venous distensibility or tissue compliance may be, remains a matter of conjecture thus far. Lucas and Floyer[101] suggest that the kidney, being the principal organ of volume homeostasis, may regulate the ability of the tissue to take up surplus fluid from the circulation by some as yet unidentified hormone. The experience with the unclipping of the kidney would require a factor which can be quickly inactivated by renal dysfunction and quickly re-activated when

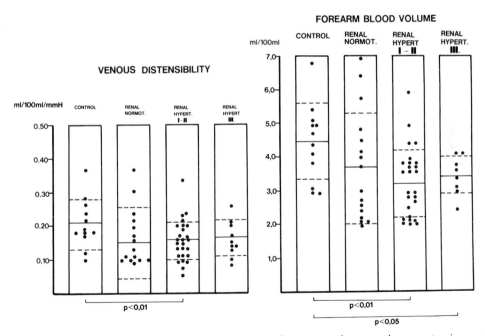

Figure 16. Venous distensibility and forearm blood volume in normotensive controls, normotensive renal subjects, and subjects with chronic renal disease and hypertension (subdivided as in Figure 5.) The decreasing trend of venous distensibility and of forearm blood volume in subjects with renal disease is obvious.[43, 44]

153

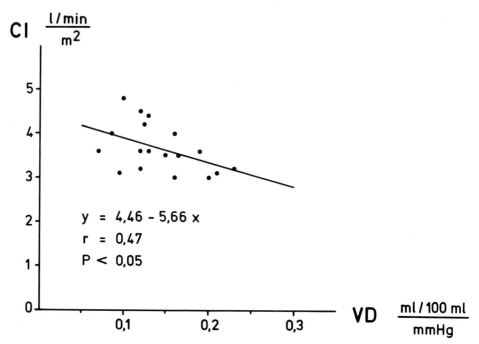

Figure 17. Correlation between the cardiac index and venous distensibility in subjects with chronic renal disease and hypertension stage I whose peripheral vascular resistance was within normal limits.[43, 44]

that function (whatever it may be) is restored. Do the renal prostaglandins fulfill this requirement? Or does the renal "natriuretic hormone" which, according to Nizet,[102] can be switched on and off at short notice not only by volume homeostasis but by renal pathology perform this function? Another possibility is that an increased amount of sodium (and water) in the interstitial spaces or in the venous walls may diminish their compliance. In experiments with acute fluid and sodium loading in man, employing an infusion of saline amounting to 10-12 percent of the extracellular fluid volume given within 20 to 30 minutes, the central venous pressure and cardiac output rose markedly and the forearm blood volume and venous distensibility were initially decreased, at least in some experiments. This investigation has not yet been completed and should be repeated after chronic sodium loading.

Venous distensibility underlies alpha-sympathetic control, as was shown in studies with acute emotional stress in which the venous compliance decreased.[103] Although earlier we could not find any reason for sympathetic activation in chronic renal disease, evidence of an increase in catecholamine forming enzymes in the vicinity of the centers controlling blood pressure in the medulla has recently been discovered in spontaneously hypertensive rats and in DOCA-salt hypertension.[104] Whether this also occurs in human disease, and what the effect on venous compliance may be, is unknown as yet. It was mentioned earlier that the veins are highly sensitive to minute amounts of angiotensin.[105] Further work will be necessary to determine whether angiotensin in very minute amounts, which would be barely detectable as an increased plasma angiotensin concentration, could stiffen the veins, shift blood centrally and raise the cardiac output while leaving the arterial site virtually unaffected. Thus far, however, our studies with the angiotensin antagonist Saralasin have not shown any effect on the venous distensibility in patients with chronic renal disease and early hypertension.

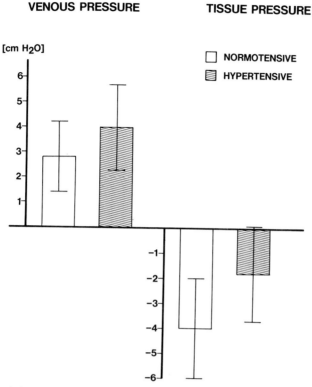

VENOUS PRESSURE　　　　　**TISSUE PRESSURE**

Figure 18. Venous and tissue pressure in rats before and 60 days after unilateral nephrectomy and renal artery constriction (after Lucas and Floyer, 1974).[101]

RENOVASCULAR HYPERTENSION

It was thought until recently that renovascular hypertension was fully explained by an oversecretion of renin by the kidney as the result of reduced blood flow. It was mentioned earlier, however, that plasma renin activity and angiotensin concentration may be, with the exception in cases of malignant hypertension, within the normal range and Saralasin may not affect the blood pressure. It is clear that the stenosed renal artery can, by lowering the renal perfusion pressure, interfere with homeostatic volume regulation in the manner suggested by Figure 19.

The original view that renal artery constriction in an experimental animal raises the total peripheral vascular resistance while leaving the cardiac output unchanged[106] supported a renin-angiotensin genesis of Goldblatt hypertension. Ledingham and Pelling[107] established, however, that this sequence occurs only if the constriction is severe. With moderate constriction, the blood pressure rise during the initial hours is due to an increase in the total peripheral vascular resistance which is accounted for by the release of renin from the ischemic kidney. From the second day, however, the body fluid volume starts to rise, the plasma renin activity and the total peripheral vascular resistance decrease, and hypertension is now sustained by a high cardiac output. Only after a week or two does a new rise in the total peripheral vascular resistance, independent of the plasma renin and due to the mechanisms discussed earlier, assume again the leading role.[108-110] This is in accord with the finding of an initially high cardiac output under-

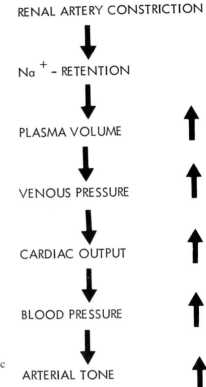

RENAL ARTERY CONSTRICTION

Na^+ - RETENTION

PLASMA VOLUME

VENOUS PRESSURE

CARDIAC OUTPUT

BLOOD PRESSURE

ARTERIAL TONE

Figure 19. Schematic representation of pathophysiologic changes induced by renal artery constriction.

lying hypertension in patients with fibromuscular hyperplasia of the renal artery.[111]

A similar interference with renal volume homeostasis will be produced by an aldosterone secreting (Conn) tumor, upsetting the glomerulotubular balance in such a way that more sodium must be filtered by the glomeruli in order to maintain sodium balance in the body. It even follows that renal vasoconstriction produced by sympathetic overactivity in the early phase and by arteriosclerotic narrowing of the afferent arterioles in the late phase of essential hypertension may, by interference with the renal adjustment to the volume homeostatic requirements of the body, add a renal element to the pathogenesis of the latter disorder. Thus, as indicated in Figure 14, the renal function curve must be shifted to the right in order to achieve a new balance between the sodium intake and output.

LATE STAGE OF RENAL PARENCHYMAL DISEASE

The course of the late stage of renal parenchymal disease has been mentioned earlier. Although the anemia of chronic renal failure tends to increase the cardiac output, its correction by transfusion of packed red cells reduces the cardiac output to normal while the high blood pressure remains unaffected, being sustained by the increased total peripheral vascular resistance[29, 30] (Fig. 6).

With progressive reduction of the glomerular filtering surface, even extreme elevation of blood pressure will eventually be ineffective in re-establishing normal fluid balance.[112] Hypervolemia with threatening pulmonary edema will subsequently follow. In

156

these patients there is a good correlation between the circulating blood volume and the blood pressure (Fig. 20). However, a good correlation has also been found at this stage between the diastolic blood pressure and the plasma renin activity.[113-119] By repeated hemodialysis it is possible, with normalization of weight and body water and salt content, to reduce the blood pressure to normotensive levels in most patients. In some cases, however, severe hypertension will persist despite considerable weight reduction. Vertes and associates[119] found that these latter patients have very high plasma renin levels in spite of their waterlogging. Conversely, Safar and coworkers[120] did not find any dividing line between these patients, and they believe that the blood pressure normalizing effect of repeated hemodialysis depends on the original severity of hypertension. The data in Figure 20 suggest in addition that the presence of renin in the plasma enhances the blood pressure dependency on plasma volume, probably by stiffening of the capacitance system.

Ledingham[112] is probably correct when concluding that in some patients with chronic renal failure the plasma renin activity is inappropriately high relative to the amount of exchangeable sodium. Progressive sodium and fluid depletion by repeated hemodialysis will elevate plasma renin activity still further so that hypertension will now be sustained by a direct pressor action of angiotensin. These are the patients whose severe hypertension can be cured only by bilateral nephrectomy.[116, 120-125] Mimran and coworkers[126] recently found that 8 of 10 such subjects, among all their patients on chronic intermittent hemodialysis, responded to Saralasin infusion by marked reduction or even normalization of blood pressure. It appears therefore that in this small group of subjects

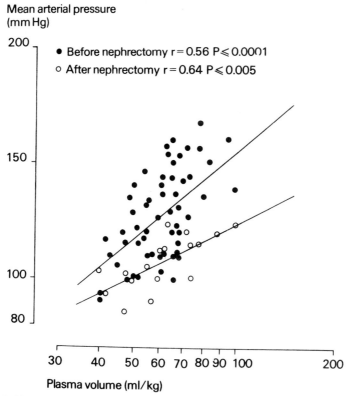

Figure 20. Correlation between mean arterial pressure and plasma volume in subjects with end-stage renal disease, before and after nephrectomy (courtesy of Dr. Safar et al.[120]).

157

with end-stage renal disease, the renin-angiotensin system plays a major role in the maintenance of their hypertension.

TREATMENT

Regarding the therapy of renal parenchymal hypertension, it should be borne in mind that high blood pressure produces pathological changes in the renal arterioles and thus contributes to the deterioration of renal function. Effective management of hypertension will therefore not only spare the heart and the extrarenal vessels from damage but simultaneously will slow down the progress of the renal disease. Specific therapeutic steps should be directed against the individual factors of the pathogenetic chain discussed earlier.

The tendency to positive sodium and water balance should be counteracted by diuretic drug therapy and reduction of salt intake to 5 grams per day. This approach may entail the risk of dehydration in patients with sodium-losing nephropathies and in all renal patients whose glomerular filtration rate has fallen below 30 ml./min. and who develop the well known polyuria of end-stage renal disease. In such instances, frequent patient followup is mandatory; and the therapeutic approach must be moderated at the slightest sign of dehydration as this may lead in turn to a total breakdown of the remaining renal function. Of the various diuretics, thiazides with their slower mode of action are preferred in the nonuremic hypertensives to the more drastic loop diuretics, i.e., furosemide or ethacrynic acid. The latter are mainly reserved for the oliguric patient with end-stage disease. Precautions must be taken also against undue potassium losses provoked by these diuretics. It should be recalled that potassium retention is the exception in chronic renal disease until the terminal oliguric or anuric phase is reached. As a rule, dietary potassium, such as is contained in fruit, will suffice as an adequate replacement. An alternative approach is to administer spironolactone or triamterene; these drugs are contraindicated, however, when the glomerular filtration rate has fallen below 20 to 30 ml./min. (because of the potential danger of hyperkalemia).

The diminished venous compliance can probably be increased by the vasodilator drugs, hydralazine and minoxidil. They will simultaneously reduce arteriolar tone which is relatively high, even early when the high cardiac output initiates the hypertension, and which subsequently assumes a dominant role. We have found hydralazine to be a safe drug, if titration is done slowly (in 25 mg./day increments, increased weekly) and if the total daily dose does not exceed 150 to 200 mg. Minoxidil, on the other hand, may produce unpleasant hypertrichosis which limits its usefulness.

Vasodilator drugs tend to mobilize the sympathetic nervous system, and this may offset the desired effect on the veins[127] and to some extent also on the arterial side of the circulation. In addition, the cardiac output may rise reflexly. Hence it is reasonable to prescribe these drugs along with both alpha- and beta-sympathetic blocking agents. The latter, in addition to preventing the cardiac output from rising will also inhibit renin secretion[128-132] which plays an important role at least in the late stage of renal parenchymal disease. Bühler[133] found an especially favorable effect of the beta-blocking agents in patients with high plasma renin activity. It is probable that they also lower alpha-sympathetic discharge by their central nervous system action on the blood pressure regulating center, thus reducing both venous and arteriolar tone. This is also the reason for prescribing agents such as clonidine, reserpine and methyldopa.

In renal patients with hypertensive crisis, the intervenous administration of diazoxide (300 mg.) or an infusion of sodium nitroprusside may produce a prompt and substantial lowering of blood pressure. However, since both substances are vasodilators, the sympathetic nervous system will be reflexly activated during the fall of blood pressure.

In end-stage kidney disease with normal plasma renin activity, the therapy of choice is repeated hemodialysis with ultrafiltration until dry body weight is achieved. In the smaller group of patients with high plasma renin values, bilateral nephrectomy is indicated; but occasionally even in these patients, hemodialysis and the administration of beta-blockers will eventually lead to a normalization of blood pressure.

SUMMARY AND CONCLUSIONS

1. Plasma renin activity and plasma angiotensin concentrations are almost never increased in the initial phase of hypertension of chronic renal parenchymal disease.

2. The hemodynamic pattern of the early stage of renal hypertension consists of a high cardiac output, normal total peripheral vascular resistance, and normal vascular resistance in most of the hemodynamically important regions. This is unlike the hemodynamic changes produced by a mildly pressor infusion of angiotensin which, in spite of its relative complexity, almost invariably raises the total peripheral vascular resistance and reflexly depresses the cardiac output.

3. The diseased kidney has a reduced ability to cope with the requirements of volume homeostasis at a normal level of blood pressure. The homeostatic feedback mechanism, by raising the blood pressure, restores the disturbed fluid balance.

4. The initally high cardiac output will subsequently fall and the hypertension will be maintained by an increased total peripheral vascular resistance.

5. A stiffening of the capacitance system, which occurs in the early stages of chronic renal disease, contributes to or in some cases may even be fully responsible for the early increase in cardiac output.

6. In the late stages of chronic renal disease, when an extreme reduction of the glomerular filtration rate occurs, even a marked rise of the blood pressure will be ineffective in re-establishing fluid balance. These patients are threatened by pulmonary congestion, and their hypertension can be reduced only by repeated hemodialysis with ultrafiltration.

7. A small group of patients with chronic renal failure have high plasma renin activity, and any attempt to reduce the volume of extracellular fluid will increase blood pressure and renin activity further. Their grave hypertension can be cured only by bilateral nephrectomy.

8. Treatment of hypertension in chronic renal disease, although in many ways still empirical, should start from these aforementioned pathogenetic considerations. In this regard, a tentative therapeutic program is suggested.

REFERENCES

1. GOLDBLATT, H., LYNCH, J., HANZAL, R. F., ET AL.: *Studies on experimental hypertension. I. The production of persistent elevation of systolic blood pressure by means of renal ischemia.* J. Exp. Med. 59: 347, 1934.

2. TIGERSTEDT, R., AND BERGMANN, P. G.: *Niere und Kreislauf.* Skand. Arch. Physiol. 8:223, 1898.

3. LANDIS, E. M., MONTGOMERY, H., AND SPARKMAN, D.: *The effects of pressor agents and of saline kidney extracts on blood pressure and skin temperature.* J. Clin. Invest. 17:189, 1938.

4. PICKERING, G. W., AND PRINZMETAL, M.: *Some observations on renin, a pressor substance contained in normal kidney, together with a method for its biological assay.* Clin. Sci. 3:211, 1938.

5. PAGE, I. H.: *On the nature of the pressor action of renin.* J. Exp. Med. 70:521, 1939.

6. BRAUN-MENÉNDEZ, B., FASCIOLO, J. C., LELOIR, L. F., ET AL.: *The substance causing renal hypertension.* J. Physiol. (Lond.) 98:283, 1940.

7. VOLHARD, F., AND FAHR, T.: *Die Bright'sche Nierenkrankheit. Klinik, Pathologie und Atlas.* Berlin, Springer, 1914.

8. HARRISON, H. E., BLALOCK, A., AND MASON, M. F.: *Effects on blood pressure of injection of kidney extracts of dogs with renal hypertension.* Proc. Soc. Exp. Biol. Med. 35:38, 1936.

9. PRINZMETAL, M., AND FRIEDMAN, B.: *Pressor effects of kidney extracts from patients and dogs with hypertension.* Proc. Soc. Exp. Biol. Med. 35:122, 1936.

10. HOUSSAY, B. A., AND TAQUINI, A. C.: *Spécificité de l'action vasoconstrictrice du sang veineux du rein ischémié.* C. r. Séanc. Soc. Biol. 129:5, 1938.

11. BRAUN-MENÉNDEZ, B., AND FASCIOLO, J. C.: *Acción vasoconstrictora e hipertensora de la sangre venosa del rinón en isquemia incompleta aguda.* Revta Soc. Argent. Biol. 15:161, 1939.

12. CASTLEMAN, B., AND SMITHWICK, R. H.: *The relation of vascular disease to the hypertensive state.* N. Engl. J. Med. 239:732, 1948.

13. TALBOTT, J. H., CASTLEMAN, B., SMITHWICK, R. H., ET AL.: *Renal biopsy studies correlated with renal clearance observations in hypertensive patients treated by radical nephrectomy.* J. Clin. Invest. 22:387, 1943.

14. SMITH, H. W., GOLDRING, W., AND CHASIS, H.: *Role of the kidney in the genesis of hypertension.* Bull. N.Y. Acad. Med. 19:449, 1943.

15. BRADLEY, E. M., CHASIS, H., GOLDRING, W., ET AL.: *Hemodynamic alterations in normotensive and hypertensive subjects during the pyrogenic reaction.* J. Clin. Invest. 24:749, 1945.

16. RATNER, N. A.: *O roli počečnogo faktora v patogeneze gipertonii.* Vest. Akad. Med. Nauk SSSR 10:39, 1958.

17. BROD, J., AND FENCL, V.: *Diurnal variations of systemic and renal haemodynamics in normal subjects and in hypertensive disease.* Cardiologia 31:494, 1957.

18. SMITH, H. W.: *Hypertension and urologic disease.* Am. J. Med. 6:724, 1948.

19. FITZ, A.: *Renal venous renin determinations in the diagnosis of surgically correctable hypertension.* J. Clin. Invest. 36:942, 1967.

20. MASSANI, Z. N., FINKIELMAN, S., WORCEL, M., ET AL.: *Angiotensin blood levels in hypertensive and non-hypertensive diseases.* Clin. Sci. 30:473, 1966.

21. CATT, K. J., CRAN, E., ZIMMET, P., ET AL.: *Angiotensin II blood levels in human hypertension.* Lancet 1:459, 1971.

22. BOYD, G. W., JONES, M. B., AND PEART, W. S.: *The radioimmunoassay of angiotensin II and plasma renin activity in human hypertension,* in GENEST, J. AND KOIW, B. (EDS.) *Hypertension.* Springer, Berlin, 1972, p. 583.

23. PEART, W. S.: *Hypertension and the kidney,* in BLACK, D. (ED.): *Renal Disease,* ed. 3. Blackwell, Oxford, 1972, p. 705.

24. STREETEN, D. H., ANDERSON, G. H., FREIBERG, J. M., ET AL.: *Use of an angiotensin II antagonist (Saralasin) in the recognition of "angiotensinogenic" hypertension.* N. Engl. J. Med. 292:617, 1975.

25. BRUNNER, H. R., GAVRAS, H., LARAGH, J. H., ET AL.: *Angiotensin II blockade in man by sar¹-ala⁸-angiotensin II for understanding and treatment of high blood pressure.* Lancet 2:1045, 1973.

26. BROD. J., FENCL, V., HEJL, Z., ET AL.: *General and regional haemodynamic pattern underlying essential hypertension.* Clin. Sci. 23:339, 1962.

27. BROD. J., HEJL, Z., HORNYCH, A., ET AL.: *Comparison of haemodynamic effects of equipressor doses of intravenous angiotensin and noradrenalin infusions in man.* Clin. Sci. 36:161, 1969.

28. BROD, J.: *The Kidney.* Butterworth, Inc., Woburn, Mass., 1973.

29. NEFF, M. S., KIM, K. E., PERSOFF, M., ET AL.: *Hemodynamics of uremic anemia.* Circulation 43:876, 1971.

30. KIM, K. E., ONESTI, G., SCHWARTZ, A. B., ET AL.: *Hemodynamics of hypertension in chronic end-stage renal disease.* Circulation 46:456, 1972.

31. BROWN, J. J., DAVIES, D. L., LEVER, A. F., ET AL.: *Plasma renin concentration in human hypertension. II. Renin in relation to aetiology.* Br. Med. J. II:1215, 1965.

32. DUSTAN, H. P., TARAZI, R. C., AND FROHLICH, E. D.: *Functional correlates of plasma renin activity in hypertensive patients.* Circulation 41:555, 1970.

33. WARREN, D. J., AND FERRIS, T. F.: *Renin secretion in renal hypertension.* Lancet 1:159, 1970.

34. LILJESTRAND, G., AND STENSTRÖM, N.: *Work of heart during rest; blood flow in increased arterial blood pressure with influence of pregnancy on blood flow.* Acta Med. Scand. 63:142, 1925.

35. HAYASAKA, E.: *Minute volume of heart in hypertension.* Tohoku J. Exp. Med. 9:401, 1927.

36. LAUTER, S., AND BAUMANN, H.: *Über den Kreislauf bei Hochdruck, Arteriosklerose und Apoplexie.* Z. Klin. Med. 109:415, 1928.

160

37. ERNST, C., AND WEISS, R.: *Über das zirkulatorische Minutenvolumen bei der Hypertonie.* Z. Ges. Exp. Med. 68:126, 1929.

38. KROETZ, C.: *Messung des Kreislaufminutenvolumens mit Acetylen als Fremdgas. Ihre bisherigen Ergebnisse bei arteriellem Hochdruck und bei Dekompensation des Kreislaufs.* Klin. Wschr. 9:966, 1930.

39. EWIG, H., AND HINSBERG, K.: *Kreislaufstudien. Neue Methode zur Bestimmung des Herzminutenvolumens.* Z. Klin. Med. 115:677, 1935.

40. FROHLICH, E. D., TARAZI, R. C., AND DUSTAN, H. P.: *Re-examination of the hemodynamics of hypertension.* Am. J. Med. Sci. 257:9, 1969.

41. BROD, J., HEJL, Z., ULRYCH, M., ET AL.: *Hemodynamický podklad renální hypertense.* Csl. Fysiol. 10: 228, 1961.

42. BROD, J., FENCL, V., AND ULRYCH, M.: *General and regional hemodynamics in hypertension in chronic renal disease.* Clin. Nephrol. 5:175, 1975.

43. BROD, J.: *Chronic renal parenchymal disease and hypertension.* Kidney Int. 8:235, 1975.

44. BROD, J., CACHOVAN, M., BAHLMANN, J., ET AL.: *Haemodynamic basis of hypertension in chronic nonuraemic parenchymatous renal disease.* Proc. 6th Intern. Congr. Nephrol., Florence, 1975. Karger, Basel, 1976, p. 305.

45. ONESTI, G., KIM, K. E., FERNANDES, M., ET AL.: *Hemodynamic alterations in hypertension of renal parenchymal diseases,* in MILLIEZ, E. P. AND SAFAR, M. (EDS.): *Recent Advances in Hypertension, 2,* Laboratories Boehringer, Ingelheim, France, 1975, p. 227.

46. BOHR, D. F.: *Individualities of vascular smooth muscles from different sites in their responsiveness to angiotensin.* Symposium on Renal Hypertension, Cleveland, 1966.

47. BRADLEY, S. E., AND PARKER, G.: *The hemodynamic effects of angiotonin in normal man.* J. Clin. Invest. 20:715, 1941.

48. MIDDLETON, S., AND WIGGERS, C. J.: *The effects of renin and angiotonin on cardiac output and total peripheral resistance.* Am. J. Physiol. 141:128, 1944.

49. JOHNSON, W. P., AND BRUCE, R. A.: *Hemodynamic and metabolic effects of angiotensin II during rest and exercise in normal healthy subjects.* Am. Heart J. 63:212, 1962.

50. PIPPIG, L., AND SCHNEIDER, K. W.: *Hämodynamische Untersuchungen mit Angiotensin.* Z. Klin. Med. 157:197, 1962.

51. McQUEEN, E. G., AND MORRISON, R. B. I.: *The effects of synthetic angiotensin and noradrenaline on blood pressure and renal function.* Br. Heart J. 23:1, 1961.

52. FINNERTY, F. A.: *Hemodynamics of angiotensin in man.* Circulation 25:255, 1962.

53. DE PASQUALE, N. P., AND BURCH, G. E.: *Effect of angiotensin II on the intact forearm veins of man.* Circ. Res. 13:239, 1963.

54. PŘEROVSKÝ, I., ULRYCH, M., LINHART, J., ET AL.: *Combined plethysmographic and isotope method for the evaluation of venous circulation,* in *Proceedings of the International Congress of Clinical Evaluation of Testing Methods of Vasoactive Drug Effects and Indication of Surgical Angiological Therapy.* Rome, 1974, p. 245.

55. PIXBERG, H. U., ECKHARDT, W., AND CACHOVAN, M.: *Blutvolumenbestimmung in definierten Körperregionen mit ^{113m}In-(III)-chlorid.* Nucl. Med. 11:132, 1972.

56. BICKERTON, B. K., AND BUCKLEY, J. P.: *Evidence for a central mechanism in angiotensin induced hypertension.* Proc. Soc. Exp. Biol. Med. 106:834, 1961.

57. LAVERTY, R.: *A nervously-mediated action of angiotensin in anaesthetized rats.* J. Pharm. Pharmacol. 15:63, 1963.

58. BERRY, W. B., AUSTEN, W. G., AND CLARK, W. D.: *Studies on the relative cardiac and peripheral actions of angiotensin.* Ann. Surg. 159:520, 1964.

59. SCROOP, G. P., AND WHELAN, R. F.: *A central vasomotor action of angiotensin in man.* Clin. Sci. 30: 79, 1966.

60. GILDENBERG, P. L.: *Site of angiotensin vasopressor activity in the brain stem.* Fed. Proc. 30:432, 1971.

61. AMES, R. P., BORKOWSKI, A. J., SICINSKI, A. M., ET AL.: *Prolonged infusions of angiotensin II and norepinephrine and blood pressure, electrolyte balance, and aldosterone in normal man and in cirrhosis with ascites.* J. Clin. Invest. 44:1171, 1965.

62. CHINN, R. H., AND DUSTERDIECK, G.: *The response of blood pressure to infusion of angiotensin II; relation to plasma concentrations of renin and angiotensin II.* Clin. Sci. 42:489, 1972.

63. OELKERS, W., SCHÖNESHÖFER, M., SCHULTZE, G., ET AL.: *Effect of prolonged low-dose angiotensin II infusion on the sensitivity of adrenal cortex in man.* Circ. Res. (Suppl.) 36 & 37: I-49, 1975.

64. Cuesta, V., Bianchi, G., Brown, J. J., et al.: *Arterial pressure and plasma angiotensin II concentration in renal hypertension*, in *Proceedings of the 6th International Congress of Nephrology*, Florence, 1975. Karger, Basel, 1976, p. 243.

65. Grollman, A., and Krishnamurthy, S. R.: *Nephrotensin, a newly-described renal pressor agent.* Fed. Proc. 30:432, 1971.

66. Grollman, A., and Rule, C.: *Experimentally induced hypertension in parabiotic rats.* Am. J. Physiol. 138:587, 1943.

67. Tobian, L., and Ishii, M.: *Interstitial cell granules and solutes in renal papilla in post-Goldblatt hypertension.* Am. J. Physiol. 217:1699, 1969.

68. Azar, S., Tobian, L., and Ishii, M.: *Prolonged water diuresis affecting solutes and interstitial cells of renal papilla.* Am. J. Physiol. 221:75, 1971.

69. Hickler, R. B., Kamm, D. E., and Thorn, G. W.: *Studies on a vasodepressor and antihypertensive lipid of rabbit renal medulla*, in Milliez, P. and Tcherdakoff, P. (eds.): *L'hypertension Artérielle.* Club International sur L' hypertension Artérielle, p. 188. L'expansion Scientifique Française, Paris, 1966.

70. Lee, J. B.: *Chemical and physiological properties of prostaglandins: The antihypertensive effects of medullin in essential hypertension*, in Bergstrom, S. and Samuelson, B. (eds.): *Nobel Symposium II. Prostaglandins*, Interscience Publ., New York, 1967, p. 197.

71. Edwards, P. R., Strong, C. G., and Hunt, J.: *A vasodepressor lipid resembling prostaglandin E_2 (PGE$_2$) in the renal venous blood of hypertensive patients.* J. Lab. Clin. Med. 74:389, 1969.

72. Muirhead, E. H., Daniels, E. G., and Hinman, G. W.: *Renomedullary antihypertensive principle*, in Milliez, P. and Tcherdakoff, P. (eds.): *L'hypertension Artérielle.* Club International sur L'-hypertension Artérielle. p. 177, 1966. L'expansion Scientifique Française, Paris.

73. McGiff, J. C., Crowshaw, K., Terragno, N. A., et al.: *Release of a prostaglandin-like substance into renal venous blood in response to angiotensin II.* Circ Res. (Suppl. 1) 26 & 27:I-121, 1970.

74. Muirhead, E. E., Brooks, B., Kosinski, M., et al.: *Renomedullary antihypertensive principle in renal hypertension.* J. Lab. Clin. Med. 67:778, 1966.

75. McGiff, J. C., Nasyletti, A., Terragno, D. A., et al.: *Polypeptides: vascular actions as modified by prostaglandins.* 4th Meeting of the International Society for Hypertension, Sydney, 1976, p. 11.

76. Lee, J. B.: *Clinical studies with prostaglandin A, indomethacin, and furosemide in normotensive and hypertensive humans.* Proceedings of the 6th International Congress of Nephrology, Florence, 1975, Karger, Basel, 1976, p. 348.

77. Hornych, A., Bedrossian, J., Bariéty, J., et al.: *Prostaglandins and hypertension in chronic renal disease.* Clin. Nephrol. 4:144, 1975.

78. Ambard, L., and Beaujard, E.: *La rétention chlorurée sèche.* Semaine Méd., Paris, 25:133, 1905.

79. Dahl, L. K.: *Possible role of salt intake in the development of essential hypertension*, in Bock, K. D. and Cottier, P. T. (eds.): *Essential hypertension. An International Symposium.* Springer, Berlin, 1960, p. 53.

80. Dahl, L. K.: *Effects of chronic excess salt ingestion—experimental hypertension in the rat: correlation with human hypertension*, in Stamler, J., Stamler, R., and Pullman, T. N. (eds.): *The Epidemiology of Hypertension.* Grune & Stratton, New York, 1967, p. 218.

81. Meneely, G. R.: *The experimental epidemiology of sodium chloride toxicity in the rat*, in Stamler, J., Stamler, R., and Pullman, T. N. (eds.): *The Epidemiology of Hypertension.* Grune & Stratton, New York, 1967, p. 240.

82. Starling, E. H.: *The Fluids of the Body.* London, 1909.

83. Richardson, T. Q., Stallings, J. O., and Guyton, A. C.: *Pressure-volume curves in live, intact dogs.* Am. J. Physiol. 201:471, 1961.

84. Guyton, A. C., Coleman, T. G., Cowley, A. W., et al.: *Role of renal salt and water clearance in renal hypertension* in: *Proceedings of the 5th International Congress of Nephrology*, Mexico, 1972. Karger, Basel, 1974.

85. Langston, J. B., Guyton, A. C., Douglas, B. H., et al.: *Effect of changes in salt intake on arterial pressure and renal function in partially nephrectomized dogs.* Circ. Res. 12:50, 1963.

86. Coleman, T. G., and Guyton, A. C.: *Hypertension caused by salt loading in the dog. III. Onset transients of cardiac output and other circulatory variables.* Circ. Res. 25:153, 1969.

87. Conway, J.: *Cardiovascular response to sustained hypervolemia in the unanesthetized dog.* Circulation 28:706, 1963.

88. Folkow, B., Grimsby, G., and Thulesius, O.: *Adaptive structural changes of the vascular walls in hypertension and their relation to the control of the peripheral resistance.* Acta Physiol. Scand. 44:255, 1958.

89. FOLKOW, B., HALLBÄCK, M., JONES, J. S., ET AL.: *Effects of noradrenaline on consecutive vascular segments at low or normal calcium concentrations in controls and spontaneously hypertensive rats.* Clin. Sci. Mol. Biol. 51 (Suppl. 3):53s, 1976.

90. GUYTON, A. C., AND COLEMAN, T. G.: *Long term regulation of the circulation. Interrelationships with body fluid volumes,* in REEVES, B. B., AND GUYTON, A. C. (EDS.). *Physical Basis of Circulatory Transport: Regulation and Exchange.* W. B. Saunders, Philadelphia, 1967, p. 179.

91. BORST, J. G. G., AND BORST-DE-GEUS, A.: *Hypertension explained by Starling's theory of circulatory homeostasis.* Lancet 1:677, 1963.

92. REUBI, F., GOSSWEILER, N., AND GÜRTLER, R.: *Renal circulation in man studied by means of a dye-dilution method.* Circulation 33:426, 1966.

93. AGREST, A., AND FINKIELMAN, S.: *Hemodynamics in acute renal failure. Pathogenesis of hyperkinetic circulation.* Am. J. Cardiol. 19:213, 1967.

94. DE FAZIO, V., CHRISTENSEN, R. C., REGAN, T. J., ET AL.: *Circulatory changes in acute glomerulonephritis.* Circulation 20:190, 1959.

95. BIRKENHÄGER, W. H., SCHALEKAMP, M. A. D. H., SCHALEKAMP-KUYKEN, M. P. A., ET AL.: *Interrelations between arterial pressure, fluid-volumes, and plasma-renin concentration in the course of acute glomerulonephritis.* Lancet 1:1086, 1970.

96. DUSTAN, H. P., TARAZI, R. C., BRAVO, E. L., ET AL.: *Plasma and extracellular fluid volumes in hypertension.* Circ. Res. (Suppl. 1) 23 & 24:I-73, 1973.

97. EDER, H. D., LAUSON, H. D., CHINARD, F. P., ET AL.: *A study of the mechanism of edema formation in patients with the nephrotic syndrome.* J. Clin. Invest. 33:636, 1954.

98. OVERBECK, H. W.: *Hemodynamics of early experimental renal hypertension in dogs.* Circ. Res. 31:653, 1972.

99. SNASHALL, P. D., LUCAS, J., GUZ, A., ET AL.: *Measurements of interstitial "fluid" pressure by means of a cotton wick in man and animals: an analysis of the origin of the pressure.* Clin. Sci. 41:35, 1971.

100. LUCAS, J., AND FLOYER, M. A.: *Renal control of the compliance of the interstitial space; a factor in the aetiology of renoprival hypertension.* Clin. Sci. 44:379, 1973.

101. LUCAS, J., AND FLOYER, M. A.: *Changes in body fluid distribution and interstitial tissue compliance during the development and reversal of experimental renal hypertension in the rat.* Clin. Sci. 47:1, 1974.

102. NIZET, A., TOST, A., AND FOIDART-WILLEMS, J.: *Control of sodium excretion following saline infusion in dogs: Natriuretic factors and blood dilution.* Pflügers Arch. 350:287, 1974.

103. BROD, J., CACHOVAN, M., BAHLMANN J., ET AL.: *Hemodynamic response to an acute emotional stress (mental arithmetic) with special reference to the venous side.* Aust. N. Z. J. Med. 6 (Suppl. 2):19, 1976.

104. AXELROD, J.: *Catecholamines and hypertension,* 4th Meeting of the International Society for Hypertension, Sydney, 1976.

105. CACHOVAN, M., BROD, J., BAHLMANN, J., ET AL.: *The effect of intravenous angiotensin on the peripheral circulation with particular reference to its bearing on the general haemodynamics,* 4th Meeting of the International Society for Hypertension, Sydney, 1976, p. 96.

106. HOLMAN, D. V., AND PAGE, I. H.: *The cardiac output in arterial hypertension. II. A study of arterial hypertension produced by constricting the renal arteries in unanaesthetized and anaesthetized (pentobarbital) dogs.* Am. Heart J. 16:321, 1938.

107. LEDINGHAM, J. M., AND PELLING, D.: *Cardiac output and peripheral resistance in experimental renal hypertension.* Circ. Res. (Suppl. 2) 20 & 21:II-187, 1967.

108. BIANCHI, G., TENCONI, L. T., AND LUCCA, R.: *Effect on the conscious dog of constriction of the renal artery to a sole remaining kidney on haemodynamics, sodium balance, body fluid volumes, plasma renin concentration and pressor responsiveness to angiotensin.* Clin. Sci. 38:741, 1970.

109. BIANCHI, G., BALDOLI B., LUCCA, R., ET AL.: *Pathogenesis of arterial hypertension after the constriction of the renal artery leaving the opposite kidney intact both in the anaesthetised and in the conscious dog.* Clin. Sci. 42:651, 1972.

110. FERRARIO, C. M.: *Contribution of cardiac output and peripheral resistance to experimental renal hypertension.* Am. J. Physiol. 226:711, 1974.

111. FROHLICH, E. D., ULRYCH, M., TARAZI, R. C., ET AL.: *A hemodynamic comparison of essential and renovascular hypertension.* Circulation 35:289, 1967.

112. LEDINGHAM, J. M.: *Blood-pressure regulation in renal failure.* J. R. Coll. Physicians Lond. 5:103, 1971.

113. TRAEGER, J., ZECH, P., FRANÇOIS, B., ET AL.: *L'hypertension artérielle des insuffisants rénaux chroniques traités par épurations extra-reńales. Acquisitions Médicales Récentes,* L'expansion Scientifique Française, 1969, p. 261.

163

114. WEIDMANN, P., MAXWELL, M. H., LUPU, A. N., ET AL.: *Plasma renin activity and blood pressure in terminal renal failure.* N. Engl. J. Med. 285:757, 1971.

115. BROWN, J. J., DUSTERDIECK, G. O., FRASER, R., ET AL.: *Hypertension and chronic renal failure.* Br. Med. Bull. 27:128, 1971.

116. DATHAN, J. R. E., AND GODWIN, F. J.: *The relationship between body fluid compartment volumes, renin and blood pressure in chronic renal failure.* Clin. Sci. 42:2P, 1972.

117. SAFAR, M., LONDON, G., BEDROSSIAN, J., ET AL.: *The role of kidneys in hypertension in chronic renal failure,* in *Proceedings of the 5th International Congress of Nephrology, 3.* Mexico, 1972. Karger, Basel, 1974, p. 91.

118. GOODWIN, F. J., DATHAN, J. R. E., GREENWOOD, R. H., ET AL.: *Influence of renin and volume on the blood pressure,* in *Proceedings of the 5th International Congress of Nephrology, 3.* Mexico, 1972. Karger, Basel, 1974, p. 81.

119. VERTES, V., CANGIANO, J. L., BERMAN, L. B., ET AL.: *Hypertension in end-stage renal disease.* N. Engl. J. Med. 280:978, 1969.

120. SAFAR, M. E., LONDON, G. M., WEISS, Y. A., ET AL.: *Overhydration and renin in hypertensive patients with terminal renal failure: a hemodynamic study.* Clin. Nephrol. 5:183, 1975.

121. MAXWELL, M., AND WEIDMANN, P.: *Hypertension in chronic bilateral renal disease,* in *Proceedings of the 5th International Congress of Nephrology, 3.* Mexico, 1972. Karger, Basel, 1974, p. 66.

122. KOLFF, W. J., SETO, D., AND NAKAMOTO, S.: *Bilateral nephrectomy and changes in sodium and water content in hypertension,* in *Comptes Rendus du 2e Congr. Intern. de Nephrol.,* Prague, 1963. Publ. House Czechosl. Acad. Sci. and Excerpta Med. Found., Amsterdam, 1964, p. 374.

123. TOUSSAINT, C., CREMER, M., HEUSE, A., ET AL.: *L'hypertension artérielle maligne, incontrôlable, indication a la néphrectomie bilaterale dans le mal de Bright au stade ultime.* Proc. Eur. Dial. Transpl. Assoc. 3:65, 1966.

124. VERNIORY, A., POTVLILÈGE, P., van GAERTRUYDEN, J. J., ET AL.: *Renin and control of arterial blood pressure during terminal renal failure treated by haemodialysis and by transplantation.* Clin. Sci. 42:685, 1972.

125. BIANCHI, G., PONTICELLI, C., BARDI, U., ET AL.: *Role of the kidney in "salt water dependent hypertension" of end-stage renal disease.* Clin. Sci. 42:47, 1972.

126. MIMRAN, A., SHALDON, S., MATHIEU, M. N., ET AL.: *Effect of Saralasin on the hypertension of hemodialysis patients.* 4th Meeting International Society for Hypertension. Sydney, 1976. p. 48.

127. BROD, J., CACHOVAN, M., BAHLMANN, J., ET AL.: *Clinical and haemodynamic study of a new vasodilator drug L 6150. (3-[bis(2-hydroxaethyl) amino]-6-hydrazinopyridazine) in man.* Clin. Sci. Mol. Biol. 51 (Suppl. 3):601s, 1976.

128. WINER, N., CHOKSI, D. S., YOON, M. S., ET AL.: *Adrenergic receptor mediation of renin scretion.* J. Clin. Endocr. 29:1168, 1969.

129. WINER, N., WALKENHORST, W. G., HELMAN, R., ET AL.: *Effects of adrenergic antagonists in states of increased renin secretion,* in *Proc. Workshop,* Santa Ynez, Calif., 1971. Plenum Press, New York, 1972, p. 65.

130. ASSAYKEEN, T. A., CLAYTON, P. L., GOLDFIEN, A., ET AL.: *Effect of alpha-and beta-adrenergic blocking agents on the renin response to hypoglycemia and epinephrine in dogs.* Endocrinology 87:1318, 1970.

131. ALEXANDRE, J. M., MENARD, J., CHEVILLARD, C., ET AL.: *Increased plasma renin activity induced in rats by physostigmine and effects of alpha- and beta-receptor blocking drugs thereon.* Europ. J. Pharmacol. 12:127, 1970.

132. MEURER, K. A.: *Die Bedeutung des sympathico-adrenalen Systems für die Reninfreisetzung.* Klin. Wschr. 49:1001, 1971.

133. BÜHLER, F. R.: *Renin-aldosterone interaction, beta-blockade, and differing antihypertensive efficacy of beta-blockers in high, normal or low renin essential hypertension,* in SCHWEIZER, W. (ED.): *Beta-blockers-present status and future prospects.* Huber, 1974, p. 68.

Renal Arterial Hypertension: Diagnosis and Management

Ross M. Tucker, M.D.

Approximately 1 in every 10 or 12 patients who seek medical care is likely to have hypertension.[1] Physicians involved in the practice of clinical medicine are called upon to make many decisions regarding these patients, especially whether to prescribe anti-hypertensive medication without extensive evaluation or the contrary. Since renovascular disease is by far the most common single group of the surgically correctable types,[2] a major effort should be directed to identify patients with this problem. Once found, it may be hard to know how to deal with them. I hope to provide information in this chapter which will assist the process. This will include a discussion of screening procedures such as angiotensin II antagonists and angiotensin I converting enzyme inhibitors as well as the conventional procedures, i.e., excretory urography, renal angiography, renal vein renin assay, radioisotope renography, and split renal function tests. When surgical therapy is suggested by these studies, we shall see how often the outcome is successful. Perhaps there is even a place for medical antihypertensive treatment rather than surgery in some patients with proven renovascular hypertension. The decision between surgical or medical therapy may be more difficult to make than any diagnostic decisions. It is my hope that this chapter will prove to be of some benefit to those who are faced with these clinical dilemnas.

THE INCIDENCE OF RENOVASCULAR HYPERTENSION

If we are to have some idea of the likelihood that any individual patient will have this condition, we need to know the occurrence rate of hypertension caused by renal artery stenosis in the population of hypertensives. Does 10 percent, 1 percent, or less of the hypertensive population have renovascular hypertension? Table 1 summarizes the reported incidence of renovascular hypertension in a number of large series.

The percentage of hypertensive patients having renal artery stenosis amenable to surgical correction for relief of hypertension varies from less than 1 percent to 5 percent. There are many patients with renal artery narrowing who have essential hypertension or normal blood pressure.[8] Those selected as candidates for surgical therapy would ideally exclude this latter group.

A recent review of the Mayo Clinic experience in the years 1973, 1974, and 1975 suggests that the incidence of renovascular hypertension in our patients, defined as those who had surgical repair of stenotic renal arteries, nephrectomy, or both, was somewhat less than reported in most series in Table 1. On the average, there were 47 patients operated per year for this disorder, with an estimated occurrence rate of about

165

Table 1. Quoted incidence of renovascular hypertension (a literature resume)

Author	Year	Ref. No.	Incidence, %	Data Base/Comments
Hunt	1974	3	5	214 with RVH out of ? hypertensives.
Gifford	1969	2	4*	5000 patients screened. 220 renal artery stenoses, 67 repaired.
Swales	1976	4	3	161 patients; 5 surgeries in two years.
Bech	1975	5	1	482 patients screened. 5 surgeries in 15 years.
Maronde	1975	6	<1	Patient data base not given.
Atkinson	1974	7	0†	985 urograms, 20 arteriograms.

*Only 1.4% of 5000 screened were operated on for renovascular repair on nephrectomy.

†No renovascular hypertension detected in series reported.

0.2 percent of all patients who had a diagnosis of hypertension at the Mayo Clinic.[9] At our institution, renovascular hypertension is actively sought with nearly 200 renal arteriograms performed per year for hypertension diagnostic purposes. This represents approximately one-fifth of the total angiographic procedures performed.

If our calculated incidence of renal artery stenosis causing hypertension is correct, it would explain why many physicians with active practices look for, but seldom find, operable renovascular hypertension. It is not a reflection on their diagnostic acumen but rather the expression of a low frequency of occurrence. If the condition is so scarce, one should seek it only in those most likely to have it. The clinical characteristics of patients with renovascular hypertension will assist in the search. These are presented in the next section.

CLINICAL CHARACTERISTICS OF PATIENTS WITH RENOVASCULAR HYPERTENSION

On review of 140 patients operated on for renovascular hypertension in three recent years we found those with fibromuscular and atherosclerotic renal artery lesions tended to be separated by characteristics of age and sex. Whereas fibromuscular renal artery stenosis patients had a mean age of 36 years (81 percent were women), those with atherosclerotic renal artery lesions were approximately 20 years older (mean age 55) and slightly more than half were male (55 percent).[9]

One characteristic finding in renovascular hypertension is the continuous, high-pitched abdominal murmur reported to occur in one-third of a small series of patients with fibromuscular disease.[10] An additional one-fourth had low-pitched continuous abdominal bruits. Other series have reported a greater incidence of these continuous bruits in the epigastrium, often heard over the upper quadrants as well. The quadrant of radiation tends to correspond to the side of most severe renal artery stenosis.[11, 12, 13] Continuous epigastric bruits are heard most frequently in patients with fibromuscular renal artery disease, a group having an excellent rate of surgical cure or improvement. Therefore, it is most important to listen for them.[14, 15, 16]

The technique of listening to the abdomen for these abdominal bruits may be a mundane subject for the average reader, but I will mention the procedure for those not familiar with it. The patient should be in the supine position with the knees flexed somewhat and the abdominal muscles relaxed. Place the diaphragm of the stethoscope just below the xyphoid process on the abdominal wall and begin to press down with the palm of the hand until the stethoscope head significantly indents the skin. Ordinarily, a

166

systolic murmur from the abdominal aorta can be heard with increasing compression. Repeat the same process by advancing along one subcostal margin and then the other. The stethoscope diaphragm should always be placed just below the rib margin (Figs. 1, 2). If present, the continuous or systolic/diastolic faint blowing murmur of renal artery stenosis will be louder in systole, trailing off into diastole. Few are very loud, so it is essential that outside noise be kept to a minimum by closing doors and turning off background music. Hearing the first continuous murmur of renal artery stenosis makes subsequent ones much easier to appreciate.

Hypertensive funduscopic changes give the examiner prognostic information, particularly if there are exudates (Keith, Wagener, and Barker Group III) or papilledema (Group IV). These two groups are present twice as often in renovascular hypertension as in essential hypertension (15 percent vs. 7 percent).[13] This finding, as well as shorter duration of hypertension and possibly higher blood pressure levels may direct the physician to apply more vigorous diagnostic efforts in patients with these clinical characteristics.[13]

EXCRETORY UROGRAPHY

The excretory urogram, with films taken sequentially within the first two, three, and four minutes after the completion of contrast injection, is used extensively as a screening procedure in the diagnosis of renovascular hypertension. The criteria used most often for diagnosing unilateral renal artery stenoses are as follows:

1. Pole to pole diameter differences of 1.5 cm. or greater.
2. Delay in appearance of contrast in the calyces or pelvis on one side.[17]

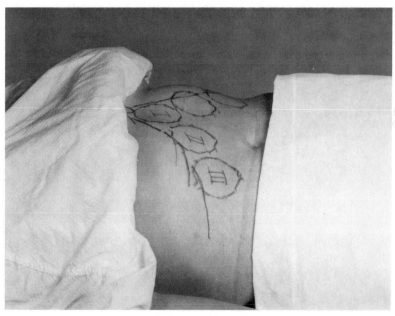

Figure 1. Technique for finding abdominal bruits. I, II, and III represent listening posts for the auscultation of renal artery bruits using the stethoscope diaphragm. Position I is over the epigastrium just below the xyphoid process; II and III, below the costal margins, advancing laterally from the epigastric position. This is the usual sequence of examination.

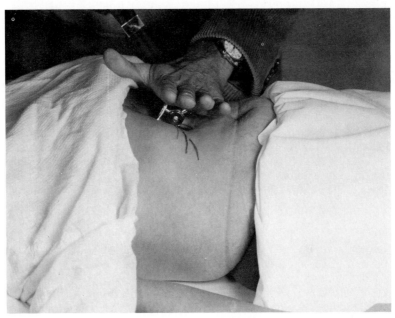

Figure 2. Technique for finding abdominal bruits. The stethoscope diaphragm is placed high in the apex of the epigastrium. Gentle pressure is used to progressively indent the abdominal wall while carefully listening for the high-pitched continuous murmur of renal artery stenosis. With increased amounts of pressure a low-pitched murmur may be produced by compressing the abdominal aorta. This is ordinarily heard in systole only.

In order to assess the value of this procedure as a screening test, I reviewed several large series with the results reported in Table 2.

Erikson[21] found 16 patients with renovascular hypertension in 102 patients who had routine angiograms for hypertension. Approximately half had falsely negative excretory urograms. Strong[20] reported 54 patients whose hypertension was cured or improved by surgery. He found about one quarter of their excretory urograms were nondiagnostic. Several authors report using the excretory urogram as a screening test for hypertensives. In one series of almost 1,000 patients, only three were found to have diseases related to hypertension, consisting of unilateral pyelonephritis in two and polycystic renal disease in one.[7] Twenty renal arteriograms were done in these 1,000 patients, but no renovascular hypertension found. In another smaller series, 80 hypertensives had excretory urograms but no curable hypertension was diagnosed.[19] Based on the rela-

Table 2. Excretory urography in hypertensive patients

Author	Ref. No.	No. Patients	RVH Patients With True Positive Ex.U.	RVH Patients With False Negative Ex.U.
Co-op	18	880	83% (128/154)	13% (26/154)
Erikson	21	102	53% (7/13)	47% (6/13)
Atkinson	7	952	0%* (0/0)	0% (0/0)
Bailey	19	80	0%* (0/0)	0% (0/0)
Strong	20	54	74% (40/54)	26% (14/54)

*No renovascular hypertension detected in series reported.

tively high incidence of reported false negatives (13 to 47 percent) the excretory urogram does not seem to be a very good screening procedure since it may be negative in a significant fraction of the patients with surgically curable renovascular hypertension. Even if it were not expensive, there are serious allergic reactions and some deaths associated with the procedure.

RADIOISOTOPE RENOGRAPHY

The radioisotope renogram enjoys a varying degree of regard as a screening procedure for the detection of renovascular hypertension. Ortho iodohippuran, containing the 125 or 131 isotope of iodine as the radioactive tag, is both filtered at the glomerulus and secreted by the renal tubule. Its clearance rate approximates that of the effective renal plasma flow. Detection probes placed over each renal area in the loins record radioactivity levels above background created by the radioactive ortho iodohippuran contained within the renal parenchyma and collecting system. These activity levels are continuously plotted against time and curves drawn on chart paper accordingly. The normal curve has an early rapid rise representing delivery of the isotope to the renal parenchyma by blood flow. This rise is terminated by a peak followed by a gradual decline, approaching the baseline asymptotically 20 to 30 minutes after the initial injection. The peak and decline occur as the isotope is cleared from the renal parenchyma and collecting system down the ureters to the bladder.

Patterns of the peak and slope seen in renovascular hypertension include unilateral elevation of the excretion phase slope, reduced height of the peak, or even failure to achieve a significant peak, the so-called nephrectomy pattern. One author[3] reports an abnormal radioisotope renogram with features to suggest unilateral disease in 72 percent of 180 patients who had renal artery stenosis and hypertension. This amounts to a 28 percent incidence of false negative tests.

As a screening procedure the radioisotope renogram has the advantage of using tiny amounts of iodine as a tracer and, therefore, few if any patients develop reactions of the sort seen with excretory urographic contrast media. Also, some evidence of separated renal function can be estimated from the renogram as there is an individual probe over each kidney recording separately. On the other hand, approximately one out of four tests are falsely negative in renovascular hypertensives, a figure not particularly impressive for a screening procedure. In my own practice, the radioisotope renogram is of minor importance in renovascular hypertension evaluation. It is certainly not a substitute for excretory urography except in the patient who is hypersensitive to iodine.

RENAL ANGIOGRAPHY

With reported cures of hypertension by removing atrophic kidneys in the 1930s[22] there followed a rash of similar surgeries in hypertensive patients hoping for cure. None had prior renal arterial studies, and the results were dismal with only about one-fifth receiving benefit by cure of their hypertension.[23, 24, 25] Therefore, many investigators began to seek more definitive ways of diagnosing renal ischemia than the urogram. In the 1950s renal angiography became routinely available in more centers for diagnostic purposes. Initially, the contrast medium was injected into the abdominal aorta by inserting the needle through the posterior lumbar approach. This was supplanted by the transfemoral technique[26], having the obvious advantage of allowing selective injection of contrast into individual visceral arteries through the manipulation of the flexible catheter. This selective technique reduced the confusing background vessel opacification seen with the midstream aortic injections.

Unfortunately, the angiographic procedures are not without risk as evidenced by the reports of iatrogenic arterial dissections[27] and renal failure.[28]

The renal artery lesions causing reduced renal blood flow can be divided into categories which have significant diagnostic angiographic characteristics. They are listed in Table 3.

Atherosclerotic lesions begin in the aorta and extend out into the proximal third of the main renal artery.[8] Fibromuscular stenoses classically originate in the distal two thirds of the main renal artery and frequently extend distally to involve the primary and the secondary branches.[29] The medial fibroplasia variety of fibromuscular disease is the most common of that category and produces typical alternating beading and sharply narrowed areas. There are other types of fibromuscular stenoses which may consist of single discrete narrowing or long smooth constrictions. A more detailed description of the classification of fibromuscular lesions can be found elsewhere.[29] The extrinsic compression lesions are less common than the atherosclerotic and fibromuscular disease types and may be produced by tumor, fibrous brands, surgical ligatures, or crura of the diaphragm.[30, 31]

A number of other renal artery lesions are associated with hypertension. They include macro-aneurysms without dissection,[32, 33, 34] aortic dissection,[35] traumatic renal artery occlusion,[36, 37, 38] AV fistula,[39] and embolic renal artery occlusion.[40] These conditions are interesting but rare, making them less relevant than the more common atherosclerotic or fibromuscular types. Representative renal artery lesions are portrayed in Figures 3, 4, 5, 6, and 7.

The presence of renal artery stenosis does not necessarily imply that there is a relation between it and coexistent hypertension. Many such lesions are even found in normotensive patients.[8, 41, 42] However, hemodynamic significance is almost always caused by those lesions with greater than 50 percent stenosis on visual estimate and seldom when the stenosis is adjudged to be less than 50 percent.[43] Studies which characterize the lesions causing significant interruption of renal perfusion are of great importance as these patients will most often benefit from surgical repair. There may be little benefit accrued by repairing nonsignificant lesions. Several such test procedures follow.

PLASMA RENIN ACTIVITY

Most investigators assume that the pathophysiology of blood pressure elevation associated with hemodynamically significant renal artery stenosis has at least some relationship to increased renin release by the renal juxtaglomerular cells.[44, 45, 46] When peripheral venous plasma renin measurements became generally available clinically, there

Table 3. Characteristics of renovascular lesions associated causally with hypertension

Type	Portion of Renal Artery Compromised	Associated Aortic Disease
Atherosclerosis	Proximal one-third	Usual
Fibromuscular	Distal two-thirds and branches	Seldom
Dissection	Distal two-thirds — See FMD	Seldom
Aneurysm	Distal two-thirds	Variable
Thrombosis	Proximal one-third	Variable
Embolism	Variable	Variable
Extrinsic Compression	Variable	Variable

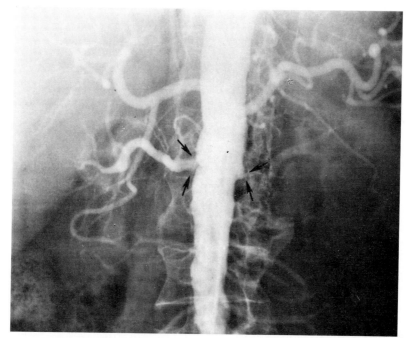

Figure 3. Midstream abdominal aortogram. The arrows indicate bilateral atheromatous renal artery stenosis, moderately severe on the right and almost 100 percent on the left.

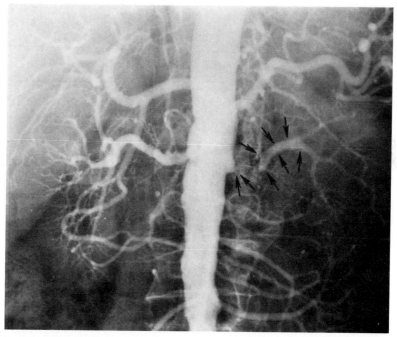

Figure 4. Midstream abdominal aortogram. This is a delayed film from the same patient as Figure 3. The left renal artery can now be seen filling in a delayed fashion. The left kidney was nonfunctioning by excretory urography. This patient underwent successful aorto-left renal artery saphenous vein bypass grafting and had cure of severe hypertension as well as the nephrotic syndrome. (Preoperative urinary protein excretion was 11.8 gm. per 24 hours.)

171

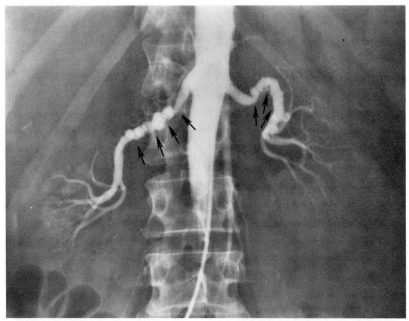

Figure 5. Midstream abdominal aortogram. The arrows point to the typical beaded appearance of fibromuscular renal artery stenosis. It is bilateral, but more severe on the right.

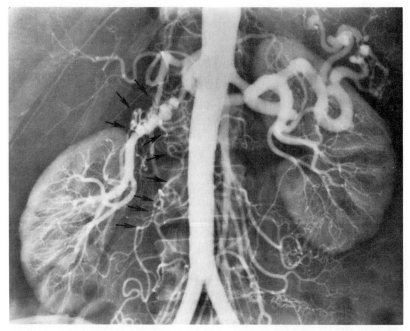

Figure 6. Midstream abdominal aortogram. Delayed film from same patient as Figure 5. The arrows point to extensive collateral arteries arising from the lumbar and ureteral circulation, a common finding in severe renal artery stenoses. This young woman underwent successful aortobilateral renal artery saphenous vein bypass graft and was normotensive almost immediately postoperatively.

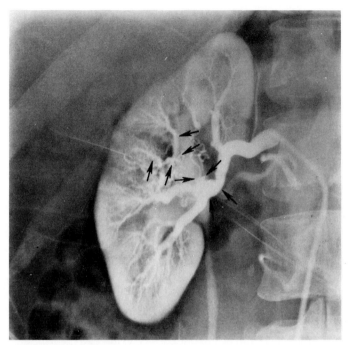

Figure 7. Selective right renal arteriogram. There is a medium-sized noncalcified aneurysm at the second branching point. Arrows point to occlusion of the proximal portion of a branch arising from this aneurysm with a distal continuation of this occluded vessel filling by intrarenal collaterals. This is probably congenital fibromuscular dysplasia, first diagnosed in a young man at age 14 years. As nephrectomy would have been the only possible surgical procedure, it was elected to control his blood pressure with medication.

was initial enthusiasm that this test could be a screening procedure for detection of renovascular hypertension or as the procedure for predicting blood pressure response to surgical renal artery repair or nephrectomy. Presumably those patients with elevated plasma renin activities would have renovascular hypertension. Unfortunately, this assumption has been followed by conflicting reports.[47, 48, 49, 50, 51] Many patients with surgically curable renovascular hypertension had normal peripheral renin activity while others with essential hypertension had high values.[53] This information makes the peripheral vein renin activity measurement of questionable value in either screening for renovascular hypertensives in populations with largely essential disease or in predicting the operative result for the patient with angiographic evidence of renal artery stenosis. We do not use the procedure in this way.

RENAL VEIN RENIN MEASUREMENTS AND SEPARATED URETERAL CATHETERIZATION

Once renal artery stenosis is seen on the angiogram, the question must be answered, Is this stenotic lesion causing hypertension? As has been mentioned already, there are many who have renal artery stenosis and normal blood pressure.[8] The converse is also true, i.e., patients with essential hypertension may have renal artery narrowings not necessarily related to their hypertension. Finally, some with essential hypertension can and do develop atherosclerotic renal artery stenosis after a number of years at which time their hypertension may become more severe.

For the purpose of relating stenosis to hypertension, a variety of functional tests have been devised including the separated ureteral catheterization test of Howard[53] and Stamey.[54] Although this procedure has excellent correlation with surgical results and has the advantage of providing separated measurements of renal plasma flow and glomerular filtration rate,[55] it is a lengthy study and usually requires a spinal anesthetic. In addition, there is some associated morbidity due to the postspinal headache and also ureteral obstruction from postcatheterization edema or blood clot. Therefore, the split renal function test is not done very often anymore. It has been replaced by the renal vein renin activity determination.

In the early 1960s, Boucher and his colleagues devised a reasonably accurate bioassay for measuring renin activity.[56] At first it was used to measure peripheral venous renin activity; but soon Judson and Helmer were to report the measurement of renin activity in samples of blood drawn directly from the separate renal veins via a transfemoral vein catheter.[57] Strong,[20] among others, suggested that the sensitivity of the test could be increased by preliminary salt depletion of the patient. Using this technique, when the renal vein renin activity was increased by 50 percent in the venous effluent from the stenosed side (ratio 1.5 to 1 or greater), there was an 80 percent correlation with surgical relief of hypertension. This correlation was significantly better in patients undergoing sodium and water diuresis than in a similar group who had renal vein renin measurements under basal circumstances. There are a variety of techniques for inducing sodium depletion including a 20 mEq. sodium diet for three days in association with 1 gm. of chlorothiazide daily for the same period. We insist that all patients not take any diuretic for the previous month, using guanethidine if medical antihypertensive therapy is required.

Other authors do not think sodium depletion is necessary for enhancement of the renal vein renin sensitivity[48, 58, 59] and record a 60 to 88 percent correlation with surgical results. Marks and coworkers[60] reviewed their data and data from over 400 patients reported in the literature. When the renal vein renin ratio was 1.5 to 1 or greater, there was an 88 percent probability that there would be surgical cure or improvement by vascular repair or nephrectomy. However, there was still an overall cure or improvement rate of 80 percent when the patients were selected by arteriographic features alone. When the renal vein renin ratio was less than 1.5 to 1, surgery was successful in only 49 percent.

In summary, the renal vein renin ratio is an excellent test for predicting a cure when renal artery stenosis repair is considered. If nonlateralizing, it should not necessarily dissuade against surgical repair when the stenosis is visually severe and hypertension difficult to control. The expectation for surgical cure will not be as optimistic, but still possible. Acute sodium depletion with the goal of about 2.5 to 3 percent of body weight loss may significantly enhance the sensitivity of this test. The patient should not take diuretics for one month prior to the study, and guanethidine is preferred if medical control of hypertension is needed. A ratio of 1.5 to 1 or greater in the differential renal vein renin activities is regarded by most as a positive result.[20]

ANGIOTENSIN BLOCKADE

In accord with the continuing search for a diagnostic screening tool which would identify those with hemodynamically significant renal artery stenosis causing hypertension, investigators began to study synthetic analogues of the pressor substance angiotensin II. They hoped to find a formulation which could attach to the vascular receptor sites commonly occupied by angiotensin II, but not trigger the adenylcyclase system sufficiently to provoke vascular smooth muscle contraction.[61, 62] The production of these analogues was vastly implemented by the solid phase peptide manufacturing technique of Merrifield reported in 1963.[63] One of the first useful angiotensin II analogues had only two amino acid alterations in the usual eight amino acid sequence of the natural hormone.[64] Isoleucine was substituted for valine in the fifth position and alanine replaced phenylalanine in the eighth or C-terminal position. This compound would competitively inhibit the vascular smooth muscle contraction response to angiotensin II. Another analogue, substituting the amino acid sarcosine for aspartate in the first or N-terminal position and alanine for phenylalanine in the eighth position, was reported by Pals.[65] This compound, 1-sarcosine, 8-alanine angiotensin II (P113, Saralasin) was found to have similar but more blocking activity than the other peptide analogues of angiotensin II. It has a short half-life, approximately five to ten minutes, and some true agonist as well as antagonistic properties of angiotensin II.[66] Another analogue with roughly similar properties, but longer acting, substituted sarcosine in the 1 position and isoleucine in the 8 position of angiotensin II[67] (Fig. 8).

Both analogues will reverse the in vitro vascular smooth muscle constriction produced by angiotensin II but not by norepinephrine.[66, 67] They will normalize blood pressure in rats made acutely hypertensive by either unilateral renal ischemia (contralateral ureter ligated) or by angiotensin II infusions.

In 1973, the first human studies were reported using the sarcosine-1, alanine-8, peptide analogue of angiotensin II (Saralasin).[68, 69, 70, 71, 72, 73] Patients with renovascular hypertension or high renin essential hypertension tended to have significant reduction in blood pressure during the infusion of Saralasin. Sodium depletion prior to the study is necessary for the depressor effect to occur. Most investigators concluded that the blood pressure reduction caused by blockade of angiotensin II was strong proof for the existence of renin dependent hypertension (Fig. 9).

In 1975, a cooperative study group was organized to investigate the efficacy of Saralasin in identifying patients with renovascular hypertension by utilizing infusions of this drug and measuring the resulting blood pressure alteration. The final tabulation of data in over 300 patients is not yet completed, but in my own series of 50 patients there were 18 who had severe unilateral or bilateral renal artery stenosis. There was a significant blood pressure reduction in 14 of these 18 patients (78 percent). Of the 32 patients with essential hypertension, 7 had significant blood pressure reduction and were, therefore, falsely positive (22 percent).[74] This degree of accuracy compares favorably with that of the renal vein renin assay. Both procedures do require some degree of sodium and water depletion for enhancement. Should Saralasin become generally available in the near future, it may well provide a reasonable procedure for screening large numbers of hypertensives for the presence of renovascular hypertension. In addition, it may be valuable in selecting patients for surgical repair with known renal artery stenotic lesions in place of the renal vein renin test.

Angiotensin II

Aspartine-arginine-valine-tyrosine-isoleucine-histidine-proline-*phenylalanine*

[Sar¹,ala⁸]-Angiotensin II (Saralasin)

Sarcosine-arginine-valine-tyrosine-isoleucine-histidine-*alanine*

[Sar²,Ile⁸]-Angiotensin II

Sarcosine-arginine-valine-tyrosine-isoleucine-histidine-proline-*isoleucine*

Figure 8. Chemical structure of angiotensin II and several competitive inhibitor analogues.

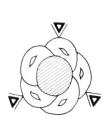

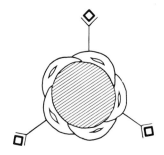

Angiotensin^{II} on
Receptors = Vasoconstriction

Angiotensin^{II} displaced by
Saralasin = Vasodilation

△ = Angiotensin^{II}

□ = Sarcosine^1 – Alamine^8 – Angiotensin^{II} (Saralasin)

Figure 9. Theoretical mechanism by which angiotensin II analogues displace the naturally occurring angiotensin II. Saralasin occupies the vascular smooth muscle receptors, reversing the smooth muscle contraction previously induced by angiotensin II.

ANGIOTENSIN CONVERTING ENZYME INHIBITION

Angiotensin I is a 10-amino-acid peptide with trivial vasoactive properties, produced by the action of renin on a plasma protein substrate, angiotensinogen. It requires the action of a converting enzyme, usually found in the lung, for the removal of two C-terminal amino acids to produce the vasoactive peptide, angiotensin II. An inhibitor of this converting enzyme was first isolated from a Brazilian snake venon *(Bothrops jararaca)*[75] and later synthesized in the laboratory (Sq 20,881). This converting enzyme inhibitor contains nine amino acids[75, 76, 77] and has a half-life of about 3 hours.[78] By preventing the transformation of angiotensin I to angiotensin II, the weakly pressor 10-amino-acid compound accumulates and the 8-amino-acid active principle is depleted. This substance may prove to have value in the treatment of renin dependent hypertensive crises such as malignant hypertensive encephalopathy or toxemia of pregnancy. In addition, it could be another screening agent for renovascular hypertension or a test for evaluation of functional significance of known renal artery stenoses. The necessary studies have not yet been reported to support these hypotheses, but they are probably in progress and almost certainly will appear in future literature (Fig. 10).

SURGICAL TREATMENT OF RENOVASCULAR HYPERTENSION

Deciding when to suggest revascularization and/or nephrectomy once the renal artery lesion is identified angiographically and characterized by differential renal vein renins with or without the Saralasin infusion response can be a trying experience. Balanced on one hand is the pain, danger, and expense of a major operation, and perhaps also the loss of functioning renal mass. On the other is the chance that hypertension might be completely relieved or partially so, with fewer drugs, less side effects, and a smaller drug bill. If each patient is selected for a renal angiogram only if he is a candidate for surgery, the decision-making process is easier. If a significant lesion is found, pre-existing medical problems, especially atherosclerotic events, prejudice the patient's chances of having a good result, defined as cure or improvement of hypertension,[14, 15, 79] and of

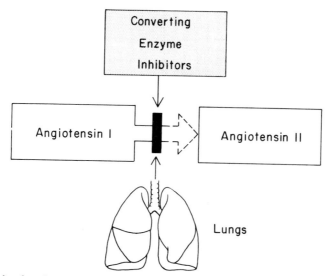

Figure 10. Blockade of angiotensin I-angiotensin II converting enzyme by an inhibitor. The effect of this inhibitor is to enhance the accumulation of nonpressor angiotensin I, while angiotensin II is depleted by the normal action of the angiotensinase systems.

surviving the procedure. In the cooperative study of renovascular hypertension reporting nearly 600 operative procedures, 34 patients died (6.8 percent).[15] Four fifths of the deaths were in the group of patients with atherosclerotic renal artery stenosis but they only comprised three fifths of the total patients operated on. Stated in another way, the mortality rate was 9.3 percent for the atherosclerotic group and only 3.4 percent for those with fibromuscular disease. An especially worrisome combination was angina pectoris and reduced glomerular filtration rate in the same patient (defined as a serum creatinine equal to or greater than 1.4 mg. percent).

The risk of losing renal mass is likewise significant when the patient has surgical therapy. This may be the case when a nephrectomy is elected rather than renal artery repair. Nephrectomy is sometimes necessary when complete renal infarction has occurred or when the renal pole to pole diameter is less than 9 cm. The gross incidence of nephrectomy varies from series to series but ranges from 16 percent[14] to as high as 35 percent.[15] Two thirds of the nephrectomies are done as an initial approach to unilateral disease, and one third as an accompanying procedure to contralateral repair. Less frequently it is a secondary operation when the initial graft failed. Nephrectomy rates in fibromuscular disease are somewhat less than in cases of atherosclerotic stenosis.[80]

There are a variety of surgical procedures devised for the repair or relief of renal artery narrowing. The technical aspects are not within the purview of this article and may be sought elsewhere if the reader is interested.[81] The result of these procedures is quite pertinent as regards the rate of cure or significant improvement. Success rate varies from series to series as does the definition of the categories "cured" and "improved". Taking each author at face value, Table 4 reports four of the larger series in the recent literature.

Most of the available data suggest that the patients under the age of 40 with fibromuscular disease are more likely to benefit from surgical repair of the renal artery lesions than their older counterparts with atherosclerotic renal artery lesions.[84] Counterbalancing the operative mortality rates, the risk of nephrectomy, and the significant incidence of improvement or failure rather than cure, is the apparent incidence of reduced survival in those patients with renovascular hypertension who were treated med-

177

Table 4. Results of renal artery repair or nephrectomy for hypertension (from the literature)

1st Author	Ref. No.	Patients Operated	% Cured	% Improved	% Cured or Improved
Hunt	82	100	61	32	93
Foster	83	162	68	23	91
McCombs	14	38	45	43	88
RVH Co-op Study	80	502	51	15	66

ically rather than surgically. In one series of patients followed from 7 to 14 years,[82] those with surgical correction of renal artery stenosis had an 84 percent survival as compared to only 60 percent for those medically treated. There lies the dilemma. Surgical intervention has its problems, but not treating surgically may adversely prejudice the patient's survival. There is no simple solution and all too often we must make decisions when there really is no perfect answer.

SUMMARY

Hidden within a large body of essential hypertensives are a rather small number of patients who have renal artery stenosis due to fibromuscular dysplasia, atherosclerotic disease, or extrinsic compression. Some, but not all, of these patients will have a causal relation between the arterial stenotic lesion and their hypertension. The physician dealing with hypertensives must try to identify those who have little likelihood of having an operable renal artery lesion or those who would not be able to tolerate any such major procedure if found. These patients should be vigorously treated medically so that their survival might be improved. The remaining patients who stand the greatest chance of having renovascular hypertension, i.e., those with brief duration, accelerated eyeground changes, or continuous epigastric and upper quadrant bruits, should be screened with a variety of procedures including excretory urography, angiotensin II blockade (in the future), and renal arteriography. Once the stenotic lesion has been identified, functional studies must be utilized so that the decision to surgically repair these lesions can be made with greater assurance of cure. The studies of value in attaching a causal relationship to the lesions are sodium depleted renal vein renin activity, Saralasin infusion, and separated ureteral urine catheterization measurements. These are most often necessary in those patients who have 50 percent or less renal artery stenosis adjudged by the arteriogram. Functional tests seem to be less important in those with greater than 50 percent stenosis. Using the best screening techniques available, we can expect a surgical cure and improvement rate of 80 percent or greater. The overall surgical mortality is highest in patients with atherosclerotic disease (9.3 percent) and lowest in those with fibromuscular disease (3.4 percent). The total surgical mortality is slightly less than 7 percent. This mortality rate appears to be more acceptable when it is seen that those patients with renal artery stenosis treated medically do not survive as long as those in which surgical intervention is chosen.

REFERENCES

1. U.S. DEPARTMENT OF HEALTH, EDUCATION, AND WELFARE: *Blood pressure of adults by race and area, United States, 1960–1962.* National Health Survey, National Center for Health Statistics Series (No. 5): 11, 1964.

2. GIFFORD, R. W., JR.: *Evaluation of the hypertensive patients with emphasis on detecting curable causes.* Milbank Mem. Fund Q. 47:170, 1969.

3. HUNT, J. C., AND STRONG, C. G.: *Hypertension Manual,* J. H. LARAGH (ED.): Dun-Donnelley Publishing Corporation, New York, 1974, p. 509.

4. SWALES, J. D.: *The hunt for hypertension.* Lancet 1:577, 1976.

5. BECH, J., AND HILDEN, T.: *The frequency of secondary hypertension.* Acta Med. Scand. 197:65, 1975.

6. MARONDE, R. F.: *The hypertensive patient, an algorithm for diagnostic work-ups.* JAMA 233:997, 1975.

7. ATKINSON, A. B., AND KELLETT, R. J.: *Value of intravenous urography in investigating hypertension.* J. R. Coll. Physicians Lond. 8:175, 1974.

8. HOLLEY, K. E., HUNT, J. C., BROWN, A. L., ET AL.: *Renal artery stenosis, a clinical-pathologic study in normotensive and hypertensive patients.* Am. J. Med. 37:14, 1964.

9. TUCKER, R. M., AND LA BARTHE, D. R.: *Incidence of surgically treated secondary hypertension at the Mayo Clinic.* Proc. Mayo Clin. 52:549, 1977.

10. EIPPER, D. S., GIFFORD, R. W., JR., STEWART, B. H., ET AL.: *Abdominal bruits in renovascular hypertension.* Am. J. Cardiol. 37:48, 1976.

11. MOSER, R. J., JR., AND CALDWELL, J. R., JR.: *Abdominal murmurs: An aid in the diagnosis of renal artery disease and hypertension.* Ann. Intern. Med. 56:471, 1962.

12. HUNT, J. C., HARRISON, E. G., JR., KINCAID, O. W., ET AL.: *Idiopathic fibrous and fibromuscular stenoses of the renal arteries associated with hypertension.* Proc. Mayo Clin. 37:181, 1962.

13. SIMON, N., FRANKLIN, S. S., BLEIFER, K. H., ET AL.: *Clinical characteristics of renovascular hypertension, cooperative study of renovascular hypertension.* JAMA 220:1209, 1972.

14. McCOMBS, P. R., BERKOWITZ, H. D., AND ROBERTS, B.: *Operative management of renovascular hypertension.* Ann. Surg. 182:762, 1975.

15. FRANKLIN, S. S., YOUNG, J. D., JR., MAXWELL, M. H., ET AL.: *Operative morbidity and mortality in renovascular disease, cooperative study of renovascular hypertension.* JAMA 231:1148, 1975.

16. FIORANI, P., BENEDETTI-VALENTINI, S., PISTOLESE, G. R., ET AL.: *Long-term results in the surgical management of renovascular hypertension due to arteriosclerosis of the renal arteries.* J. Cardiovasc. Surg. (Torino) Spec. Issue:183, 1975.

17. WITTEN, D. M., HUNT, J. C., SHEPS, S. G., ET AL.: *Excretory urography in renovascular hypertension: Minute sequence filming and osmotic diuresis.* Am. J. Roentgenol. 98:114, 1966.

18. BOOKSTEIN, J. J., ABRAMS, H. L., BUENGER, R. E., ET AL.: *Radiologic aspects of renovascular hypertension, cooperative study of renovascular hypertension. Part II: The role of urography in unilateral renovascular disease.* JAMA 220:1225, 1972.

19. BAILEY, S. M., EVANS, D. W., AND FLEMING, H. A.: *Intravenous urography in investigation of hypertension.* Lancet 2:57, 1975.

20. STRONG, C. G., HUNT, J. C., SHEPS, S. G., ET AL.: *Renal venous renin activity, enhancement of sensitivity of lateralization by sodium depletion.* Am. J. Cardiol. 27:602, 1971.

21. ERIKSON, U., HEMMINGSSON, A., LJUNGSTRÖM, A., ET AL.: *On the use of renal angiography and intravenous urography in the investigation of renovascular hypertension.* Acta Med. Scand. 198:39, 1975.

22. BUTLER, A. M.; *Chronic pyelonephritis and arterial hypertension.* J. Clin. Invest. 16:889, 1937.

23. BRAASCH, W. F.: *The surgical kidney as an etiological factor in hypertension.* Can. Med. Assoc. J. 46:9, 1942.

24. SMITH, H. W.: *Hypertension and urologic disease.* Am. J. Med. 4:724, 1948.

25. SMITH, H. W.: *Unilateral nephrectomy in hypertensive disease.* J. Urol. 76:685, 1956.

26. SELDINGER, S. I.: *Catheter placement of the needle in percutaneous arteriography, a new technique.* Acta Radiol. 39:368, 1953.

27. TALMER, L. B., McLAUGHLIN, A. P., AND BOOKSTEIN, J. J.: *Renal artery dissection: A complication of catheter arteriography.* Radiology 117:291, 1975.

28. PORT, S. K., WAGONER, R. D., AND FULTON, R. E.: *Acute renal failure after angiography.* Am. J. Roentgenol. 121:544, 1974.

29. HARRISON, E. G., AND McCORMACK, L. J.: *Pathologic classification of renal arterial disease in renovascular hypertension.* Mayo Clin. Proc. 46:161, 1971.

30. KINCAID, O. W., AND DAVIS, G. O.: *Renal arteriography in hypertension: Symposium on hypertension associated with renal artery disease.* Proc. Staff Meet. Mayo Clin. 36:689, 1961.

31. SILVER, D., AND CLEMENTS, J. D.: *Renovascular hypertension from renal artery compression by congenital bands.* Ann. Surg. 183:161, 1976.

32. STANLEY, J. C., RHODES, E. L., GEWERTZ, B. L., ET AL.: *Renal artery aneurysms: Significance of macroaneurysms exclusive of dissections and fibrodysplastic mural dilations.* J. Cardiovasc. Surg. 17:85, 1976.

33. MONTERO, G. H. G., AND BAGLEY, M.: *Renovascular hypertension secondary to renal arterial aneurysm.* J. Urol. 6:647, 1975.

34. McCARRON, J. P., MARSHALL, V. F., AND WHITSELL, J. C., II: *Indications for surgery on renal artery aneurysms.* J. Urol. 114:177, 1975.

35. SETHI, G. K., SCOTT, S. M., AND TAKARO, T.: *Renovascular hypertension and acute aortic dissection in a patient with renal transplant.* Am. Surg. 42:160, 1976.

36. STABLES, D. P., FOUCHE, R. S., VanNIEKERK, J. P. D., ET AL.: *Traumatic renal artery occlusion: 21 cases.* J. Urol. 115:228, 1976.

37. SECHIS, M. N., PLESSAS, S. N., AND SKALKEAS, G. D.: *Post-traumatic renovascular hypertension.* Surgery 76:666, 1974.

38. RICHIE, J. P., BENNETT, C. M., AND BROSMAN, S. A.: *Traumatic renal artery thrombosis with acute malignant hypertension and hyperreninemia.* Urology 6:481, 1975.

39. KIRKPATRICK, J. R.: *Traumatic arteriovenous fistula of the kidney: An unusual case of hypertensive encephalopathy.* J. Trauma. 15:363, 1975.

40. FORD, K. T., TEPLICK, S. K., AND CLARK, R. E.: *Renal artery embolism causing neonatal hypertension: A complication of umbilical artery catheterization.* Radiology 113:169, 1974.

41. LISA, J. R., ECKSTEIN, D., AND SOLOMON, C.: *Relationship between arterial sclerosis of the renal artery and hypertension: Analysis of 100 necropsies.* Am. J. Med. Sci. 205:701, 1943.

42. OPPENHEIMER, B. S., KLEMPERER, P., AND MOSCHKOWITZ, L.: *Evidence for the Goldblatt mechanism of hypertension in human pathology.* Proc. Assoc. Am. Physicians 54:69, 1939.

43. FOURNIER, A., ROMEDER, J. M., FALMON, D., ET AL.: *Predictive criteria of surgical curability of renovascular hypertension.* Acta Med. Scand. 189:391, 1971.

44. GULATI, O. M., CARRETERO, A., OZA, N. D., ET AL.: *Role of renin in the pathogenesis of renal hypertension.* Circ. Res. 36, 37(Suppl. I):I-187, 1975.

45. BRAUN-MENENDEZ, E., FASCIOLO, J. C., LELOIR, L. F., ET AL.: *Renal Hypertension.* Charles C Thomas, Springfield, Illinois, 1946.

46. LARAGH, J. H.: *Curable renal hypertension — renin, marker or cause?* JAMA 218:733, 1971.

47. BATH, N. M., GUNNELLS, J. C., JR., AND ROBINSON, R. R.: *Plasma renin activity in renovascular hypertension.* Am. J. Med. 45:481, 1968.

48. GUNNELLS, J. C., JR., McGUFFIN, W. L., JOHNSRUDE, F., ET AL.: *Peripheral and renal venous plasma renin activity in hypertension.* Ann. Intern. Med. 71:555, 1969.

49. COHEN. E. L., ROVNER, D. R., AND CONN, J. W.: *Postural augmentation of plasma renin activity: Importance in diagnosis of renovascular hypertension.* JAMA 197:973, 1966.

40. AMSTERDAM, E., COUCH, M. P., CHRISTLIEB, A. R., ET AL.: *Renal vein renin activity in the prognosis of surgery for renovascular hypertension.* Am. J. Med. 47:860, 1969.

51. HUSSAIN, R. A., GIFFORD, R. W., STEWART, B. H., ET AL.: *Differential renal venous renin activity in diagnosis of renovascular hypertension: Review of 29 cases.* Am. J. Cardiol. 32:707, 1973.

52. BRUNNER, H. R., LARAGH, J. H., BAER, L., ET AL.: *Essential hypertension: Renin and aldosterone, heart attack, and stroke.* N. Engl. J. Med. 286:441, 1972.

53. CONNOR, T. B., THOMAS, W. C., JR., HADDOCK, L., ET AL.: *Unilateral renal disease as cause of hypertension: Its detection by ureteral catheterization studies.* Ann. Int. Med. 52:544, 1960.

54. STAMEY, T. A., NUDELMAN, I. J., GOOD, P. H., ET AL.: *Functional characteristics of renovascular hypertension.* Medicine 40:347, 1961.

55. HUNT, J. C., MAHER, F. T., AND GREENE, L. F.: *Functional characteristics of the separate kidneys in hypertensive man.* Am. J. Cardiol. 17:493, 1966.

56. BOUCHER, R., VEYRAT, R., deCHAMPLAIN, J., ET AL.: *New procedures for measurement of human plasma angiotensin and renin activity levels.* Can. Med. Assoc. J. 90:194, 1964.

57. JUDSON, W. E., AND HELMER, O. M.: *Diagnostic and prognostic values of renin activity in renal venous plasma in renovascular hypertension.* Hypertension 13:79, 1965.

58. DEAN, R. H., AND FOSTER, J. H.: *Split renal function studies and renal vein renin assays, comparative analysis.* Surg. Forum 25:257, 1974.

59. SCHAEFFER, A. J., AND FAIR, W. R.: *Comparison of split function ratios with renal vein renin ratios in patients with curable hypertension caused by unilateral renal artery stenosis.* J. Urol. 112:697, 1974.

60. MARKS, L. S., MAXWELL, M. H., VARADY, P. B., ET AL.: *Renovascular hypertension: Does the renal vein renin ratio predict operative results?* J. Urol. 115:365, 1976.

61. SCHWARZ, H., BUMPUS, F. M., AND PAGE, I. H.: *Synthesis of a biologically active octapeptide similar to natural isoleucine angiotonin octapeptide.* J. Am. Chem. Soc. 79:5697, 1957.

62. RITTEL, W., ISELIN, B., KEPPLER, H., ET AL.: *Synthese eines hockwirksamen hypertensin II-amids (L-Asparaginyl-L-arginyl-L-Valyl-L-tyrosyl-L-isoleucyl-L-histidyl-L-Prolyl-L-Phenylalanin).* Helv. Chim. Acta 40:614, 1957.

63. MERRIFIELD, R. B.: *Solid phase peptide synthesis. I. The synthesis of a tetrapeptide.* J. Am. Chem. Soc. 85:2149, 1963.

64. KHAIRALLAH, P. A., TOTH, A., AND BUMPUS, F. M.: *Analogs of angiotensin II. II. Mechanism of receptor interaction.* J. Med. Chem. 13:181, 1970.

65. PALS, D. T., MASUCCI, F. D., SIPOS, F., ET AL.: *A specific competitive antagonist of the vascular action of angiotensin II.* Circ. Res. 29:664, 1971.

66. PALS, D. T., AND FULTON, R. W.: *Mechanism of the antihypertensive effect of I-Sar-8-ala-angiotensin II during the acute phase of experimental renal hypertension.* Arch. Int. Pharmacodyn. Ther. 204:20, 1973.

67. SWEET, C. S., FERRARIO, C. M., KHOSLA, M. C., ET AL.: *Antagonism of peripheral and central effects of angiotensin II by (I-sarcosine, 8-isoleucine) angiotensin II.* J. Pharmacol. Exp. Ther. 185:35, 1973.

68. BRUNNER, H. R., GAVRAS, H., LARAGH, J. H., ET AL.: *Angiotensin-II blockade in man by sar[1]-ala[8]-angiotensin II for understanding and treatment of high blood pressure.* Lancet 2:1045, 1973.

69. STREETEN, D. H. P., ANDERSON, G. H., FREIBERG, J. M., ET AL.: *Use of an angiotensin II antagonist (Saralasin) in the recognition of "angiotensinogenic" hypertension.* N. Engl. J. Med. 292:657, 1975.

70. STREETEN, D. H. P., ANDERSON, G. H., JR., AND DALAKOS, T. G.: *Angiotensin blockade: Its clinical significance.* Am. J. Med. 60:817, 1976.

71. CASE, D. B., WALLACE, J. M., KEIM, H. J., ET AL.: *Usefulness and limitations of Saralasin, a partial competitive agonist of angiotensin II, for evaluating the renin and sodium factors in hypertensive patients.* Am. J. Med. 60:825, 1976.

72. RIBEIRO, A. B., AND KRAKOFF, L. A.: *Angiotensin blockade in coarctation of the aorta.* N. Engl. J. Med. 295:148, 1976.

73. MARKS, L. S., MAXWELL, M. H., AND KAUFMAN, J. J.: *Saralasin bolus test, rapid screening procedure for renin-mediated hypertension.* Lancet 2:784, 1975.

74. TUCKER, R. M., STRONG, C. G., SHEPS, S. G., ET AL.: Saralasin infusion study. Report to medical department, c/o Dr. R. E. Keenan, Norwich Pharmacal Company, August 1976.

75. BAKHLE, Y. S.: *Conversion of angiotensin I to angiotensin II by cell-free extracts of dog lung.* Nature 220:919, 1968.

76. NG, K. K. F., AND VANE, G. R.: *Some properties of angiotensin converting enzyme in the lung in vivo.* Nature 225:1142, 1970.

77. BAKHLE, Y. S., REYNAUD, A. M., AND VANE, J. R.: *Metabolism of the angiotensins in isolated profused tissues.* Nature 222:956, 1969.

78. COLLIER, J. G., ROBINSON, B. F., AND VANE, J. R.: *Reduction of pressor effects of angiotensin I in man by synthetic nonapeptide (B.P.P. 9a or SQ 20,881) which inhibits converting enzyme.* Lancet 1:72, 1973.

79. SHAPIRO, A. P., MCDONALD, R. H., AND SCHEIB, E.: *Renal artery stenosis and hypertension. II. Current criteria for surgery.* Am. J. Cardiol. 37:1065, 1976.

80. FOSTER, J. H., MAXWELL, M. H., FRANKLIN, S. S., ET AL.: *Renovascular occlusive disease. Results of operative treatment. The cooperative study of renovascular hypertension.* JAMA 231:1043, 1975.

81. POUTASSE, A. F.: *Surgical treatment of renal hypertension.* Am. J. Surg. 107:97, 1964.

82. HUNT, J. C., SHEPS, S. G., HARRISON, E. G., JR., ET AL.: *Renal and renovascular hypertension. A reasoned approach to diagnosis and management.* Arch. Intern. Med. 133:988, 1974.

83. FOSTER, J. H., AND DEAN, R. H.: *Results of surgical treatment of renovascular hypertension.* J. Cardiovasc. Surg. (Torino) Spec. Issue:169, 1975.

84. EDITORIAL. *Renovascular hypertension and the role of surgery.* JAMA 27, 1975.

Physiologic Determinants and Clinical Applications of Angiotensin II Blockade in Hypertensive Disorders*

Jose Z. Parra-Carrillo, M.D., Leslie Baer, M.D., and Ildiko Radichevich, Ph.D.

One of the mechanisms involved in hypertension is the renal endocrine factor, first elucidated by Tigerstedt and Bergman in 1898[1] and first related to human forms of hypertension by Goldblatt.[2] The renal pressor hormonal system, i.e., the renin-angiotensin system, continues to be the focus of studies in many laboratories. Recent progress in this field has been rapid and relates to improvements in methods for measuring plasma renin activity and to new pharmacologic tools that permit specific antagonism of angiotensin II. These new methods have led to a more precise chemical identification of the renin participation in the control of blood pressure. Moreover, these new experimental procedures may help in the future to define more precisely the control of renin secretion per se and thus indirectly they will expand our understanding of the mechanisms of hypertension.

Renin secretion has been demonstrated to be controlled by a number of physiologic factors. These include the state of sodium balance and possibly tubular sodium reabsorption, potassium balance, blood pressure per se, the adrenergic nervous system and upright posture.[3] A feedback system sensitive to circulating levels of angiotensin II has also been demonstrated to regulate renin secretion.[4, 5, 6]

The physiologic determinants of the depressor response to angiotensin II blockade provide the basis for the detection of angiotensin II dependent forms of hypertension. A number of studies have demonstrated that in hypertensive patients with an elevated plasma renin activity, competitive blockade of angiotensin II[7, 8, 9] with sarcosine[1]-alanine[8]-angiotensin II (Saralasin or P113) lowers blood pressure. Plasma renin activity is not uniformly elevated, however, in renal or renovascular forms of hypertension.[6, 10] Angiotensin II blockade in the normal renin group of patients may not act as a depressor and thus may lead to the conclusion that the renin-angiotensin system is not involved in the hypertension. Alternatively, a false positive interpretation of angiotensin II blockade could result in patients with an elevated plasma renin activity secondary to appropriate physiological responses of the kidney. This phenomenon has been demonstrated during chronic vasodilator treatment of hypertension and has been related to the stimulation of plasma renin activity by these agents.[11] Thus a depressor response to competitive blockade of angiotensin II may identify either a critical pathophysiological mechanism in renal or renovascular forms of hypertension or an appropriate physiologic response to signals stimulating renin secretion.

The studies described below of the physiological determinants of depressor and renin

*This work was supported in part by General Clinical Research Center Grant No. RR. 00645.

183

responses to angiotensin II blockade provide a basis for the clinical application of this procedure. In these studies we explored the role of sodium balance and plasma renin activity on the depressor response to angiotensin II blockade in a variety of renal and nonrenal forms of hypertension. In addition, the determinants of the renin responses during angiotensin II blockade are analyzed. The stimulation of plasma renin activity during angiotensin II blockade is inversely correlated to the fall in blood pressure. This observation emphasizes the importance of the baroreceptor control of renin release and suggests that this renin response may become an additional useful index for the presence of renin-dependent forms of hypertension. The postoperative blood pressure responses in patients with renovascular hypertension exhibit a close parallelism to the preoperative assessment of patients for surgery to correct renovascular hypertension. Altogether these observations suggest that studies of angiotensin II blockade will provide new insights into the mechanism and treatment of hypertensive disorders.

MATERIALS AND METHODS

Eighty-seven studies in 46 hypertensive patients were performed in the General Clinical Research Center of the Columbia Presbyterian Medical Center, New York. The studies were approved by the Institutional Review Board responsible for the conduct of clinical investigations and in all instances patients gave their written informed consent. Hypertensive patients in whom all medication was discontinued for at least three weeks prior to admission were placed on a constant 95 to 100 mEq. sodium intake diet per day. In 2 severely hypertensive patients among the entire group of 46 patients the studies were performed only during a 10 mEq. sodium intake diet. In the first of these 2 patients, Saralasin was infused two days after stopping antihypertensive treatment and in the second all medication except alpha methyldopa was stopped three days before the study. Daily weights, 24 hour urine collections for sodium and potassium excretion measured by flame photometry, and serial blood pressure determinations were performed. Laboratory tests including 24 hour urinary metanephrine excretion and rapid sequence pyelography were obtained in all patients. Hormonal analyses including thyroid function tests and plasma or urinary corticoid levels excluded other secondary forms of hypertension. Peripheral plasma renin activity was determined after 4 hours ambulation by radioimmunoassay of angiotensin I after patients had equilibrated to the constant sodium intake.[12] In patients undergoing surgery for correction of renovascular hypertension, renin was determined under the same conditions 3 to 10 weeks postoperatively. In this group, the clinical followup ranged from 3 to 8 months after surgery.

Angiotensin II blockade was carried out using the competitive antagonist Saralasin (P113). The studies were performed in the supine position after an overnight fast. Blood pressure was monitored either manually or by an automatic blood pressure device (Arteriosonde) every 2 minutes. After a control period of 30 to 60 minutes peripheral venous blood was collected for measurement of plasma renin activity and an intravenous infusion of the angiotensin II antagonist was begun. Saralasin was infused with a constant infusion pump at rates of 2, 5 or 10 μg./kg./min. Each dose was infused for 30 minutes. Prior to the conclusion of the infusion period a second blood collection was obtained for measurement of plasma renin activity. In 38 of 46 patients the studies were repeated after 80 mg. oral furosemide was administered 14 hours prior to angiotensin II blockade. A significant depressor response was defined as a decrease in diastolic blood pressure of at least 7 mm. Hg. Diastolic blood pressures during the control period and during Saralasin infusion were averaged and compared with each other. Blood pressures during the first 4 minutes of infusion were excluded and analyzed separately. Low, normal and high plasma renin activity was defined in the ambulatory state after 4 hours of upright posture using a nomogram based on 24 hour urinary sodium excretion.[13] Statistical analyses were performed using the Fisher paired and unpaired test and Pearson's regression coefficient.[14] The results were expressed as mean ± standard error of the mean.

RESULTS

Saralasin was infused in 87 studies of 46 hypertensive patients. Thirteen of forty-six patients (19 studies) exhibited a decline of blood pressure from control values of 179 ± 7.5 mm. Hg systolic and 110 ± 4.1 mm. Hg diastolic before Saralasin to 146 ± 5.3 mm. Hg systolic and 93 ± 3.3 mm. Hg diastolic during Saralasin infusion (Fig 1). In this group, plasma renin activity prior to Saralasin infusion was 16.3 ± 3.5 ng./ml./hr. and rose strikingly during angiotensin blockade to 53.4 ± 15.2 ng./ml./hr. The changes in blood pressure and plasma renin activity during angiotensin II blockade were highly significant statistically ($p < 0.01$). The increase in plasma renin activity in renin-dependent forms of hypertension was at least 58 percent and averaged 330 percent during the depressor response. A close correlation was observed between the decline in diastolic blood pressure during Saralasin infusion and the increase in plasma renin activity ($p < 0.001$) (Fig. 2). A close relationship was also observed between control plasma renin activity and the decline of diastolic blood pressure during angiotensin II blockade ($p < 0.001$) (Fig. 3). All 13 patients exhibited renovascular abnormalities on renal arteriography. Renal vein renin ratios in 9 of the 10 in whom it was measured lateralized to the

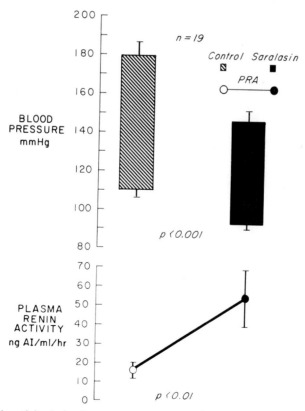

Figure 1. Plasma renin activity during depressor responses to angiotensin II blockade.

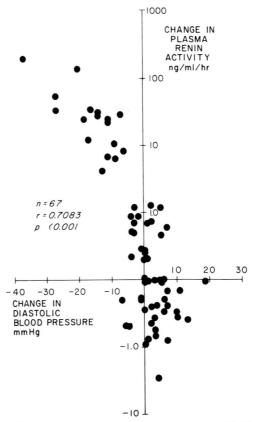

Figure 2. Correlation between the depressor responses to angiotensin II blockade and corresponding changes in plasma renin activity.

affected kidney with ratios greater than 1.6 (range 1.6 to 4.1) (Table I). In the tenth, bilateral nephrosclerosis was observed. In another patient with a single transplanted kidney with renal artery stenosis, peripheral plasma renin activity was very high. In two patients renal vein renin was not determined; one had bilateral nephrosclerosis and the second an abdominal aortic aneurysm and a small kidney on intravenous pyelography.

In 33 patients (68 studies) no depressor response to Saralasin infusion was observed (Fig. 4). Control blood pressure in this group was 155 ± 3.4 mm. Hg systolic and 99 ± 1.6 mm. Hg diastolic. During angiotensin II blockade blood pressure was 160 ± 4.3 mm. Hg systolic and 101 ± 1.6 mm. Hg diastolic. In contrast to the marked renin stimulation in the group exhibiting depressor responses to Saralasin, plasma renin activity in the nonresponders was 1.9 ± 0.3 ng./ml./hr. and was unchanged during Saralasin infusion (1.9 ± 0.2 ng./ml./hr.). In the group of nonresponders to Saralasin, renal vein renin levels were measured in six and the renal vein renin ratios did not lateralize (mean value 0.88) (see Table 1).

The initial diastolic blood pressure responses during the first 4 minutes of Saralasin infusion followed one of two different patterns (Table 2). In patients exhibiting a depressor response to angiotensin II blockade, blood pressure fell 2.2 ± 2.2 mm. Hg diastolic during the first 4 minutes of the study. In contrast, in patients without a depressor response during Saralasin infusion, diastolic blood pressure rose 17 ± 8.6 mm. Hg during the first 4 minutes of infusion. The difference in the initial blood pressure response between the two groups was highly significant statistically (p < 0.001). Furosemide

186

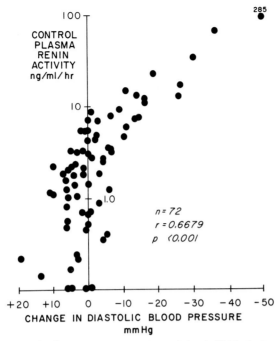

Figure 3. Correlation between the depressor responses to angiotensin II blockade and control plasma renin activity.

Table 1. Renal vein renin ratios in responders and nonresponders to angiotensin II blockade

Responders	Renal vein renin ratios affected/contralateral	Arteriographic findings
1	1.6	Left renal artery occlusion
2	1.6	Left renal artery stenosis
3	1.7	Left renal artery stenosis
4	1.6	Left renal artery stenosis
5	3.0	Right renal artery occlusion
6	4.1	Left renal artery occlusion
7	2.4	Left renal artery stenosis
8	1.8	Left renal artery stenosis
9	1.7	Right renal artery occlusion
Mean	2.2	
Nonresponders	*Left/Right*	
10	0.74	Right renal artery stenosis
11	0.92	Nephrosclerosis, small left kidney
12	0.98	Normal
13	0.83	Right renal artery stenosis
14	0.84	Right renal artery aneurysm
15	0.96	Normal
Mean	0.88	

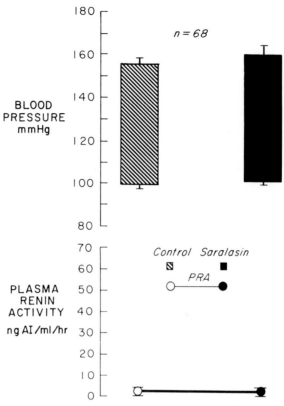

Figure 4. Plasma renin activity in nonresponders during angiotensin II blockade.

pretreatment did not modify the initial blood pressure responses to Saralasin in the two groups.

In 8 low-renin patients, blood pressure did not fall during angiotensin II blockade either before or after furosemide (Fig. 5). During the 95 to 100 mEq. sodium intake per day, control blood pressure was 166 ± 13 mm. Hg systolic and 98 ± 3.6 mm. Hg diastolic, and during Saralasin 176 ± 13 mm. Hg systolic and 104 ± 3.4 mm. Hg diastolic. After furosemide pretreatment in this same group, control blood pressure was 154 ± 12 mm. Hg systolic and 96 ± 2.7 mm. Hg diastolic, and during Saralasin 160 ± 15 mm. Hg systolic and 98 ± 4.0 mm. Hg diastolic. Three high-renin patients were studied before and after pretreatment with furosemide. Blood pressure in this group fell 24 mm. Hg systolic and 15 mm. Hg diastolic during 95 to 100 mEq. sodium intake per day in response to Saralasin infusion and 33 mm. Hg systolic and 18 mm. Hg diastolic when Saralasin infusion was repeated 14 hours after 80 mg. oral furosemide (Fig. 5).

In contrast to the homogenous response to Saralasin in the high-renin and low-renin

Table 2. Initial diastolic blood pressure responses during the first 4 minutes of angiotensin II blockade

Responders (19 studies)	− 2.2 ± 2.2 mm. Hg
Nonresponders (48 studies)	17 ± 8.6 mm. Hg
	P < 0.001

188

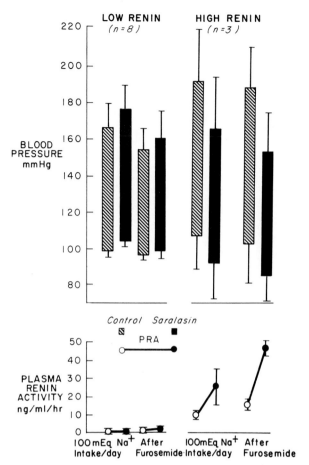

Figure 5. Blood pressure and renin responses to angiotensin II blockade during 100 mEq. Na⁺ intake/day and 14 hours after 80 mg. furosemide orally in low- and high-renin hypertension.

hypertensives, normal-renin patients exhibited 2 different responses based on their sodium balance (Fig. 6). All 14 normal-renin patients exhibited no depressor response to Saralasin when studied on the 95 to 100 mEq. sodium intake/day and 10 of 14 had similarly negative responses after pretreatment with furosemide (Fig. 6). Renal arteriography was performed in 8 of these 10 patients, and three were abnormal; one revealed a small kidney with bilateral nephrosclerosis but no renal artery stenosis (case 11, Table 1). In case 13 (Table 1) renal artery stenosis was found. In case 14 a renal artery aneurysm was present. In all three of these normal-renin patients with no depressor response to Saralasin, renal vein renin did not lateralize (Table 1); nor was lateralization present in one low-renin patient with renal artery stenosis (case 10).

In contrast, 4 other normal-renin patients exhibited a depressor response to Saralasin after furosemide pretreatment and a mean weight loss of 1.1 kg. (Fig. 6). Blood pressure fell from 153 ± 8.5 mm. Hg systolic and 104 ± 6.4 mm. Hg diastolic to 142 ± 7.9 mm. Hg systolic and 95 ± 5.4 mm. Hg diastolic, with a mean decline of 11 mm. Hg systolic and 9 mm. Hg diastolic. Three of these four patients were found to have renal artery stenosis with lateralizing renal vein renins (Table 1, cases 1, 5 and 8) and the fourth, bilateral nephrosclerosis.

Pretreatment with furosemide in the 10 normal-renin nonresponders to Saralasin

189

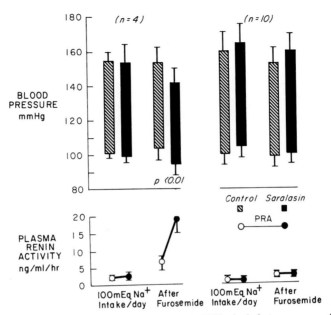

Figure 6. Blood pressure and renin responses to angiotensin II blockade in two groups of patients with normal renin hypertension. Three of four patients subsequently found to have renin-dependent hypertension only exhibited depressor responses after pretreatment with furosemide. In the 10 other normal-renin patients a depressor response was not observed even after furosemide. Renin-dependent hypertension was excluded in this latter group by renal arteriography and by renal vein renin determinations.

increased control plasma renin activity from 1.2 ± 0.3 ng./ml./hr. to 2.3 ± 0.4 ng./ml./hr. In the 4 normal-renin patients with depressor responses to Saralasin after furosemide pretreatment, control renin was 2.1 ± 0.5 and rose to 6.7 ± 1.5 ng./ml./hr. after furosemide (Fig. 6). The mean control renin in these 4 patients was only slightly higher than in the remaining 10 ($p < 0.10$) but was stimulated to significantly higher levels by furosemide ($p < 0.01$). Thus, under the conditions of this study, all 13 patients with a depressor response to Saralasin exhibited high plasma renin activity. The 4 normal-renin patients did not experience a lowered blood pressure during angiotensin II blockade until plasma renin activity was stimulated by furosemide. All 13 patients had evidence of renal or renovascular abnormalities radiologically. Renal vein renin determinations lateralized to the affected kidney in 9 patients and did not lateralize in the 6 nonresponders in whom it was measured. One responder with a single transplanted kidney and severe renal artery stenosis also exhibited high peripheral plasma renin activity.

In these studies, 2 instances of untoward responses were observed. In a patient with severe hypertension secondary to renal artery stenosis in a transplanted kidney, alpha methyldopa was continued at the time of Saralasin infusion. The depressor response during Saralasin from an initial value of 180/139 to 132/102 mm. Hg was associated with left precordial chest pain and an increase in heart rate from 110 to 130 beats/minute. The chest pain subsided after one-half hour and there was no evidence of myocardial necrosis on either serial electrocardiograms or enzyme determinations. This patient had experienced similar episodes of chest pain during prior admissions with reduction of blood pressure by vasodilators. A second patient with severe hypertension, renal artery stenosis and coexistent active ileitis experienced malaise and weakness during Saralasin infusion and a fall in blood pressure from 159/143 to 99/92

190

mm. Hg without a change in heart rate. Saralasin was stopped, isotonic saline administered and blood pressure returned to control levels within 20 minutes.

In all other studies with maximum blood pressure reductions of 60 mm. Hg systolic and 51 mm. Hg diastolic, no untoward responses were observed. Similarly, no undesirable reactions to the initial pressor responses were observed.

Surgery was performed in 6 patients: nephrectomy in 3 and saphenous vein bypass in 3. The postoperative blood pressure and renin responses are illustrated in Figure 7. Five of six patients exhibited a significant decline in blood pressure from 189/122 to 131/92 mm. Hg followed from 3 to 8 months after surgery. None of these patients was on antihypertensive medications. In this group, plasma renin activity fell from a mean of 56.7 ng./ml./hr. preoperatively to 4.8 ng./ml./hr. postoperatively. In the one patient who did not exhibit a decline of blood pressure after surgery, plasma renin activity was unchanged.

DISCUSSION

A number of recent studies have described the blood pressure responses to the competitive blockade of angiotensin II in hypertensive disorders and in normal subjects.[7, 8, 9, 15] Patients with renovascular and renal forms of hypertension exhibit a depressor response during angiotensin II blockade. The depressor response is closely related to circulating levels of renin.[16] Accordingly, hypertensive patients with high plasma renin activity tend to respond most dramatically to Saralasin while those with low and normal plasma renin activity do not. In our studies, plasma renin activity in the 13 hypertensive patients exhibiting a depressor response during angiotensin II blockade was 16.3 ± 3.5 ng./ml./hr. as compared to 1.9 ± 0.3 ng./ml./hr. in the group of patients not responding to Saralasin. All 13 patients exhibited renovascular or unilateral renal disease. Renal vein renin data in 9 of these responders lateralized to the

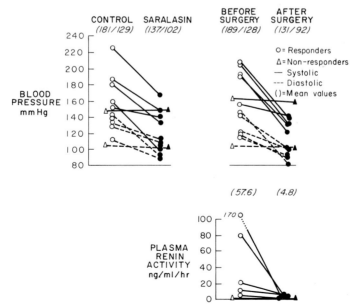

Figure 7. Blood pressure responses to angiotensin II blockade and surgery in patients with radiologic evidence of renovascular hypertension.

191

affected kidney. In contrast, in the nonresponders to Saralasin, pyelography, renal arteriography, peripheral and renal vein renin data altogether point to a non-renovascular, non-angiotensin II dependent form of hypertension. These findings in both responders and nonresponders to competitive angiotensin II blockade with Saralasin are in harmony with the pharmacologic and clinical reports of others, suggesting a high degree of specificity of this agent in detecting angiotensin II dependent forms of hypertension.

Renin secretion can be altered by a number of physiological factors as well as by renal disease.[3, 4] It seems possible therefore that stimuli leading to increased renin secretion per se could lead to depressor responses during competitive angiotensin II blockade. This phenomenon has already been observed with potent vasodilators which stimulate plasma renin activity.[11] Saralasin infusion in patients treated with Minoxidil can lead to severe hypotensive responses. Suppression of plasma renin activity by the beta adrenergic blocker, propranolol, diminishes this hypotensive action of Saralasin.[11] Thus the determinants of the state of renin secretion in hypertensive disorders may be critical for the response to competitive blockade of angiotensin II. One important determinant of renin secretion is the state of sodium balance. High sodium intake suppresses plasma renin activity while sodium depletion stimulates plasma renin activity.[3] In our studies we explored the relationship between sodium depletion induced by furosemide and competitive angiotensin II blockade.

Pretreatment with furosemide in 10 normal-renin essential hypertensive patients was associated with a mean 1.4 kg. weight loss, and an increase of plasma renin activity from 1.2 to 2.3 ng./ml./hr., but no depressor response to Saralasin was observed (Fig. 6). In striking contrast, in 4 other normal-renin patients with associated renovascular abnormalities similarly pretreated with furosemide and with a similar weight loss of 1.1 kg., plasma renin activity rose from 2.1 to 6.7 ng./ml./hr. In this group, Saralasin induced a depressor response only after furosemide. These findings are of particular interest. They indicate that renovascular hypertension may be associated with a normal plasma renin activity. These observations have been made in a number of previous studies.[7, 8, 9, 16] Detection of this group of normal-renin renovascular hypertensives with Saralasin was accomplished in our studies only after furosemide induced sodium depletion and stimulation of plasma renin activity. A mean depletion of 144 ± 19 mEq. of sodium converted these non-angiotensin II dependent hypertensives to an angiotensin II dependent state. Prior studies have demonstrated augmentation of angiotensin II pressor responses during sodium loading and a diminution of angiotensin II pressor responses by sodium depletion.[17, 18] Similarly sodium depletion has been shown to augment depressor response to Saralasin.[7] It appears that in some forms of renovascular hypertension a critical sodium mass depresses renin secretion and converts a depressor response to angiotensin II blockade into a seemingly non-angiotensin II dependent form of hypertension. In contrast, this same phenomenon was not demonstrated in our studies in other normal-renin forms of hypertension. The degree of sodium depletion in response to furosemide was similar in this latter group (159 ± 17 mEq. sodium) when compared to the normal-renin renovascular hypertensives, but renin was not stimulated to the same high level.

In experimental models of renovascular hypertension the initial hyperreninemia following placement of the renal artery clip may diminish in time and is associated with positive sodium balance.[19, 20] This phenomenon of chronic sodium retention in renovascular hypertension leading to suppression of the plasma renin activity also appears to be operating in the normal-renin renovascular group in this study. These patients only exhibit elevated plasma renin activity and an angiotensin II dependent form of hypertension after sodium depletion with furosemide. Two of these patients have subsequently been cured or their hypertension improved by surgery.

The remarkable balance between the control of blood pressure, sodium balance and renin secretion is illustrated by the normal-renin group of hypertensive patients. Despite similar sodium depletion, plasma renin activity rose only modestly and angiotensin II blockade did not produce a depressor response. The dose of furosemide and the degree of sodium depletion in these studies were purposely chosen to avoid marked sodium depletion. It seems possible that more severe sodium depletion could lead to associated depressor responses to Saralasin in normal-renin forms of essential hypertension by severely stimulating plasma renin activity.[21] However, we have not encountered this situation using the methods described above. Thus, our studies suggest that the sensitivity to Saralasin in renin-dependent forms of hypertension may be increased by pretreatment with furosemide without converting a non-depressor to a depressor response in other forms of hypertension.

An initial pressor response during the first 5 minutes of Saralasin infusion has been described in a number of studies.[9, 22] This appears related to the weak agonistic properties of this peptide. However, in our studies, patients with a depressor response during Saralasin infusion did not exhibit a pressor response. Blood pressure in this group already began to fall slightly during the first 4 minutes of the study. In contrast, in the patients without a depressor response to Saralasin diastolic blood pressure rose by 17 mm. Hg. Furosemide pretreatment did not alter this initial pressor response in the low-renin or high-renin groups. Thus, the initial pressor response to Saralasin is correlated with plasma renin activity per se. In our experience to date the pressor response is usually transient and has not led to recognizable untoward effects. We have observed 3 instances of sustained pressor response during Saralasin infusion. All 3 patients had suppressed plasma renin activity.

The depressor response to angiotensin II blockade was inversely correlated with the rise of plasma renin activity (Fig. 2). In patients not exhibiting a depressor response, plasma renin activity did not increase. These findings suggest that during angiotensin II blockade the control of renin secretion is mediated by a baroreceptor sensitive mechanism. They are in harmony with work by others emphasizing the importance of blood pressure per se in the control of renin release.[3, 4] The sensitivity of renin secretion to changes in blood pressure during angiotensin II blockade is an important additional index for the presence of renin-dependent forms of hypertension. Even when blood pressure reduction has been modest, in our experience, the stimulation of plasma renin activity during Saralasin infusion has provided additional evidence of a significant fall in blood pressure.

A second mechanism that has been found to control renin release involves circulating levels of angiotensin II. Vander and Geelhoed observed that the increased renin release induced by aortic constriction or ureteral occlusion was suppressed by small quantities of infused angiotensin II.[23] De Champlain and coworkers demonstrated that subpressor doses of angiotensin II depressed plasma renin activity during sodium depletion.[24] This negative feedback mechanism may explain the suppressed renin secretion observed in the contralateral kidney in renovascular hypertension.[6] However, in our studies negative feedback control of renin secretion does not appear to be operating in essential forms of hypertension. Even very large doses of Saralasin in this group did not stimulate plasma renin activity when blood pressure was not reduced. In contrast, the proportionality between the depressor responses to Saralasin and renin secretion in renin-dependent forms of hypertension points to the baroreceptor as the signal for renin release during angiotensin II blockade.

The blood pressure responses to angiotensin II blockade and surgery in these patients with renovascular hypertension illustrate a close parallelism. Five of six exhibited depressor responses to Saralasin and were cured of hypertension or significantly improved by renovascular repair or nephrectomy. The single patient not exhibiting a depressor response to Saralasin has also not demonstrated any improvement of hypertension after surgery. Plasma renin activity fell dramatically in the 5 patients cured or improved by surgery while in the sixth it was unchanged.

These findings support the view that angiotensin II blockade may be an additional tool to predict surgical cure of renovascular or renal hypertension.[7,8,9] Depressor responses to angiotensin II blockade may also be observed in high renin forms of essential hypertension and in the presence of bilateral renovascular disease.[25] Accordingly, Saralasin infusion complements rather than replaces existing diagnostic methods including renal vein renin determination. In the experience of most groups, renal vein renin identifies the hyper-reninemic kidney in a large fraction of cases.[6,10] However, placement of the catheter for sampling, the potential mixing of renal venous blood with that of other regional circulations, segmental renal artery abnormalities and changes in renin secretion during the sampling procedure are among the variables that may lead to erroneous conclusions when the decision to operate is based on renal vein renin alone. The lack of sensitivity of radiologic tests and their frequent application to identify renovascular hypertension together with the potential hazards of the surgical procedure point to the need for improved methods of detection and prediction of surgical cure. These studies indicate a promising role for angiotensin II blockade in the preoperative evaluation of renovascular hypertension.

REFERENCES

1. TIGERSTEDT, R., AND BERGMAN, P. G.: *Niere und Kreislauf.* Skand. Arch. Physiol. 8:223, 1898.

2. GOLDBLATT, H.: *Studies on experimental hypertension: 1. The production of persistent elevation of systolic blood pressure by means of renal ischemia.* J. Exp. Med. 59:345, 1934.

3. VANDER, A. J.: *Control of renin release.* Physiol. Rev. 47:359, 1967.

4. DAVIS, J.: *Control of renin release.* Am. J. Med. 55:333, 1973.

5. REGOLI, D., HESS, R., BRUNNER, H., ET AL.: *Interrelationship of renin content in kidneys and blood pressure in renal hypertensive rats.* Arch. Int. Pharmacodyn. Ther. 140:416, 1962.

6. VAUGHAN, E. D., JR, BUHLER, F. R., LARAGH, J. H., ET AL.: *Renovascular hypertension: renin measurements to indicate hypersecretion and contralateral suppression, estimate renal plasma flow and score for surgical curability.* Am. J. Med. 55:402, 1973.

7. BRUNNER, H. R., GAVRAS, H., LARAGH, J. H., ET AL.: *Hypertension in man. Exposure of the renin and sodium components using angiotensin II blockade.* Circ. Res. 34, 35 1-34, 1974.

8. STREETEN, D. H. P., ANDERSON, C. H., FREIBERG, J. M., ET AL.: *Use of an angiotensin II antagonist (Saralasin) in the recognition of "angiotensinogenic" hypertension.* N. Eng. J. Med. 292:657, 1975.

9. MARKS, L. S., MAXWELL, M. H., AND KAUFMAN, J. J.: *Saralasin bolus test. Rapid screening procedure for renin-mediated hypertension.* Lancet II:784, 1975.

10. AMSTERDAM, E. A., COUCH, N. P., CHRISTLIEB, A. R., ET AL.: *Renal vein renin activity in the prognosis of surgery for renovascular hypertension.* Am. J. Med. 47:860, 1969.

11. PETTINGER, W. A., AND MITCHELL, H. C.: *Renin release, Saralasin and the vasodilator-beta-blocker drug interaction in man.* N. Eng. J. Med. 292:1214, 1975.

12. SEALEY, J. E., AND LARAGH, J. H.: *Radioimmunossay of plasma renin activity.* Semin. Nucl. Med. 5:189, 1975.

13. LARAGH, J. H., BAER, L., BRUNNER, H. R., ET AL.: *Renin angiotensin and aldosterone system in pathogenesis and management of hypertensive vascular disease.* Am. J. Med. 52:633, 1972.

14. SNEDECOR, G. W., AND COCHRAN, W. G.: *Statistical Methods,* ed. 6. Iowa State University Press, Ames, Iowa, 1967.

15. HOLLENBERG, N. K., WILLIAMS, G. H., BURGER, B., ET AL.: *Blockade and stimulation of renal, adrenal and vascular angiotensin II receptors with 1-sar, 8-ala, angiotensin II in normal man.* J. Clin. Invest. 57:39, 1976.

16. BRUNNER, H. R., GAVRAS, H., AND LARAGH, J. H.: *Angiotensin II blockade in man by sar-1-ala-8-angiotensin II for understanding and treatment of high blood pressure.* Lancet II:1045, 1973.

17. AMES, R. P., BORKOWSKI, A. J. SICINSKI, A. M., ET AL.: *Prolonged infusions of angiotensin II and nor-epinephrine and blood pressure, electrolyte balance, aldosterone and cortisol secretion in normal man and in cirrhosis with ascites.* J. Clin. Invest. 44:1171, 1965.

18. PALS, D. T., MASSUCCI, F. D., DENNING, G. S., ET AL.: *Role of the pressor action of angiotensin II in experimental hypertension.* Circ. Res. 29:693, 1971.

19. GAVRAS, H., BRUNNER, H. R., VAUGHAN, E. D., ET AL.: *Angiotensin-sodium interaction in blood pressure maintenance of renal hypertensive and normotensive rats.* Science 180:1369, 1973.

20. MILLER, E. D., SAMUELS, A. I., HABER, E., ET AL.: *Inhibition of angiotensin conversion and prevention of renal hypertension.* Am. J. Physiol. 228:448, 1975.

21. ANDERSON, G. H., ELIAS, A., TOMYCZ, N., ET AL.: *Pressor response to Saralasin in hypertensives.* Clin. Res. 34:205A, 1976.

22. STREETEN, D. H. P., FREIBERG, J. M., ANDERSON, G. H., ET AL.: *Identification of angiotensinogenic hypertension in man using 1-sar-8-ala-angiotensin II (Saralasin, P-113).* Circ. Res. 36, 37:I-125, 1975.

23. VANDER, A. J., AND GEELHOED, G. W.: *Inhibition of renin secretion by angiotensin II.* Proc. Soc. Exp. Biol. Med. 120:399, 1965.

24. DE CHAMPLAIN, J., GENEST, J., VEYRATT, R., ET AL.: *Factors controlling renin release in man.* Arch. Int. Med. 117:355, 1966.

25. BAER, L., PARRA-CARRILLO, J. Z., RADICHEVICH, I., ET AL.: *Detection of renovascular hypertension with angiotensin II blockade.* Ann. Intern. Med. 86:257, 1977.

Essential Hypertension: Hemodynamics, Pressor Mechanisms, and Mechanisms of Drug Action*

Edward D. Frohlich, M.D.

Over the past 25 years the approach to the hypertensive patient has changed radically. In the 1940s there was little hope of preventing death from malignant hypertension, cardiac failure, hypertensive encephalopathy, and other major hypertensive complications. However, since then prospective studies have shown that with efficacious and safe modern antihypertensive drugs,[1, 2] cardiovascular morbidity and mortality in these hypertensive patients can be reduced dramatically (Fig. 1).[3]

This discussion elaborates upon the public health problem of hypertensive diseases, their prevalence, and how they are the major cause of two of the most common cardiac conditions encountered by the cardiologist: congestive heart failure and coronary disease.[4, 5] It will consider how therapy over this past generation has become so sophisticated that it might be well for the clinician to consider a variety of factors in order to be prepared to continue treatment of hypertensive patients effectively and safely. Updating this information will enable the physician to utilize intelligently the newer antihypertensive agents presently under study in clinical cardiovascular research laboratories.

THE PROBLEM

Diseases of the heart and blood vessels comprise the major cause of all deaths in the United States today.[6] Deaths from cardiovascular disease exceed the sum total of all other diseases and causes of death in the United States regardless of age. The most common cardiovascular disease is hypertension. Over 23 million adult Americans have arterial pressures in excess of 160 mm. Hg systolic and 105 mm. Hg diastolic. The higher the blood pressure (systolic or diastolic) the greater the chance for cardiovascular morbidity or mortality.[7] Life insurance actuarial data demonstrate that a man at age 35 years, for example, having a normal life expectancy of 76½ years will die 4 years sooner than projected if his blood pressure is 130/90 (and if he remains untreated). If his blood pressure is 140/95, life span will be reduced even more dramatically by 9 years. Further, if his blood pressure is 150/100, life expectancy will be diminished by 16½ years (Fig. 2).[8] In these hypothetical examples, the diastolic blood pressures referred to are lower than the minimum level for treatment (105 mm. Hg) recommended by the National High Blood Pressure Education Program.[9]

*This study, from the Salmen Family Hypertension Research Laboratory, was supported, in part, by a grant-in-aid from the National Heart, Lung, and Blood Institute (HL-20572).

197

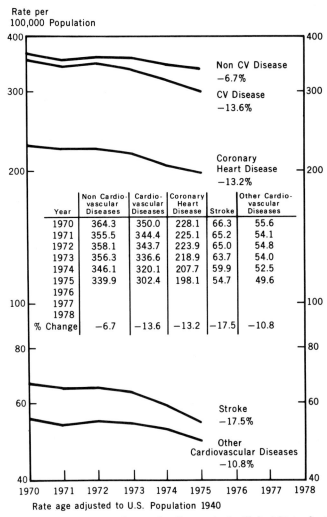

Rate per
100,000 Population

Year	Non Cardio-vascular Diseases	Cardio-vascular Diseases	Coronary Heart Disease	Stroke	Other Cardio-vascular Diseases
1970	364.3	350.0	228.1	66.3	55.6
1971	355.5	344.4	225.1	65.2	54.1
1972	358.1	343.7	223.9	65.0	54.8
1973	356.3	336.6	218.9	63.7	54.0
1974	346.1	320.1	207.7	59.9	52.5
1975	339.9	302.4	198.1	54.7	49.6
1976					
1977					
1978					
% Change	−6.7	−13.6	−13.2	−17.5	−10.8

Non CV Disease −6.7%

CV Disease −13.6%

Coronary Heart Disease −13.2%

Stroke −17.5%

Other Cardiovascular Diseases −10.8%

Rate age adjusted to U.S. Population 1940

Figure 1. Reduction in death rates from cardiovascular diseases in the United States for the period including 1970 through 1975. Note the sudden break in the curves for cardiovascular and coronary heart disease and for stroke beginning 1973. (With permission of the National Heart, Lung, and Blood Institute.)

JUSTIFICATION FOR THERAPY

The Veterans Administration Cooperative Study clearly established that effective reduction of arterial pressure—with such simple compounds as a thiazide diuretic, reserpine, and hydralazine—will result in significantly reduced morbidity and mortality.[1,2] Indeed, this prospective multiclinic study was the major impetus behind the present National High Blood Pressure Education Program, which has recommended a simple stepped-care approach to medical treatment of the hypertensive diseases, and which has been updated recently in order to include some of the newer antihypertensive compounds (Fig. 3).[10] This schema suggests a simplified standard stepped-care treatment regimen for patients with diastolic pressures in excess of 105 mm. Hg. Within

198

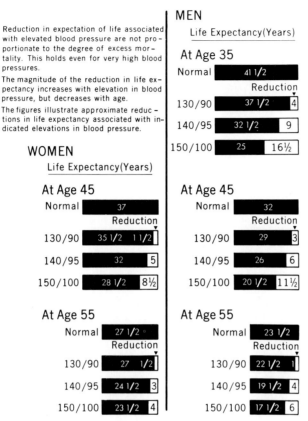

Figure 2. Projected life tables estimated by the Statistical Bureau of Metropolitan Life Insurance based on the experience of 26 life insurance companies from 1935 to 1954. These projected life tables demonstrate the effect of minimal elevation of arterial pressure in men and in women.

this approach there is laterality for the clinician not only to select several options of therapy but, through subscription of paramedical professional assistance, to treat large numbers of hypertensive patients. For the remainder of this discussion we shall present an alternative way of considering antihypertensive therapy which, in reality, is probably not very different from the former approach. However, it provides a physiologic (and pharmacologic) rationale for therapy.

THERAPY: MECHANISMS OF ACTION

The modern clinician has available a wide variety of antihypertensive compounds which literally permits pharmacologic dissection of the autonomic nervous system and nephron at any anatomic level. Autonomic nervous function can be stimulated or inhibited at any level (Table 1). Excretion of sodium and water can be increased at most levels of renal function. In recent years, as our knowledge concerning the renin-angiotensin system has burgeoned, it has become possible to stimulate or inhibit components of this system (Table 2). Therefore, remarkable pharmacologic contributions to the treatment of hypertensive patients have been made over these past 25 years.

Nevertheless, as physicians, we should not become so complacent as to assume that

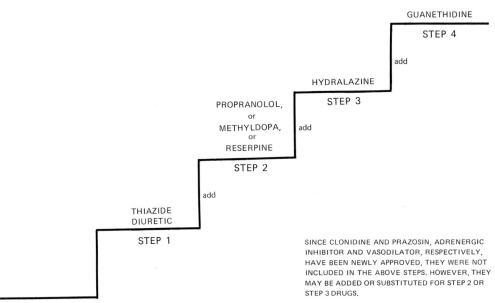

Figure 3. Stepped-care approach for the treatment of hypertension (as amended by the High Blood Pressure Education Program, 1976). This is a new version of the program originally offered by the National High Blood Pressure Education Program taking into consideration the new agents presently available in the United States. (With permission of the National Heart, Lung, and Blood Institute.)

Table 1. Drugs are presently available that can stimulate or inhibit autonomic nervous function at many anatomic levels. The following illustrates this remarkable pharmacologic achievement.

Site	Stimulant	Inhibitor
Cerebral	Amphetamines	Barbiturates Antidepressants
Hypothalamus		Methyldopa Clonidine
Medulla	Pentylenemetrazol Ethamiran	Phenylthiazines
Ganglion	Tetraethylammonium Nicotine Dimethylphenylpiperazinium	Hexamethonium Pentolinium Trimethaphan
Postganglionic adrenergic neurone	Tyramine Ephedrine Cocaine	Reserpine Methyldopa Guanethidine Bethanidine
Alpha-adrenergic receptor site	Phenylephrine Methoxamine	Phentolamine Phenoxybenzamine
Beta-adrenergic receptor site	Isoproterenol	Propranolol Oxprenolol Timolol Sotolol Practolol Tolamolol (and many others)

Table 2. The major pharmacologic agents which serve to stimulate or inhibit the major components of the renin-angiotensin system.

Factor	Stimulant	Inhibitor
Renin substrate	Estrogens Oral contraceptives	

Renin (renal)	Vasodilators:
	  hydralazine
	  prazosin
	  minoxidil
	  diazoxide
	  nitroprusside
	Diuretics (all)
	Restricted sodium dietotherapy
		Adrenergic inhibitors:
		  reserpine
		  methyldopa
		  guanethidine
		  bethanidine
		  guanethidine
		  clonidine
		Beta-adrenergic receptor site inhibitors

Converting enzyme		SQ 20,881
Angiotensin II	Vasodilators Diuretics Sodium restriction	Saralasin

present day therapy has achieved the millennium. A variety of new antihypertensive agents are "in the therapeutic wings" and under current clinical pharmacological study by cardiovascular researchers in this country and elsewhere. There are newer sympatholytic drugs (e.g., bethanidine) which work at the postganglionic nerve ending and have a more prompt onset of action and dissipation of action than guanethidine, the current major sympatholytic agent of this type. Also available are beta-adrenergic blocking drugs having both general systemic effects of inhibiting beta-adrenergic receptor sites as well as agents which are more cardiospecific. The advantage of the latter type of compound would be in the selectivity of excluding the bronchiolar smooth muscle from inhibition of its beta-adrenergic receptor sites. Diuretics are available which selectively will retain potassium or promote uricosuria.[11] Drugs are also available that inhibit adrenal steroid biosynthesis at varying levels.[12]

With this increased sophistication in our pharmacological armamentarium, certain dangers will be inherent. Medications may be more specific (e.g., beta-adrenergic and renin-angiotensin inhibiting drugs):[13-15] and with this increasing specificity, there will be, perhaps, potentially greater dangers. It may be possible to obviate some of these inherent dangers and side effects if we were to clinically "wed" the mechanism of drug action with the pressor mechanism by which the elevated arterial pressure is maintained in our hypertensive patients. Therefore, let us examine some of these mechanisms whereby arterial pressure seems to be elevated in a hypertensive patient.

PRESSOR MECHANISMS

We are all well aware of the fundamental fact that a variety of mechanisms are available (and are continually being called into play) to regulate arterial pressure at normal levels. These and several others are also operative in varying degrees in maintaining arterial pressure at abnormally elevated levels in the variety of hypertensive diseases we encounter (Table 3).[16, 17] None of these mechanisms operates alone in maintaining arterial pressure at abnormally elevated levels. For example, even when the forward flow of blood is mechanically obstructed (e.g., in a patient with aortic coarctation), the renopressor system may be stimulated. Or, with respect to the renopressor system, minute subpressor doses of angiotensin II can stimulate increased sympathetic outflow from the brain; and angiotensin can stimulate release of catecholamines from

201

Table 3. Pressor and depressor mechanisms which operate normally and in the various hypertensive diseases, including the many ways in which essential hypertension is expressed pathophysiologically

Mechanism	*Other Mechanisms Involved*
Cathecholamines	Renopressor; neural; volume
Renopressor	Aldosterone; neural; volume; renodepressor (prostaglandins)
Volume	Hormonal; electrolytes; fluid volume partition shifts; renopressor; neural
Neural	Renopressor; adenylate cyclase system; renodepressor (prostaglandins); fluid volume partition shifts
Hormonal:	
Thyroid	Sympathetic nervous system
Parathyroid	Calcium ion
Estrogens	Renopressor system; fluid volumes
Growth hormone	?
Aldosterone Compounds DEF 18-OH-DOC 16β-OH-dehydroepiandostrone	Electrolytes; fluid volume shifts; transmembrane ion gradients

the adrenal medulla.[18] Of course, the renopressor system is also known to produce secondary aldosteronism, as in renovascular hypertension. Depending upon whether the hyperaldosteronism is primary or secondary, there will be extracellular fluid volume expansion, as with primary hyperaldosteronism,[19] or plasma volume contraction, as in patients with renovascular hypertension and secondary hyperaldosteronism.[20] The role of depressor mechanisms in hypertension remains under active investigation; and we must wait for some time to learn whether the prostaglandins or other renal depressor substances (including the kinins) have any role in hypertension.[21]

A variety of other hormonal mechanisms may also participate in initiating or maintaining hypertension. The adrenal corticosteroid hormones (most notably aldosterone) and the estrogens are discussed elsewhere in this book. However, excess parathyroid hormone is associated with hypertension via calcium excess;[22] and a variety of other hypercalcemic disease states have been associated with an increased prevalence of hypertension.[23, 24] Thyroid hormone, perhaps through its interrelationship with the sympathetic nervous system, is associated with systolic hypertension in hyperthyroidism.[25, 26] However, there seems to be a less tangible explanation for the association of hypothyroidism and hypertension. That catecholamines elevate arterial pressure has been repeatedly demonstrated in patients having pheochromocytoma. Less known, however, is the role of catecholamines in stimulating the release of renin from the kidney,[27] the release of catecholamines from the adrenal medulla by angiotensin,[28] and the relationship of catecholamines to essential hypertension either by excessive levels[29, 30] or via altered catecholamine metabolism.[31] It seems clear that neural mechanisms must play a most important role in maintaining arterial pressure in many patients with established essential hypertension since those antihypertensive compounds which inhibit neural actions have played a major part in the reduction of morbidity and mortality. Even early in the development of hypertension, neural (adrenergic) mechanisms seem to play a major role.[32-34] Rather than further discussing these secondary forms of hypertension, I shall emphasize how these pressor mechanisms seem to participate in the patient with essential hypertension that we commonly encounter in our clinical practice.

ESSENTIAL HYPERTENSION: MECHANISMS AND THERAPY

Mild Severity

An appropriate place to consider this concept might be with those patients in whom neural mechanisms are associated with the milder degrees of severity of hypertension. In the Middle Ages, Avicenna, in his *Ad Medicorum Principis,* described the patient who is fearsome, having a rapid heart rate, an increased body temperature, and what he described as a hyperdynamic circulation. Perhaps this description is one which preceded by many hundred years Da Costa's description of "soldier's heart" during the Civil War,[35] the description of neurocirculatory asthenia,[36] or even Gorlin's more recent description of the hyperkinetic heart syndrome.[37] The patient that these descriptions seem to refer to is one with an arterial pressure that is intermittently or possibly persistently elevated.[32] Associated with this pressure elevation is a hyperdynamic apical cardiac impulse characterized by a rapid upswing of the ventricular impulse and its prompt dissipation. The cardiac rate, while not true sinus tachycardia, is nevertheless faster than that of a normotensive individual who is in a fasting, untreated basal state.

These patients with labile or mild essential hypertension usually present no symptoms; however, they may have palpitations and tachycardia. When studied hemodynamically, they have evidence of a hyperkinetic circulation and increased adrenergic participation; effective therapy is usually achieved with adrenergic inhibitors or perhaps diuretics.[38-40]

One such group of hypertensive patients with a hyperkinetic circulation may demonstrate a *hyperdynamic beta-adrenergic circulatory state.*[41, 42] These patients, I believe, merely represent one segment of the individuals we have just described. They all have symptoms of disabling palpitations and tachycardia, evidence of a hyperkinetic circulation manifested by a faster heart rate, increased cardiac output, and increased left ventricular ejection rate. They may have mildly or moderately severe hypertension or they may be normotensive.[41] When challenged with an isoproterenol infusion (isoproterenol is the specific beta-adrenergic receptor site agonist), their cardioaccelerator response is far more rapid than a normotensive individual or other hypertensive patients having the same arterial pressure elevation but without these symptoms.[42] Isoproterenol may also evoke an emotional response; all of these findings can be blocked completely by treatment with a beta-adrenergic blocking compound.

That these findings in one segment of the hypertensive population seem to be but an exaggeration of normal function—a state of disregulation, if you will—may be shown by the work of Tarazi, Ibrahim, and Dustan.[43] In their studies they demonstrated that in the patient with mild essential hypertension, the relationship between the volume of blood in the central circulation and the cardiac output is shifted upward, but in a parallel fashion, from the normotensive subject or patient with more established essential hypertension—but not so high as the normotensive subject receiving beta-adrenergic stimulation with isoproterenol. Thus, the patient with mild hypertension demonstrates an upward or abnormal shift in cardiac function, much as if a normal myocardium were stimulated by the specific beta-adrenergic agonist, isoproterenol. Nevertheless, whether these patients have mild essential hypertension, labile hypertension, or demonstrate the characteristics of a hyperdynamic beta-adrenergic circulatory state, when they are treated with beta-adrenergic receptor inhibiting compounds (such as propranolol) there usually is a rather significant fall in the systolic, diastolic, and mean arterial pressures, whether these pressures are taken at home or in the office.[40, 44-46]

When we first reported our experiences with beta-adrenergic blocking therapy in hypertension, we demonstrated that the reduction of arterial pressure was directly related to the height of the pretreatment cardiac output.[40, 44] Thus, after patients had been treated with propranolol for as long as 14 months, the reduced arterial pressure was associated with a fall in heart rate, cardiac index, and left ventricular ejection rate. However, at that time we were at a loss to offer an explanation for our reported observation that plasma renin activity was directly proportional to the height of their cardiac output in these essential hypertensive patients.[48] Later, however, Bühler and his co-workers suggested that elevated plasma renin activity provided an excellent basis for selection of patients for beta-blocking therapy.[49] It seems likely that the rationale for these two physiological means of preselection of hypertensive patients for beta-blocking therapy might rest in the fact that both increased cardiac output and plasma renin activity can be elevated by enhanced adrenergic activity.

Nevertheless, the mechanism whereby arterial pressure is reduced in patients with essential hypertension by beta-blocking drugs still remains unexplained. Some investigators have suggested that the reduction in blood pressure may result from a resetting of baroreceptors.[50] However, mechanoreceptors respond to changes in pressure rather than to flow changes. Although we had suggested earlier that there may be an adaptation of the circulation produced via myogenic[51] or metabolic mechanisms, at present this mechanism remains purely speculative. In any event, vascular resistance does not seem to fall below pretreatment levels despite prolonged reduction of blood pressure with propranolol;[52] and so a mechanism involving an adaptation of the circulation to the decrease in blood pressure remains possible.[51] It is also possible that beta-blocking drugs have a direct action on the central nervous system.[53] Another possibility is that certain metabolites of the beta-blocking drugs act as antipressor agents per se.[54]

Moderate Severity

The pathophysiological mechanisms which seem operative in patients with moderately severe essential hypertension are somewhat different. Some of these patients also are asymptomatic; others may complain of cardiac awareness, shortness of breath, and angina pectoris.[55] The latter may result either from coexistent atherosclerosis or from the increased myocardial oxygen demand associated with the increased pressure and myocardial tension of hypertensive cardiovascular disease;[56] more commonly, these two factors coexist clinically. Treatment of these patients obviously should be directed at reduction of the elevated arterial pressure and vascular resistance. It is most important to remember that as arterial pressure is reduced by antihypertensive agents which either inhibit adrenergic function or produce vasodilation, diuretic therapy becomes mandatory due to sodium retention associated with the fall in arterial pressure.[57, 58]

Cardiac Involvement in Hypertension

In understanding the rationale for meaningful antihypertensive therapy, it is useful to review the pathophysiological alterations associated with progressive vascular involvement in hypertensive disease. All clinicians are aware of the radically different apical precordial findings characterizing the patient with milder essential hypertension and a hyperkinetic precordium versus the patient with more severe hypertension with left ventricular hypertrophy and a left ventricular lift which is characterized by a prolonged and forceful apical beat. These findings obviously can be confirmed by the electrocardiogram and the chest x-ray,[59, 60] preferably when interpreted simultaneously.[61] Thus, when these two clinical tools are used together for a prognostic index of morbidity and mortality from hypertension, approximately 90 percent of patients with cardiac enlargement by chest x-ray and electrocardiogram die within five years if they are not treated; in contrast, if the heart is perfectly normal by chest x-ray and electrocardiogram, the five-year mortality rate is only 10 percent.[61]

Falling somewhere in between in this wide spectrum of patients with hypertension having a normal size heart and those with obvious left ventricular hypertrophy are other patients with essential hypertension who have evidence of left atrial abnormality by ECG but no definite findings of obvious ventricular hypertrophy.[62, 63] These hypertensive patients were first described by Potain in 1875 when he described the "bruit d'gallop" (the fourth heart sound or atrial diastolic gallop) in patients with hypertension.[64] This fourth heart sound is highly concordant with at least two electrocardiographic criteria of left atrial abnormality.[63] It is important to realize that these patients with left atrial abnormality do not actually have atrial disease; the left atrium only reflects decreased left ventricular compliance, as ventricular hypertrophy is taking place. The hypertrophy, however, is not yet obvious enough to be detected by the electrocardiogram or the chest x-ray; hemodynamically, the atrium is providing an extra "kick" to ventricular pumping performance.[65]

Hemodynamics

To bring the foregoing concept into clearer focus, we have studied a series of approximately 100 untreated essential hypertensive patients by hemodynamic techniques and compared the findings with normal subjects (Fig. 4).[59] In this study, arterial pressure progressively and significantly (the probability factor between each succeeding group was $p < 0.001$) increased from the normal subjects (Group N) to patients with no cardiac involvement (Group I), to those with left atrial abnormality (Group II), and then to those patients with obvious left ventricular hypertrophy (Group III). Resting heart rate was significantly faster in all patients with essential hypertension, regardless of severity of cardiac involvement. The cardiac index was normally maintained in all hypertensive patients until left ventricular hypertrophy developed (Group III). However, even before cardiac output significantly fell in the patients with left ventricular hypertrophy, impaired left ventricular function was demonstrable in patients with left atrial abnormality (Group II), as indicated by a significant reduction in left ventricular ejection rate. Derived data of left ventricular function (i.e., stroke work, power, tension time index, and pressure time per beat) also demonstrated progressive impairment with progressive increase in afterload. These findings were confirmed recently in our laboratory by means of noninvasive echocardiographic studies demonstrating progressively increased left ventricular wall thickness and diminished left ventricular fiber shortening in Group II patients.[66]

Hypertensive Encephalopathy

The therapeutic implications of these findings are now apparent. If a patient has severe arterial vascular disease with vasospasm and hypertensive encephalopathy, we would expect the hemodynamics to be characterized by very high vascular resistance and a cardiac output which is not increased. The antihypertensive agent selected should produce a prompt and immediate fall in vascular resistance via a reduction in vascular smooth muscle tension. Such therapy might be provided by sodium nitroprusside or diazoxide, since these agents produce an immediate fall in arterial pressure following intravenous infusion or bolus injection. With the onset of hypotension, headache, restlessness, somnolence, coma, nausea, and vomiting promptly disappear, only to reoccur if the infusion is discontinued or when arterial pressure rises. With

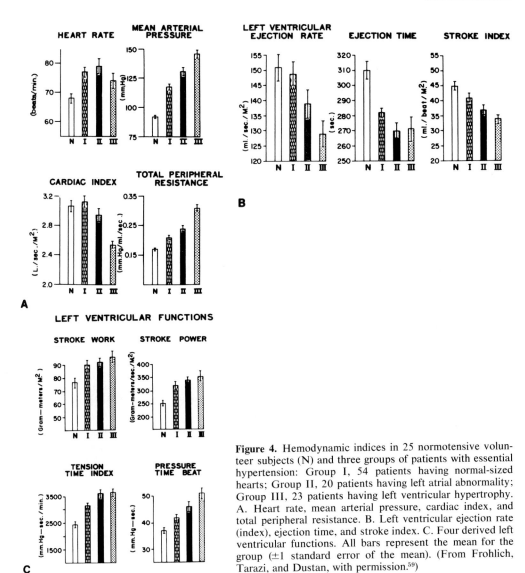

Figure 4. Hemodynamic indices in 25 normotensive volunteer subjects (N) and three groups of patients with essential hypertension: Group I, 54 patients having normal-sized hearts; Group II, 20 patients having left atrial abnormality; Group III, 23 patients having left ventricular hypertrophy. A. Heart rate, mean arterial pressure, cardiac index, and total peripheral resistance. B. Left ventricular ejection rate (index), ejection time, and stroke index. C. Four derived left ventricular functions. All bars represent the mean for the group (±1 standard error of the mean). (From Frohlich, Tarazi, and Dustan, with permission.[59])

reinstitution of therapy and reduction in arterial pressure, symptoms will once again remit.

Malignant Hypertension

Another expression of severe vasoconstrictor disease is seen in the patient with malignant hypertension. This patient will demonstrate exudative retinopathy (hemorrhages and exudates) and papilledema associated with secondary hyperaldosteronism. If *immediate* pressure reduction is necessary (e.g., associated with intracranial hemorrhage), therapy with nitroprusside may be initiated with further addition of a diuretic to maintain a reduced arterial pressure and to prevent intravascular volume expansion. Intravenous medications should be discontinued as soon as oral therapy is feasible. If the need for therapy is less urgent (e.g., malignant or accelerated hypertension without acute central nervous system or cardiac findings), oral antihypertensive agents may be selected in conjunction with a diuretic agent. However, because malignant hypertension is associated with severe secondary hyperaldosteronism, it is important to prevent potassium wastage; under these circumstances the renal aldosterone antagonist, spironolactone, may be used alone or in conjunction with another diuretic, such as a thiazide or furosemide. Upon reduction of arterial pressure in these patients there may be some impairment in renal function; this can be expected to improve with continued and persistent treatment and therapy should not be withdrawn.

As already indicated, any potent antihypertensive drug which reduces arterial pressure via vasodilation or adrenergic inhibition will be associated with sodium retention and an expanded intravascular and extracellular fluid volume. This is due to a variety of factors including reduced renal perfusion pressure and decreased capillary hydrostatic pressure. These events indicate a concept of the role of plasma volume changes in the hypertensive disorders.

Plasma Volume

Several years ago we studied the relationship of plasma volume and diastolic pressure in patients with essential hypertension.[20, 67] When untreated essential hypertensive men had their plasma volume measured in the supine position resting early in the morning in the fasting state, an inverse relationship of diastolic pressure with plasma volume was demonstrated. Thus, when their arterial pressure was high their intravascular volume was proportionally low; and similarly, the higher the vascular resistance to blood flow the lower the intravascular volume. One explanation for this phenomenon may be understood by applying knowledge of the Starling forces on the fluid movement at the capillary level.[68] In this respect, the higher the intravascular hydrostatic pressure the greater the force will be for movement of the intravascular fluid (plasma) to enter the interstitial compartment. Conversely, as hydrostatic pressure falls (with treatment) there is a tendency for that fluid to return to the intravascular compartment. Therefore, perhaps one of the explanations for the sodium retention associated with antihypertensive therapy with vasodilators and antiadrenergic therapy is the fall in pressure and the alteration of the Starling forces on transcapillary fluid migration at the capillary level. Other factors may also participate, such as decreasing renal perfusion pressure, which tends to promote sodium and water retention[69] and may also provoke secondary hyperaldosteronism consequent to a release of renin.

Plasma Renin Activity

This inverse relationship between intravascular volume and arterial pressure is also consistent with the finding of higher plasma renin activity in those essential hypertensive patients having a more contracted intravascular volume.[48] Therefore, those patients that have the higher peripheral plasma renin activity seem to be those with the lower or more contracted intravascular volume. And, as we have indicated, those patients with the lowest plasma (or total blood) volume would be those with the higher plasma renin activity and arterial pressure. These findings relating high plasma renin activity and severity of vascular disease in essential hypertension were also reported by Brunner and his associates.[70] It is therefore not surprising that patients with hypertension and *lower* plasma renin activity might be those patients with expanded intravascular volume. This explains the low plasma renin activity in primary aldosteronism,[71] low-renin essential hypertension,[70] and those patients with essential hypertension who might respond better to diuretic therapy.[14] Consequently, it is also not at all surprising to see why those patients with high-renin essential hypertension have the greatest vascular disease, the highest arterial pressures, and favorable response to drugs that inhibit adrenergic function.[14]

With these concepts in mind, it is now possible to explain the mechanism for the development of "pseudotolerance" to antihypertensive drug therapy. Initially, arterial pressure falls with effective vasodilator or adrenolytic therapy (alone or with inadequate diuretic dosages), but subsequently returns to or toward pretreatment levels. Responsiveness to this treatment can be restored with addition or institution of full dosages of diuretic therapy or more vigorous control of dietary sodium intake.[58]

CONCLUSION

It is now possible, with the variety of antihypertensive drugs available, to appraise our essential hypertensive patients from the viewpoint of which physiological mechanisms seem to be participating most in the maintenance of elevated arterial pressure. If blood volume seems normal, inappropriately normal, or expanded, therapy might be initiated with a variety of diuretics and/or sodium dietotherapy. If hormonal mechanisms seem involved, it is possible to specifically inhibit those hormones that seem to be most operative — spironolactone for aldosterone, thyroid hormone inhibitors, or inhibitors of adrenal biosynthesis. With respect to the renopressor system, it is also possible (with methyldopa, propranolol, clonidine, or other sympatholytic drugs) to inhibit renin release, and the generation or responsiveness of vessels to angiotensin II. Finally, there are a variety of drugs which permit inhibition of autonomic nervous activity at a variety of neural levels, from subcortical to adrenergic receptor sites.

Continued and vigorous antihypertensive therapy is essential if we expect to reverse the severe morbidity and mortality that is associated with the very common problem of hypertensive cardiovascular disease. A simple and practical standard (stepped-care) treatment program may be used. Its feasibility has been popularized through the Veterans Administration Cooperative Study and the High Blood Pressure Education Program. However, in this regard, it is most important to understand those mechanisms which are operative in the maintenance of the elevated pressure in the patient with hypertension and to recognize the specificity of present day therapy and those newer agents which will become available.

This mechanistic concept of hypertension is not new. It has been described earlier by Page in his mosaic theory.[72] He indicated a variety of factors which interrelate and participate in maintaining arterial pressure either at normal levels in normotensive individuals or at elevated levels in hypertensive patients. Page, therefore, suggested that hypertension may be considered a disease of disregulation. It seems to me that this concept is an extremely valuable one for the practicing physician in understanding the interrelationships of the pathophysiological aspects of this disease, in applying present day therapy, and in anticipating the antihypertensive drugs of the future.

REFERENCES

1. VETERANS ADMINISTRATION COOPERATIVE STUDY GROUP ON ANTIHYPERTENSIVE AGENTS: *Effects of treatment on morbidity in hypertension. I. Results in patients with diastolic blood pressure averaging 115 through 129 mm Hg.* JAMA 208:1028, 1967.

2. VETERANS ADMINISTRATION COOPERATIVE STUDY GROUP ON ANTIHYPERTENSIVE AGENTS: *Effects of treatment on morbidity in hypertension. II. Results in patients with diastolic blood pressure averaging 90 through 114 mm Hg.* JAMA 213:1143, 1970.

3. NATIONAL HEART, LUNG, AND BLOOD INSTITUTE: *Annual Report 1976.*

4. KANNEL, W. B., SCHWARTZ, M. J., AND McNAMARA, P. M.: *Blood pressure and risk of coronary heart disease: The Framingham study.* Dis. Chest. 56:43, 1969.

5. KANNEL, W. B., GORDON, T., CASTELLI, W. P., ET AL.: *Electrocardiographic left ventricular hypertrophy and risk of coronary heart disease. The Framingham study.* Ann. Intern. Med. 72:813, 1970.

6. *Heart Facts.* American Heart Association, Dallas, Texas, 1975, 29 pages.

7. KANNEL, W. B., GORDON, T., AND SCHWARTZ, M. J.: *Systolic versus diastolic blood pressure and risk of coronary heart disease.* Am. J. Cardiol. 27:335, 1971.

8. SOCIETY OF ACTUARIES: *Build and Blood Pressure Study, Vol. 1.* Society of Actuaries, Chicago, 1959.

9. NATIONAL HIGH BLOOD PRESSURE EDUCATION PROGRAM, NATIONAL HEART AND LUNG INSTITUTE: *Professional Education.* Report of Task Force II to the Hypertension Information and Education Advisory Committee, September 1, 1973.

10. MOSER, M. (CHAIRMAN): *Report of the Joint National Committee on Education, Evaluation, and Treatment of High Blood Pressure.* JAMA 237:255, 1977.

11. DE CARVALHO, J. G. R., DUNN, F. G., CHRYSANT, S. G., ET AL.: *Ticrynafen: A novel uricosuric antihypertensive natriuretic agent.* Arch. Intern. Med., in press.

12. WOODS, J. W., LIDDLE, G. S., STOUT, E. G., JR., ET AL.: *Effect of an adrenal inhibitor in hypertensive patients with suppressed plasma renin.* Arch. Intern. Med. 123:366, 1969.

13. FROHLICH, E. D., TARAZI, R. C., AND DUSTAN, H. P.: *Beta-adrenergic blocking therapy in hypertension: Selection of patients.* Internat. J. Pharm. Therap. Toxicol. 4:151, 1970.

14. LARAGH, J. H.: *Vasoconstriction-volume analysis for understanding and treating hypertension: The use of renin and aldosterone profiles.* Am. J. Med. 55:261, 1976.

15. STREETEN, D. H. P., FREIBERG, J. M., ANDERSON, G. H., ET AL.: *Identification of angiotensinogenic hypertension in man using 1-Sar-8-Ala-angiotensin II.* Circ. Res. 36 (Suppl. 2):125, 1975.

16. FROHLICH, E. D.: *Hypertension and hypertensive heart disease,* in CHUNG, E. K. (ed.): *Quick Reference to Cardiovascular Disease.* J. B. Lippincott Company, Philadelphia, in press.

17. FROHLICH, E. D.: *Cardiovascular pathophysiology of essential hypertension,* in ZELIS, R. (ed.): *The Peripheral Circulations.* Grune & Stratton, Inc., New York, 1975, p. 261.

18. DUNN, F. G., DE CARVALHO, J. G. R., KEM, D. C., ET AL.: *Pheochromocytoma crisis induced by Saralasin: Relationship of angiotensin analog to catecholamine release.* N. Engl. J. Med. 295:605, 1976.

19. SLATON, P. E., AND BIGLIERI, E. G.: *Hypertension and hyperaldosteronism of renal and adrenal origin.* Am. J. Med. 38:324, 1965.

20. TARAZI, R. C., DUSTAN, H. P., FROHLICH, E. D., ET AL.: *Plasma volume and chronic hypertension. Relationship to arterial pressure levels in different hypertensive diseases.* Arch. Intern. Med. 125:835, 1970.

21. MCGIFF, J. C., AND VANE, J. R.: *Prostaglandins and the regulation of blood pressure,* Kidney Int. 8:5262, 1975.

22. HELLSTRÖM, J., BIRKE, G., AND EDVALL, C. A.: *Hypertension in hyperparathyroidism.* Br. J. Urol. 30:13, 1958.

23. EARLL, J. M., KURTZMAN, N. A., AND MOSER, R. H.: *Hypercalcemia and hypertension.* Ann. Intern. Med. 64:378, 1966.

24. WEIDMANN, P., MASSRY, S. G., COBURN, J. W., ET AL.: *Blood pressure effects of acute hypercalcemia.* Ann. Intern. Med. 76:741, 1972.

25. GRISWALD, D., AND KEATING, J. H., JR.: *Cardiac dysfunction in hyperthyroidism.* Am. Heart J. 38:818, 1949.

26. BREWSTER, W. R., JR., AND ISAACS, J. P.: *The hemodynamic and metabolic interrelationships in the activity of epinephrine, norepinephrine, and the thyroid hormones.* Circulation 13:1, 1956.

27. WINER, N., CHOKSKI, D. S., AND WALKENHORST, W. G.: *Effects of cyclic AMP, sympathomimetic amines, and adrenergic receptor antagonists on renin secretion.* Circ. Res. 29:239, 1971.

28. PEACH, M. J.: *Adrenal medullary stimulation induced by angiotensin I, angiotensin II, and analogues.* Circ. Res. 28 (Suppl. 2):107, 1971.

29. LOUIS, W. J., DOYLE, A. E., AND ANAVEKAR, S.: *Plasma norepinephrine levels in essential hypertension.* N. Engl. J. Med. 288:599, 1973.

30. DEQUATTRO, V., AND CHAN, S.: *Raised plasma catecholamines in some patients with primary hypertension.* Lancet 1:806, 1972.

31. MANGER, W. M., GIFFORD, R. W., JR., FROHLICH, E. D., ET AL.: *Norepinephrine infusion in normal subjects and patients with essential or renal hypertension: Effect on blood pressure, heart rate, and plasma catecholamine concentrations.* J. Clin. Pharmacol. 16:129, 1976.

32. FROHLICH, E. D., KOZUL, V. J., TARAZI, R. C., ET AL.: *Physiological comparison of labile and essential hypertension.* Circ. Res. 27 (Suppl. 1): 55, 1970.

33. FROHLICH, E. D., AND PFEFFER, M. A.: *Adrenergic mechanisms in human and SHR hypertension.* Clin. Sci. Mol. Med. 48:225s, 1975.

34. FROHLICH, E. D.: *Adrenergic nervous system and hypertension.* Proc. Mayo Clinic 52:361, 1977.

35. DA COSTA, J. M.: *On irritable heart, a clinical form of functional cardiac disorder and its consequences.* Am. J. Med. Sci. 61:17, 1971.

36. COHEN, M. E., AND WHITE, P. D.: *Life situations, emotions, and neurocirculatory asthenia (anxiety neurosis, neurasthenia, effort syndrome).* Psychosom. Med. 13:336, 1951.

37. GORLIN, R.: *The hyperkinetic heart syndrome.* JAMA 182:823, 1962.

38. FROHLICH, E. D.: *Beta-adrenergic blockade in the circulatory regulation of hyperkinetic states.* Am. J. Cardiol. 27:195, 1971.

39. FROHLICH, E. D.: *Hyperdynamic circulation and hypertension.* Postgrad. Med. 52:68, 1972.

40. FROHLICH, E. D.: *Clinical significance of hemodynamic findings in hypertension.* Chest 64:94, 1973.

41. FROHLICH, E. D., DUSTAN, H. P., AND PAGE, I. H.: *Hyperdynamic beta-adrenergic circulatory state.* Arch. Intern. Med. 117:614, 1966.

42. FROHLICH, E. D., TARAZI, R. C., AND DUSTAN, H. P.: *Hyperdynamic beta-adrenergic circulatory state: Increased beta receptor responsiveness.* Arch. Intern. Med. 123:1, 1969.

43. TARAZI, R. C., IBRAHIM, M. M., DUSTAN, H. P., ET AL.: *Cardiac factors in hypertension.* Circ. Res. 34 (Suppl. I):213, 1974.

44. FROHLICH, E. D., TARAZI, R. C., DUSTAN, H. P., ET AL.: *The paradox of beta-adrenergic blockade in hypertension.* Circulation 37:417, 1968.

45. FROHLICH, E. D., TARAZI, R. C., AND DUSTAN, H. P.: *Use of beta-adrenergic blockade in hypertensive disease,* in KATTUS, A. A. ET AL. (EDS.): *Cardiovascular Beta-Adrenergic Responses.* UCLA Forum in Medical Sciences, No. 13. University of California Press, Los Angeles, 1970, p. 223.

46. FROHLICH, E. D.: *The use of beta-adrenergic blockade in hypertension,* in ONESTI, G. ET AL. (EDS.): *Hypertension: Mechanisms and Management.* Grune & Stratton, Inc., New York, 1973, p. 333.

47. FROHLICH, E. D.: *Beta-adrenergic inhibition in hypertension associated with renal arterial disease,* in FISCHER, J. W. AND CAFRUNY, E. J. (EDS.): *Renal Pharmacology.* Appleton-Century-Crofts Publishing Co., New York, 1971, p. 241.

48. DUSTAN, H. P., TARAZI, R. C., AND FROHLICH, E. D.: *Functional correlates of plasma renin activity in hypertensive patients.* Circulation 41:555, 1970.

49. BÜHLER, F. R., LARAGH, J. H., BAER, L., ET AL.: *Propranolol inhibition of renin secretion.* N. Engl. J. Med. 287:1209, 1972.

50. PRICHARD, B. N. C., AND GILLAM, P. M. S.: *Treatment of hypertension with propranolol.* Br. Med. J. 1:7, 1969.

51. FROHLICH, E. D., AND PAGE, I. H.: *The clinical meaning of cardiovascular beta-adrenergic receptors.* Physiol. Pharmcol. Physicians 1, 1966.

52. TARAZI, R. C., AND DUSTAN, H. P.: *Beta-adrenergic blockade in hypertension. Practical and theoretical implications of long-term hemodynamic variation.* Am. J. Cardiol. 29:633, 1972.

53. LAVERTY, R., AND TAYLOR, K. M.: *Propranolol uptake into the central nervous system and the effect on rat behavior and animal metabolism.* J. Pharm. Pharmacol. 20:605, 1968.

54. ISHIZAKI, T., PRIVITERA, P. H., WALLE, T., ET AL.: *Cardiovascular actions of a new metabolite of propranolol: Isopropylamine.* J. Pharmacol. Exp. Ther. 189:626, 1974.

55. FROHLICH, E. D.: *The practical management of hypertension.* Curr. Probl. Cardiol. 1:1, 1976.

56. FROHLICH, E. D.: *Hypertension and angina pectoris: pathophysiology and treatment.* JAMA, in press.

57. FROHLICH, E. D.: *Hypertension,* in CONN, H. F. (ED.): *Current Therapy 1976.* W. B. Saunders Company, Philadelphia, 1976, p. 208.

58. DUSTAN, H. P., TARAZI, R. C., AND BRAVO, E. L.: *Dependence of arterial pressure on intravascular volume in treated hypertensive patients* N. Engl. J. Med. 286:861, 1972.

59. FROHLICH, E. D., TARAZI, R. C., AND DUSTAN, H. P.: *Clinical-physiological correlations in the development of hypertensive heart disease.* Circulation 44:446, 1971.

60. FROHLICH, E. D.: *Clinical physiological classification of hypertensive heart disease in essential hypertension,* in ONESTI, G. ET AL. (EDS.): *Hypertension: Mechanisms and Management.* Grune & Stratton, Inc., New York, 1973, p. 181.

61. SOKOLOW, M., AND PERLOFF, D.: *Five-year survival of consecutive patients with malignant hypertension treated with antihypertensive agents.* Am. J. Cardiol. 6:858, 1960.

62. TARAZI, R. C., MILLER, A., FROHLICH, E. D., ET AL.: *Electrocardiographic changes reflecting left atrial abnormality in hypertension.* Circulation 34:818, 1966.

210

63. TARAZI, R. C., FROHLICH, E. D., AND DUSTAN, H. P.: *Left atrial abnormality and ventricular pre-ejection period in hypertension.* Dis. Chest 55:214, 1969.

64. POTAIN, P. C.: *Du Rhythme Cardiaque Appelée Bruit de Galop. De Son Mécanisme et de sa Valeur Séméiblogique.* Bull. et Mem. Soc. med. hôp., Paris, 2nd series 12:137, 1875.

65. BRAUNWALD, E., AND FRAHM, C. J.: *Studies on Starling's law of the heart. IV. Observations on the hemodynamic functions of the left atrium in man.* Circulation 24:633, 1961.

66. DUNN, F. G., CHANDRARATNA, P. N., BASTA, L. L., ET AL.: *Pathophysiological assessment of hypertensive heart disease by echocardiography.* Am. J. Cardiol. 37:133, 1976.

67. TARAZI, R. C., FROHLICH, E. D., AND DUSTAN, H. P.: *Plasma volume in men with essential hypertension.* N. Engl. J. Med. 278:762, 1968.

68. STARLING, E. H.: *On the absorption of fluids from the connective tissue space.* J. Physiol. (London) 19:312, 1896.

69. SHIPLEY, R. E., AND STUDY, R. S.: *Changes in renal blood flow, extraction of inulin, glomerular filtration rate, tissue pressure, and urine flow with acute alterations of renal artery blood pressure.* Am. J. Physiol. 167:676, 1951.

70. BRUNNER, H. R., LARAGH, J. H., BAER, H., ET AL.: *Essential hypertension: renin and aldosterone, heart attack, and stroke.* N. Engl. J. Med. 286:441, 1972.

71. CONN, J. W., COHEN, E. L., AND ROVNER, D. R.: *Suppression of plasma renin activity in primary aldosteronism.* JAMA 190:213, 1964.

72. PAGE, I H.: *The mosaic theory of arterial hypertension—its interpretation.* Perspect. Biol. Med. 10:325, 1967.

Long-Term Management of Hypertension

Marvin Moser, M.D.

Hypertension remains a major solvable public health problem. It affects approximately one in five or six adult Americans and contributes significantly to approximately 55 percent of all deaths annually in the United States. The risks of having elevated blood pressure have been clearly defined.[1, 2] Its complications are well known. Encouraging results of therapy been widely publicized,[3, 4, 5] yet management of hypertension has not been satisfactory in many areas until recent years. A major reason for this is not necessarily a lack of knowledge, but rather the improper application of appropriate methods of treatment and followup techniques. It is useful, therefore, to review some reasons for these failures before outlining specific treatment methods that are simple, cost-effective, and have proved to be successful over a long-term period.

POSSIBLE REASONS FOR PHYSICIAN FAILURE IN TREATING HYPERTENSION

During the past four or five years, there has been a definite increase in the number of people aware that they have elevated blood pressure and receiving effective medical management, but a significant number of patients with known hypertension are still being inadequately treated (Fig. 1). Part of the problem relates to physician education and reflects the fact that throughout their medical training experience, physicians are oriented toward high technology, crisis care, or end-stage intervention. The management of the stroke patient is complicated and expensive; the treatment of acute pulmonary edema is dramatic; whereas the management of the average asymptomatic hypertensive patient *before* he develops target involvement or end-stage disease is relatively simple. Many medical schools, because of their orientation toward institutional in-patient medicine and, until recent years, their relative neglect of the management of chronic illness in its early stages, have done a relatively poor job in training physicians in this area. Outpatient experience is viewed as a chore, and the best teachers rarely spend a great deal of time teaching in the clinic.

Other basic reasons why some physicians have failed to treat high blood pressure more effectively are: (1) Until recent years, some of them have not taken the data seriously that indicate that a single, casual elevated blood pressure, *either systolic or diastolic*, is of significance in prognosis, Too often a physician will take a blood pressure during an insurance or routine examination when the patient is "nervous," find it elevated, and dismiss the patient with no followup. Available data indicate clearly that a transiently elevated blood pressure is of significance and that such patients are at

213

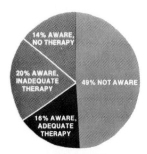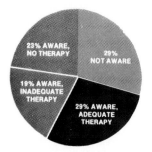

HEALTH AND NUTRITION
EXAMINATION SURVEY
1971 (Preliminary Data)
Computed from
Unpublished Preliminary Data
Furnished by the National
Center for Health Statistics

FOURTEEN COMMUNITIES
FEBRUARY, 1973–JUNE, 1974
Hypertension Detection and
Follow-Up Study, National
Heart and Lung Institute

Figure 1. Percent of hypertensives aware, treated and controlled; National Health Examination Survey, 1971, and followup study, 1973–74. Although the number of adequately treated hypertensive patients almost doubled between 1971 and 1974, over 40 percent of patients who know about their hypertension are still either not being treated or are inadequately treated.

greater risk for developing cardiovascular complications.[6] These individuals should be followed and not ignored. (2) Many physicians are not convinced by the abundantly available data indicating that treatment is effective in reducing the incidence of cardiovascular complications directly related to elevated blood pressure;[3, 4] until they are, they obviously will not be motivated to undertake long-term treatment programs with their patients. (3) The nature of hypertension is such that the patient rarely seeks medical care. Unlike the patient with painful arthritis who will accept the use of medications with potentially serious side effects or injections of steroids into a joint, the patient with hypertension is usually asymptomatic and may not be willing to become involved in a costly or uncomfortable program of treatment. The physician, on the other hand, is concerned about producing side effects in a relatively asymptomatic patient and frequently waits until cardiac enlargement or other complications occur before beginning therapy. (4) Physicians have not been trained to be health educators and often neglect to motivate patients to continue therapy. Motivation of the patient is largely the physician's or health care provider's responsibility. Patients frequently discontinue treatment of high blood pressure because they are unaware of the risk, because they have no symptoms, and because no one has provided them with the basic information that is necessary in the treatment of any chronic illness.

A physician (as a health educator) has the opportunity to provide information, to arrange for proper followup, to control at least partially the expense of a treatment program, and to monitor any drug side effects. He should provide the patient with the following information before any treatment program is instituted: (1) how the patient feels does not always correlate with blood pressure levels; (2) high blood pressure is a life-long condition requiring ongoing treatment; medication cannot usually be stopped after blood pressure is normalized; (3) untreated high blood pressure is a major cause of stroke, heart failure and kidney disease, but it can usually be controlled and the complications prevented in most cases; (4) treatment need not be complicated, costly, or involve a major change in lifestyle.

Although these simple, almost self-evident instructions may not appear to be of importance, they must in fact become an integral part of any treatment program. Long-

214

term management will not usually succeed without both physician and patient motivation. For the past 20 years, I have been using a booklet entitled "How You Can Help Your Doctor Treat Your High Blood Pressure" (available through local American Heart Associations) as an adjunct to the physician's instructions.

HOW DO WE INCREASE THE PERCENTAGE OF EFFECTIVELY TREATED PATIENTS?

Stress Treatment — Not Diagnosis

In many medical centers the obligation to the patient appears to be discharged after diagnostic studies are done. Too many patients are admitted to the hospital or required to return for clinic or office visits four, five or six times to undergo extensive diagnostic studies that are expensive and time consuming. The patient is pleased to learn that no treatable cause has been found for the high blood pressure. Some physicians still believe that "completeness" is necessarily good medical care; some patients equate "thoroughness" with "lots of testing." The patient and the physician have expended much time and effort, but the patient remains untreated.

An example of this type of problem is that of a 49-year-old physician who in 1970 had a blood pressure of 180–200/100–115 mm. Hg and was extensively studied during an 8-day hospitalization at a major medical center. A report to his referring physician from the center stated, "We are pleased to report that all studies were negative for secondary hypertension. If blood pressure remains high, we recommend treatment with a diuretic such as hydrochlorothiazide, 50 mg. a day. As you know, all antihypertensive drugs should be used with care in view of the elevated creatinine level of 1.6–1.8 mg. percent." Six months later, when first seen by us, his blood pressure was 250/140 mm. Hg, and creatinine was 2.5 mg. percent. In view of previous advice, a great deal of persuasion was necessary to convince him and his physician that large dosages of antihypertensive drugs were necessary. On 100 mg. of hydrocholorthiazide, 150 mg. of guanethidine, and 250 mg. of hydralazine daily, blood pressure was normalized. Five years later, the creatinine level was 1.6 mg. percent and the patient normotensive on less medication.

This type of problem will rarely occur if treatment, rather than diagnosis, is emphasized.

A recent report of the Joint National Committee on Detection, Evaluation and Treatment of Hypertension[7] has suggested the following simple, relatively inexpensive, basic workup in the management of hypertension: (1) history and physical exam, (2) urinalysis, (3) hematocrit, (4) blood creatinine or blood urea nitrogen, (5) serum potassium, (6) electrocardiogram, and in many cases, blood sugar, serum cholesterol, uric acid, and chest x-ray. I have followed this simple procedure for over 20 years in both private and clinic practice. Hospitalization has rarely been necessary for a "workup" and cannot be justified merely because the cost is reimbursable in the hospital — reimbursable but at least four to five times as expensive as a simple, outpatient approach. In all cases, where clues from the history, physical examination or laboratory studies suggest secondary hypertension, where an inappropriate response to therapy occurs, or where rapidly progressive hypertension is present, additional studies, such as an intravenous urogram and/or vanillylmandelic acid (VMA), catecholamine and metanephrine levels, can be obtained. In my opinion, peripheral renin levels and 24-hour sodium output are not routinely required prior to starting therapy.

The history and physical exam can be extremely helpful in making an accurate diagnosis. Specifically, what does one look for (Fig. 2)? Essential hypertension is relatively

STUDY	RULES OUT	ESTABLISHES
HISTORY	MOST CASES OF PHEOCHROMOCYTOMA SOME CASES OF ALDOSTERONISM	
PHYSICAL EXAM	COARCTATION OF AORTA MOST CASES OF CUSHINGS DISEASE	SEVERITY OF HYPERTENSION
URINE EXAM	PARENCHYMAL–RENAL DISEASE OF ANY SIGNIFICANCE	
BUN	RENAL FAILURE	
BLOOD POTASSIUM	MOST CASES OF ALDOSTERONISM	
ELECTROCARDIOGRAM		TARGET ORGAN INVOLVEMENT

Figure 2. Outpatient evaluation of the hypertensive patient.

asymptomatic. Conversely, pheochromocytoma patients usually present with symptoms. Also, such patients are rarely obese. Therefore, if a patient has high blood pressure and symptoms, especially episodic "attacks" of headaches, palpitations, nervousness, tremor or excessive sweating, further studies (urinary VMA, catecholamines and/or metanephrines) for pheochromocytoma are indicated. Obviously, only a very small percentage of such symptomatic, thin patients will have a pheochromocytoma, but these are the individuals on whom studies should be done. Furthermore, if there is an inappropriate response to therapy or significant postural hypotension, pheochromocytoma should be suspected.

Most cases of surgically curable aldosteronism occur in young females between the ages of 20 and 40. Many of these patients are symptomatic, especially with polyuria, weakness and muscle cramps. Obviously, these symptoms are not diagnostic, since patients with diabetes or other diseases, such as hyperparathyroidism, may also have them; but they are suggestive of aldosterone excess.

A serum potassium determination will rule out the presence of primary aldosteronism in most cases. This diagnosis should be strongly suspected if the potassium is below 3.2 to 3.5 mEq./L. without therapy or consistently low (below 3.0 mEq./L.) while on diuretics. A simple 24-hour urine collection will help clarify the diagnosis. The presence of hyperaldosteronism would be most unusual if the total urinary potassium output is below 30 to 35 mEq. in the presence of a low serum potassium and an adequate dietary sodium intake of 90 to 100 mEq./day.

Specific diagnostic tests for renovascular disease are reviewed elsewhere. There are certain clinical clues, however, that may help to exclude significant renovascular disease or to suggest those patients who require further study or surgery. For example: (1) Renovascular disease is rare in blacks. (2) Patients who respond best to surgery are those in whom the disease is of relatively short duration. (3) Elderly patients do not do as well when treated surgically as they do on medication. In these patients (over age 50 or 55 years), therefore, it is usually not useful to obtain expensive and time consuming procedures. (4) The presence of a high-pitched, holosystolic murmur with a short diastolic component, heard best to the left or right of the umbilicus, is highly suggestive of a renovascular lesion; in young females, it suggests fibromuscular dysplasia.

A careful history and physical examination, and certain basic tests, therefore, are all that are necessary before undertaking treatment of the average hypertensive patient.

Gifford[8] reported that 94 percent of all patients examined at a hypertension clinic had primary hypertension or chronic renal parenchymal disease which was easily diagnosed by a urinalysis and/or blood urea nitrogen test (Table 1). Only 6 percent, therefore, had potentially curable causes of hypertension. Outside of referral centers, the percentage

Table 1. Frequency of various diagnoses among 4,939 patients seen at the Cleveland Clinic during 1966–1967*

Diagnosis	Percent
Essential hypertension	89
Chronic renal disease	5
Renovascular disease	4
Coarctation	1
Primary aldosteronism	0.5
Cushing's syndrome	0.2
Pheochromocytoma	0.2

*Gifford, R. W.[8]

of secondary hypertension is considerably smaller. Exact figures are not known, but probably the incidence of pheochromocytoma and hyperaldosteronism combined is less than 0.5 percent. Renovascular disease may conceivably account for 1 percent; but even if many of these cases are "missed," medical therapy is often effective.

It is cost-ineffective and may actually represent poor medical practice to submit all hypertensives to exhaustive "workups." This would be true even if the patient's time and resources were unlimited. Perhaps, someday, we will be able to define the exact etiology of hypertension by performing a few simple tests; but at present we must approach treatment in a simple pragmatic way, an approach which has proved to be clinically effective.[9]

TREATMENT OTHER THAN DRUG THERAPY

Many physicians routinely suggest that hypertensive patients be placed on a low-salt diet, obesity be corrected, certain lifestyle changes such as "taking it easy" be implemented, and sedatives or tranquilizers be tried before specific drug therapy is begun. This approach may appear to be correct but is rarely effective in controlling elevated blood pressure other than the mildest forms. Although obesity is more common in hypertensive patients, the prognosis of obese hypertensives may actually be better than that of thin hypertensives. Furthermore, although significant weight loss will lower blood pressure in some obese patients with mild hypertension, it is probable that less than 15 or 20 percent of obese patients will have lost weight at the end of six months to a year, or more importantly, will have sustained the weight loss for any length of time. Therefore, depending upon weight reduction *alone* in the treatment of hypertension is often ineffective and frequently delays necessary therapy. It is important for obese people to lose weight, but while weight is being lost, blood pressure should be treated more specifically with antihypertensive drugs.

There is little doubt that reducing salt intake from the American average of 10 to 12 grams daily to below half a gram per day will lower the blood pressure in a significant number of people. However, this too is impractical, and few patients will remain on this type of rigid diet for longer than a few weeks, *even* if they are well motivated and convinced that this procedure is life-saving. Therefore, it is usually impractical to depend solely on a low-sodium diet for effective management of hypertension. There are some data that demonstrate that the reduction of salt from the usual 10 to 12 grams to 5 or

217

6 grams per day will aid specific drug regimens and may be of some benefit in achieving satisfactory blood pressure control.[10] Patients, therefore, might appropriately be placed on a modified, easily tolerated 5 to 6 gram salt diet, eliminating obviously salty foods such as pretzels, peanuts, bacon, ham, and processed foods.

Too often, patients with hypertension are advised to "change their lifestyle" and their job; yet it has been demonstrated that control of blood pressure can be achieved without dramatic shifts in occupations and the like. In fact, patients rarely can quit their jobs, take longer vacations, take an hour a day off, etc. It has not been necessary, in my experience, to suggest significant changes in lifestyle in order to achieve good treatment results. Obviously, moderation of smoking, lowering high-fat intakes, avoidance of excessive alcohol intake, etc. should be discussed with the patient prior to and during a treatment program for high blood pressure.

Tranquilizers and sedatives should not be depended upon as definitive therapy. There are also no data that transcendental meditation, biofeedback or other types of behavior modification techniques result in significant, permanent lowering of blood pressure other than in a small percentage of patients with mild hypertension.

GUIDELINES FOR TREATMENT

After a patient's blood pressure has been found to be elevated, the following guidelines are useful in determining when specific treatment should be begun.

It is apparent that not everyone with blood pressures greater than 140/90 mm. Hg needs treatment with medication. On the other hand, all patients with diastolic blood pressures higher than 105 mm. Hg should be placed on antihypertensive drug therapy. There are good data to demonstrate that therapy is clearly indicated in the latter patients. Although data are not so definite for patients with diastolic pressures between 90 and 105 mm. Hg, it is appropriate, in my opinion, to treat many of these patients with antihypertensive drugs, especially if they are male, black, or have other risk factors for cardiovascular disease such as diabetes, obesity, or hypercholesterolemia. Patients with high systolic and normal diastolic pressures should also be treated, although there are few studies validating the results of treatment in these patients. Nonetheless, systolic blood pressure elevations increase the risk for cardiovascular disease and should not be ignored.

It should be carefully explained to the patient that medication must be taken indefinitely but that he may not need to be examined more than three or four times a year once blood pressure is controlled. This *seeming* neglect decreases expense of care and has actually resulted in good patient adherence to therapy programs over a 23-year experience in both private and clinic practice. It represents the current recommendation of the Joint National Committee on Hypertension regarding followup patient visits.

ANTIHYPERTENSIVE DRUG THERAPY

Once the diagnosis has been confirmed, after two or more blood pressure readings of 140/90 mm. Hg or higher, and after careful instructions have been given to the patient with "enthusiasm and a 'positive' approach" and a decision to use specific therapy has been made, a wide variety of drugs are available for treatment. Table 2 summarizes the more commonly used antihypertensive drugs and their potential side effects. It is apparent that medications are available that may influence plasma volume (diuretics), vascular resistance (hydralazine), and/or cardiac output (guanethidine, propranolol), specific factors that are believed to be of importance in the pathogenesis of primary hyperten-

Table 2. Characteristics of commonly used oral antihypertensive drugs

Drug	Trade name	Dosage (mg. day)	Side effects
Diuretics			Serum chemistry abnormalities
			↓ Potassium
Hydrochlorothiazide	Hydrodiuril		↑ Uric acid
	Esidrix	50–100	↑ Urea nitrogen
Chlorthalidone	Hygroton	50–100	↑ Blood glucose
Methyclothiazide	Enduron	5–10	Blood dyscrasias, photosensitivity
			Gastrointestinal upsets, pancreatitis*
Rauwolfia derivatives			Sedation, bradycardia, nasal congestion, night-
Reserpine	Serpasil	0.1–0.25	mares
Whole root	Raudixin	50–100	Depression
			Activation of gastric ulcer
Hydralazine	Apresoline	100–250	Headaches, tachycardia, nausea } when used alone
			Increase in angina pectoris
			Rheumatoid-like syndrome, lupus reaction†
Guanethidine	Ismelin	10–150 or more	Weakness, diarrhea, loss of ability to ejaculate
			Orthostatic hypotension
Methyldopa	Aldomet	500–2500	Drowsiness, depression, edema, impotence
			Abnormal liver function tests, fever
			Orthostatic hypotension
Propranolol	Inderal	40–480	Insomnia, bradycardia, bronchospasm, heart failure, sedation
Clonidine	Catapres	0.1–1.5	Drowsiness, fatigue, dry mouth
Prazosin	Minipress	1–10	Syncope (first or second dose)

*Many side effects, for example, blood dyscrasias and pancreatitis, are rare with diuretics.
†Rare with doses under 300 mg.

sion. Figure 3 outlines the approach to therapy that we have used successfully for many years. Most cases of mild to moderate hypertension should be started on a thiazide or thiazide-like diuretic (Step 1 drug).

Diuretic agents represent a cost-effective, simple approach to therapy in the vast majority of cases. Approximately 30 to 40 percent of all patients with mild to moderate hypertension will respond to these drugs alone. In a recent series from the Bahamas, approximately 70 percent of patients achieved and maintained normotensive blood pressure levels on diuretic therapy alone.[11] Most of these patients were black, where the incidence of low-renin, diuretic-responsive hypertension is somewhat higher than in the general population. Despite the fact that diuretics are so effective, approximately 25 to 30 percent of all prescriptions in the United States for initial treatment are written for second-step drugs such as alpha methyldopa, rauwolfia, or propranolol. If, after an appropriate time, depending upon the severity of the disease, blood pressure is not reduced to normotensive levels by a diuretic drug alone, the addition of one of several drugs is appropriate (Step 2). Whole root rauwolfia, in doses of 50 to 100 mg. daily (or reserpine 0.1 to 0.25 mg. per day), alpha methyldopa, in graduating doses from 500 mg. to as high as 2500 mg. daily, or propranolol, in doses of 40 mg. to as high as 480 mg. per day, are possible additions to diuretic therapy. If one of these combinations is not effective (they will be in over 60 to 70 percent of cases), the addition of hydralazine, in dosages between 25 and 300 mg. daily, to the rauwolfia-thiazide, propranolol-thiazide, or methyldopa-thiazide combination is indicated (Step 3). In a recent report, 88 percent

SEVERITY	DRUGS OF CHOICE	ADDITIONAL PRESCRIPTION IF NEEDED
GRADE I, WITH NO ORGAN SYSTEM INVOLVEMENT A. DIASTOLIC BP >90–<110 mmHg	1. ORAL DIURETIC	2. RAUWOLFIA OR 3. HYDRALAZINE OR 4. PROPRANOLOL OR 5. ALPHAMETHYLDOPA
B. DIASTOLIC BP >110 mmHg	1 AND 2 ABOVE PLUS HYDRALAZINE	PROPRANOLOL OR ALPHAMETHYLDOPA OR GUANETHIDINE OR CLONIDINE
GRADE II OR III, WITH HEART KIDNEY OR BRAIN INVOLVEMENT DIASTOLIC BP'S USUALLY >110 mmHg	1. ORAL DIURETIC 2. RAUWOLFIA 3. GUANETHIDINE	PROPRANOLOL HYDRALAZINE ALPHAMETHYLDOPA ADDITIONAL DIURETICS CLONIDINE

Figure 3. Recommended drug therapy for ambulatory patients with hypertension.

of male patients with mild to moderately severe hypertension responded satisfactorily to a rauwolfia-thiazide regimen; 81 percent responded to propranolol-thiazide therapy.[20] If normotensive or near normotensive blood prssure levels are not obtained with triple drug therapy, the addition or substitution of guanethidine for one of the other sympathetic blocking drugs, such as alpha methyldopa, is frequently effective (Step 4). The use of guanethidine, in dosages between 10 and 200 mg. per day, will frequently change a poor result to a good one in the more severe cases.

Clonidine, a centrally acting sympathetic blocking drug, and prazosin, a vasodilator, have recently been approved for use as antihypertensive drugs. They are moderately potent and can be substituted for one of the Step 2 or Step 3 drugs.

Treatment must be pursued in all cases to a goal of normotensive or near normotensive levels, keeping in mind the benefits of therapy versus the risks of uncontrolled hypertension. In some elderly patients, it may be necessary to accept a less than optimal fall in blood pressure. For example, it is frequently impossible to lower a 70-year-old patient's blood pressure from 200/90 mm. Hg to normotensive levels; 160–170/80 mm. Hg may have to be accepted as "optimal therapy" because of side effects.

Patients with substantial blood pressure elevation (diastolic pressure greater than 115 mm. Hg) should probably be seen at 1- to 2-week intervals while drug therapy is being adjusted. Patients with blood pressures between 140/90 and 170–180/110–115 mm. Hg may be seen every 2 to 4 weeks until blood pressure is regulated.

PROBLEM OF DRUG SIDE EFFECTS

Since concern about producing side effects is one of the causes of poor physician adherence in treatment programs and a major reason why some patients discontinue therapy, it is appropriate to review the more significant side effects of antihypertensive drugs (Table 2).

Diuretics are frequently withheld because of the fear of producing hypokalemia. The average decrease in serum potassium while on thiazide therapy is approximately 0.5 mEq. (from a range of 4.2–4.5 to 3.7–4.0 mEq./L.). The majority of patients who experience this mild reduction, however, remain asymptomatic over many years. The initial fear that hypokalemic myocardiopathy or renal tubular damage would occur in these patients has proved to be unfounded. In elderly patients, in patients receiving digitalis, or in patients with renal disease, this degree of potassium loss may be significant, and dietary or drug supplements or potassium-sparing drugs may be required to either prevent or correct it. In the majority of patients, dietary supplements at the beginning of treatment, before depletion occurs, plus moderate sodium restriction, which decreases the amount of sodium available for distal renal tubular potassium-sodium exchange, are usually effective in preventing significant hypokalemia. Patients are given a simple diet sheet to follow (Table 3). In patients who develop significant hypokalemia (below 3.3 mEq./L.) and/or patients who develop symptoms of weakness, fatigue, muscle cramps, etc., with less severe degrees of hypokalemia, the use of potassium supplements in the form of tablets or liquid (K Lyte, Kaon, Slow K, etc.) may be necessary. In some instances, the use of potassium-sparing agents such as triamterene is necessary. The fear of producing hypokalemia should not deter the physician from treating all hypertensive patients with diuretic drugs.

Pretreatment hyperuricemia, or a history of gout, should also not prevent physicians from treating hypertensive patients with diuretic agents. An example of how this concern resulted in a poor treatment result is that of a 58-year-old male with long-standing hypertension (Fig. 4).

The patient was treated over a 2-year period of time on many different medications in small doses, with a poor blood pressure response. Adequate diuretic therapy was not used by his physician because of an initially elevated uric acid level. In 1972 therapy was increased as noted, with a prompt fall in blood pressure. Pressures have remained normal for four years with treatment. Side effects from thera-

Table 3. Diet, potassium and blood pressure lowering drugs

Your high blood pressure is being treated with a medication called a diuretic. This drug increases the amount of salt or sodium that is washed out of your body. Diuretics may also cause a decrease in the body stores of another mineral called potassium. Most of the time, an adequate diet will prevent excess potassium loss. In some cases, especially when symptoms of muscle cramps or weakness occur, it may be necessary to give extra potassium as a tablet or liquid, or use medications that will prevent potassium loss.

The following lists may give you an idea of which foods to eat or stay away from in order to keep your potassium intake high and your salt or sodium intake low.

Foods relatively high in potassium but also high in sodium or salt (should be avoided, if possible):

Tomato juice, canned	Peas, frozen
Clams, raw	Spinach, canned
Sardines	Carrots, canned
Lima beans, frozen	

Foods relatively high in potassium and low in sodium (extra amounts will prevent a potassium deficiency):

Fruits	Fruit Juices	Vegetables
Apples	Apple	Asparagus
Apricots	Grapefruit	Beans, white or green
Avocado	Prune	Brussels sprouts
*Banana	*Orange	Cabbage
Cantaloupe		Cauliflower
Dates		Corn on the cob
Grapefruit		Lima beans, fresh, cooked
Nectarines		Peas, green, cooked
Orange		Peppers
Prunes		*Potato, baked or boiled
*Raisins		Radish
Watermelon		Squash

*Especially helpful.

221

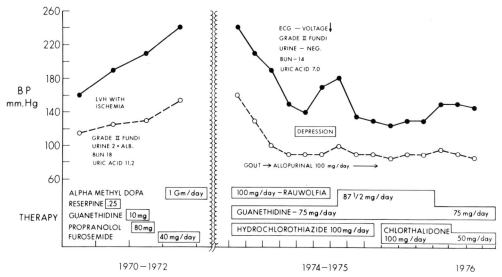

Figure 4. Dramatic improvement in results of treatment when adequate dosages of antihypertensive drugs were used.

py included a depressive reaction (rauwolfia was stopped) and an episode of gout (uric acid levels were reduced by use of allopurinal). Despite these problems, there is little question that the benefit of blood pressure lowering in a patient with this severe degree of hypertensive vascular disease is greater than the risk of therapy.

I have frequently observed such patients who were not treated adequately because of the fear of producing gout and who progressed to experience a significant complication of hypertension.

Rauwolfia drugs are frequently not employed because of their potential depressant effect. In some cases, this effect is dose related. It has been relatively uncommon in our experience when only 50 mg. of whole root rauwolfia or 0.1 mg. of reserpine per day has been used. The addition of rauwolfia to diuretic therapy has often made management simpler, especially in those cases with an initially high systolic blood pressure, i.e., the labile hypertensive with a "hyperkinetic" heart. If dreams, nightmares or insomnia occur, rauwolfia should be discontinued. The drug should not be used in patients with a history of emotional illness.

Some investigators favor the use of the beta blockers, such as propranolol, as the Step 2 drug of choice in patients with tachycardia and/or a relatively high systolic blood pressure. While this drug is often effective with a thiazide diuretic, it is relatively costly and at least 2 to 4 tablets/day are usually necessary.

Some physicians no longer prescribe rauwolfia drugs in women, following reports of an association between breast cancer and rauwolfia use.[12] Recent data, however, have failed to substantiate this association.[13, 14] At present there is little reason to withhold the use of this drug in women. Additional studies are underway in an effort to clarify this issue.

Alpha methyldopa will occasionally produce depression, fatigue, and rarely a high fever and abnormal liver function tests. If a patient experiences these manifestations, the drug should be discontinued and another drug substituted. Fortunately, there are

222

many different drugs available; it is uncommon for a patient not to be controlled on one or another combination.

Propranolol is the only beta blocking agent available in the United States for treatment of hypertension. It is most effective in patients with tachycardia and, in combination with a thiazide and hydralazine, will lower blood pressure in a high percentage of patients regardless of the initial severity of their hypertension. Troublesome side effects include marked bradycardia and insomnia. The drug should be used with care or avoided in patients with a history of asthma or congestive heart failure. It is frequently necessary to use large doses of this drug to achieve an effect (320 mg./day or more). This must be kept in mind when planning a treatment program, especially since cost and a large number of pills frequently deter patients from continuing treatment.

Hydralazine is a relatively safe drug and an effective vasodilator. It should usually be used with a rauwolfia drug or a beta blocker such as propranolol so that possible secondary effects on the cardiovascular system, i.e., reflex tachycardia and/or increase in cardiac output, will not occur. The fear of producing a lupus-like syndrome should not prevent the use of this drug, since these reactions are extremely rare with doses of 300 mg./day or less.

Clonidine can produce a dry mouth and drowsiness. Frequently, this is not tolerated by the patient, and the drug must be stopped. Initial doses of *prazosin* may produce severe hypotension and syncope. The drug should be used in small initial dosage of 1.0 mg., but may be increased to as high as 10 to 15 mg./day.

Guanethidine is an extremely effective antihypertensive drug. In my experience, it is not used frequently enough or in appropriate dosages. Postural hypotension may occur, but this represents a physiologic and not a toxic effect of the drug. It often signals the fact that blood pressure has been lowered significantly. Frequently, the physician stops the drug immediately when the patient complains of postural hypotension or dizziness, instead of readjusting the dosage. In my experience, this drug is generally safe to use if dosage is gradually increased and if the patient is told to reduce the dosage himself should early morning dizziness occur.

Ejaculatory impotence is a significant side effect of guanethidine. Impotence may occur with any of the antihypertensive agents except possibly propranolol and hydralazine. If this occurs in a patient with marked pretreatment hypertension, it is often necessary to convince him to tolerate the side effect for at least a short period of time in the hope that blood pressure will be lowered and drug dosage reduced at a later date. If the patient initially has only mild hypertension and this is not controlled by thiazides, a combination of medications can usually be found that does not have a significant effect on potency. (Intermittent drug intake may be effective in this situation).

A major mistake in the medical management of hypertension, in addition to making management too complex and expensive, is that medication is not changed or altered until a goal of normotensive or near normotensive blood pressure levels is achieved.

An example of a good long-term result in a patient who "battled through" side effects is that of a 42-year-old asymptomatic male who was discovered to be hypertensive in 1953 during a routine insurance examination (Fig. 5). Blood pressures of 240–250/140–150 mm. Hg were recorded, to his amazement. Left ventricular hypertrophy was noted; funduscopic examination showed Grade 2 retinopathy; and BUN of 13.6 mg. percent was recorded. The patient was treated with rauwolfia, 50 mg. per day, and hydralazine in increasing dosages up to 600 mg. per day (doses considerably higher than are now recommended). Mecamylamine, a ganglion blocker no longer in use except in rare cases, was added to the regimen and blood pressure was gradually reduced as noted. The patient developed a syndrome

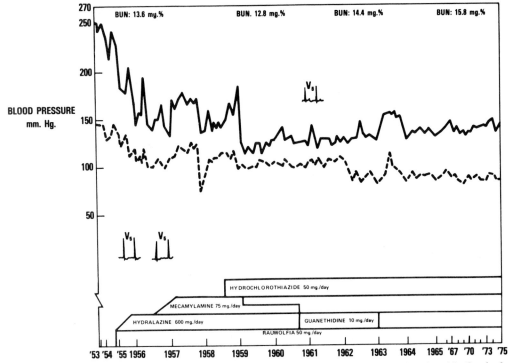

Figure 5. Long-term response to adequate antihypertensive therapy of 42-year-old male with Grade 2 retinopathy.

of fever, pleuritic pain, and abnormal liver function tests with a positive lupus prep; and hydralazine was discontinued. He was maintained on steroid therapy for approximately six weeks before symptoms cleared. When thiazide diuretics were introduced in 1957, the patient was placed on chlorothiazide, 1 gram per day, and later on hydrochlorothiazide, 50 mg./day. Since that time he has been maintained on thiazide therapy, guanethidine in dosages between 10 and 30 mg./day, and rauwolfia, 50 mg./day. He has remained normotensive for approximately 17 years and is asymptomatic. A marked decrease in voltage on the electrocardiogram and improvement in the previously abnormal ST segments and T waves have occurred. The tracing is now normal. Kidney function has remained within normal limits.

This patient demonstrates an excellent long-term response to adequate antihypertensive therapy. A mortality rate of 50 percent within five years would have been expected in a similar patient who had remained untreated. The patient experienced significant side effects but was able to tolerate them because of a high degree of motivation. His prognosis now is excellent.

HOME BLOOD PRESSURE READINGS

Some investigators have advocated the use of home blood pressure recordings as an important factor in increasing patient adherence to therapy. Knowledge of the blood pressure levels is intended to motivate patients to continue with treatment. While there are some patients (about 10 percent in my experience) who benefit from this approach, I do not believe that in the majority of cases home recording is necessary for effec-

224

tive management. Home monitoring of patients with more serious degrees of hypertensive vascular disease who may be on multiple drugs may be useful until blood pressure control is achieved; in the majority, however, it tends to increase blood pressure consciousness. Home recordings are useful in patients who live far from a source of medical care or whose occupation may put them at some risk if blood pressure were to be lowered excessively.

RESULTS OF EFFECTIVE MANAGEMENT

In a series of 242 hypertensive patients followed over a 19-year period of time (average 8.9 years), 85 percent were controlled using the aforementioned approach (Table 4).[15] Data from the Veterans Administration study and others[16-19] have clearly established the fact that blood pressure control over a long period of time will: (1) reduce both morbidity and mortality of hypertension; (2) dramatically increase survival from zero percent to more than 40 percent over a 5 to 10 year period of time in patients who present with malignant hypertension; (3) prevent accelerated or malignant hypertension if blood pressure is treated early; (4) reduce recurrence rates in patients with pretreatment cerebrovascular accidents from an average of 45 to 50 percent over a 5-year period of time to less than 20 to 25 percent; and (5) reduce the incidence of angina pectoris and decrease evidence of left ventricular hypertrophy on x-ray or the electrocardiogram in more than 50 percent of cases.

Most studies have failed to demonstrate a statistically significant reduction in the incidence of myocardial infarction in treated patients. No data are available, however, on a group of male patients whose treatment was begun during the first few years of blood pressure elevation and continued over a long period of time. These data are presently being accumulated.

Another unanswered question relates to the results of treatment of the less severe hypertensive. Are they sufficiently encouraging to warrant therapy of all patients with mildly elevated blood pressure? The answer to this question is also being sought in a multicenter long-term clinical trial.

SUMMARY

The ambulatory management of hypertension is relatively simple. A key factor in the success of any program is motivation of both the physician and the patient. Workup should be limited to a few simple tests as outlined; need rarely, if ever, involve hospitalization; and can be completed in one or two office or clinic visits. Treatment of hyper-

Table 4. Effect of antihypertensive drug therapy on blood pressure*

	Number of patients	Pretreatment diastolic blood pressure level (mm. Hg)	Blood pressure results		
			Excellent	Fair	Poor
	51	115+	40	4	7
	128	105–114	112	10	6
	63	90–104	54	6	3
Total	242		206 (85%)	20 (8%)	16 (7%)

*Moser, M.[15]

tension over a long-term period involves the use of specific drug therapy, although some slight modification of lifestyle or diet is occasionally helpful. There are numerous drugs available, and in over 80 to 85 percent of cases, an effective combination can be found. Drug therapy must be continuous; it is rare, in our experience, that medication can be completely discontinued. Data available from the Veterans Administration study, as well as my own, clearly indicate that effective lowering of blood pressure over a long period of time is cost-effective and delays or prevents numerous complications that are frequently noted in untreated patients.

REFERENCES

1. SOKOLOW, M., AND PERLOFF, D.: *The prognosis of essential hypertension treated conservatively.* Circulation 23:697, 1961.
2. KANNEL, W. B., WOLF, P. A., VERTER, J., ET AL.: *Epidemiologic assessment of the role of blood pressure in stroke. The Framingham study.* JAMA 214:301, 1970.
3. MOSER, M.: *Management of essential hypertension,* in MOSER, M. (ED): *Hypertension: A Practical Approach.* Little, Brown and Co., Boston, 1975, pp. 115–142.
4. VETERANS ADMINISTRATION COOPERATIVE STUDY: *Effects of treatment on morbidity in hypertension.* JAMA 202:116, 1967.
5. PERRY, M.: *Survival of treated hypertensive patients.* JAMA 210:890, 1969.
6. PAFFENBARGER, R. S., THORNE, M. C., AND WING, A. L.: *Chronic disease in former college students.* Am. J. Epidemiol. 88:25, 1968.
7. Report of the Joint National Committee on Detection, Evaluation and Treatment of High Blood Pressure, available through National High Blood Pressure Information Center, National Institutes of Health, Bethesda, Md.
8. GIFFORD, R. W.: *Evaluation of the hypertensive patient with emphasis on detecting curable causes.* Milbank Mem. Fund Q. 47:170, 1969.
9. MOSER, M.: *A simplified approach to hypertension.* Am. Fam. Physician 7:117, 1973.
10. PARIJS, J.: *Moderate sodium restriction and diuretics in the treatment of hypertension.* Am. Heart J. 85: 22, 1973.
11. LUNN, J., AND MOSER, M.: Unpublished observations.
12. BOSTON COLLABORATIVE DRUG SURVEILLANCE PROGRAM: *Reserpine and breast cancer.* Lancet 2:669, 1974.
13. O'FALLON, W. M., LABARTHE, D. R., AND KURLAND, L. T.: *Rauwolfia derivatives and breast cancer.* Lancet 2:292, 1975.
14. LASKA, E. M., SIEGEL, C., MEISNER, M., ET AL.: *Matched-pairs study of reserpine use and breast cancer.* Lancet 2:296, 1975.
15. MOSER, M.: *Office management of hypertension.* Am. Fam. Physician 10:152, 1974.
16. MARSHALL, J.: *A trial of long-term hypotensive therapy in cerebrovascular disease.* Lancet 1:10, 1964.
17. BARNETT, A. J., AND SILBERBERG, F. G.: *Long-term results of treatment of severe hypertension.* Med. J. Aust. Nov. 24, 1973, p. 960.
18. BEEVERS, D. G., HAMILTON, M., FAIRMAN, M. J., ET AL.: *Antihypertensive treatment and the course of established cerebral vascular disease.* Lancet 1:1407, 1973.
19. POBLETE, P. F., KYLE, M. C., PIPBERGER, H. V., ET AL.: *Effect of treatment on morbidity in hypertension.* Circulation 48:481, 1973.
20. VETERANS ADMINISTRATION COOPERATIVE STUDY GROUP ON ANTIHYPERTENSIVE DRUGS: *Propranolol in the treatment of essential hypertension.* JAMA 237:2303, 1977.

Management of Complicated Hypertension Including Hypertensive Emergencies

David W. Richardson, M.D., and A. Jarrell Raper, M.D.

The primary goal in management of high blood pressure is its detection and elimination before onset of complications produced by hypertensive damage to the heart or to the arterial blood vessels such as:

1. Encephalopathy and the renal and retinal ravages of fibrinoid necrosis of the small arterial vessels.
2. Intracerebral hemorrhage, subarachnoid hemorrhage, and dissecting aortic hematoma, all the result of rupture of arteries.
3. Ischemic myocardial and cerebral disease, the result of narrowing or blockage of larger arteries.
4. Heart failure, the result of increased load on the left ventricle, often with added narrowing of the coronary arteries.

The management of uncomplicated hypertension and of renal failure produced by hypertension is presented in other chapters. Here we discuss the complications listed above with special attention to hypertensive emergencies, i.e., those conditions defined arbitrarily as requiring reduction of blood pressure within a few hours (Table 1).

When blood pressure is very high, e.g., above 240/140 mm. Hg, with or without clinical evidence of fibrinoid necrosis, intracranial hemorrhage is the only irreparable catastrophe preventable by abrupt reduction in pressure. The risk of bleeding into the brain in the ensuing two days probably does not exceed the troubles produced by sudden lowering of pressure (cardiac or cerebral ischemia), and achievement of a lowered blood pressure within 48 hours rather than in two hours seems reasonable in the absence of the complications listed in Table 1.

Subsequent sections of this review consider the definition, pathogenesis, diagnosis, and management of these complications of hypertension.

ACCELERATED PHASE (MALIGNANT PHASE) OF HYPERTENSION
Definition

The accelerated (malignant) phase of hypertension is a clinical diagnosis, suspected when patients with very high blood pressure show the clinical findings listed below, and confirmed by disappearance of these manifestations when blood pressure is reduced. The manifestations may be ocular (acute hypertensive retinopathy), renal (malignant nephrosclerosis), or may involve the central nervous system (hypertensive encepha-

Table 1. Common hypertensive emergencies

Emergency	Underlying anatomic defect	Underlying functional abnormality	Drugs of choice	Goal* mm. Hg
A. Rapid Reduction of Elevated Pressure of Proven Benefit				
1. Hypertensive, encephalopathy	Fibrinoid arteriolar necrosis	Cerebral edema?	Nitroprusside Diazoxide	150/95
2. Dissection of aorta	Medial necrosis?	Unknown	Trimethaphan	110/70
3. Pulmonary edema	None, or coronary or valvar	Left ventricular failure	Nitroprusside Diazoxide Diuretic	150/95
B. Rapid Reduction of Pressure Rational, Not of Proven Benefit				
1. Intracranial hemorrhage	Cerebral microaneurysm?	Weakened wall of cerebral artery?	Nitroprusside	20% Reduction?
2. Catecholamine excess	Pheochromocytoma	MAO inhibitor Clonidine withdrawal	Phentolamine	150/95
3. Acute myocardial infarction	Coronary artery narrowing	Coronary occlusion?	Nitroglycerin	20 mm. Hg Reduction

*To be achieved in first six hours. Subsequent further reduction in blood pressure may be desirable.

lopathy). In time, all three organ systems will be affected, but in early stages, only one or two may be abnormal.[1]

Acute Hypertensive Retinopathy

This manifestation of accelerated hypertension is recognized by linear striate or flame-shaped hemorrhages oriented with their long axis radiating out from the optic disc, or fluffy irregular exudates, with long axis similarly placed. The diagnosis is made certain by disappearance of these lesions upon successful lowering of the blood pressure to the normal range (see below) and by clinical evaluation excluding other causes (bacterial endocarditis, gastrointestinal hemorrhage, blood dyscrasias). Papilledema may occur, but is not necessary to make the diagnosis.

Hypertensive Encephalopathy

This is characterized by generalized cerebral dysfunction, i.e., lethargy, somnolence, coma, or convulsions, and sometimes by fleeting subtle neurological deficits in various locations. Marked or stable neurological deficit is not present. Other causes for similar dysfunction should be ruled out (drugs, severe uremia). The diagnosis is made certain when the cerebral state returns to normal after successful control of the blood pressure (see below).

Malignant Nephrosclerosis

This diagnosis is suspected when severe hypertension is accompanied by otherwise unexplained hematuria and proteinuria. Late in the patient's course, the creatinine clearance may be markedly reduced and BUN and creatinine elevated (these abnormalities are not necessary to make the diagnosis). The diagnosis is made certain by gradual clearing of the urinary findings (proteinuria and hematuria) after adequate control of the blood pressure. The subsequent behavior of renal function is variable (see below).[2]

Pathogenesis of Accelerated Phase

Pickering has shown that the changes of the accelerated phase may occur in hypertension of *any* etiology, as long as the hypertension is severe.[1] Diastolic blood pressures of 125 to 135 mm. Hg or more are necessary; the presence of milder hypertension should lead one to suspect that the diagnosis is mistaken. The vascular walls undergo progressive damage in which protein-rich material leaks from the blood stream into the muscular layers, culminating in fibrinoid necrosis of small arteries and arterioles (the material labelled "fibrinoid" is in actuality fibrin). These vessels then leak red cells and protein, and may thrombose. The lesions seen with the ophthalmoscope in acute retinopathy have been shown at autopsy in the brains of victims of hypertensive encephalopathy and in the kidneys at autopsy or on renal biopsy.[3] Whether arteriolar spasm or dilation produce the loss of integrity of the vessels is still controversial. See Gifford for thoughtful review.[4]

Recognition and Differential Diagnosis

In patients whose blood pressure is well controlled, little attention need be placed upon recognition of the above manifestations — as they do not occur. In a patient with markedly elevated blood pressure, evidence of acute retinopathy, cerebral dysfunction, and altered renal function or hematuria should be sought frequently.

It is evident that other conditions may mimic each of the aforementioned clinical syndromes. Thus, acute hypertensive retinopathy can be mimicked (though not exactly) by hemorrhagic disorders, by endocarditis, or by gastrointestinal hemorrhage; hypertensive encephalopathy can be mimicked by subarachnoid hemorrhage or metabolic or chemical brain disorders; and malignant nephrosclerosis can be mimicked by tumor, stone, infection, or renal inflammation of other causes.

Management of Accelerated Hypertension

How Rapidly Should Blood Pressure Be Reduced?

Clinical evidence of fibrinoid arteriolar necrosis is an urgent indication for reduction of blood pressure within one or two days. Renal function deteriorates rapidly in the untreated malignant phase, and prognosis for survival is greatly decreased by the presence of renal failure.[5] Reduction of blood pressure lessens the likelihood that renal failure will develop,[6] and prevents encephalopathy. Presentation with encephalopathy is usually considered to demand reduction in pressure within a few hours, though complete recovery has occurred after many days of encephalopathy. There is no clear evidence that very rapid lowering of pressure is of special benefit for encephalopathy, but the dramatic return of sanity which follows within a few hours after reduction of pressure is gratifying to all concerned. Worry about cerebral or myocardial ischemia[7, 8] produced by instant fall in blood pressure in the unrecognized presence of narrowing by plaques of cerebral or coronary arteries has led clinicians in large medical centers to prefer intravenous nitroprusside, with which pressure can be gradually lowered over several hours. Nitroprusside requires the continual presence of nurse or physician as long as it is used, to observe blood pressure and readjust infusion rate. Diazoxide, despite the rapidity with which its maximum antihypertensive effect occurs, 1 or 2 minutes after rapid intravenous injection, has an impressive safety record[9, 10] and is the drug of first choice when intensive care is not easily available. Alternatively, the aim of good control of blood pressure within 72 hours using oral drugs is also reasonable, but there are no comparisons of regimens with differing rates of reduction in blood pressure on the prognosis of patients who have entered the accelerated phase of hypertension.

How Far Should Blood Pressure Be Reduced?

Nitroprusside or diazoxide can lower arterial pressure within minutes or hours to any desired level. Should blood pressure be reduced to normal? The retinal signs of the malignant phase may disappear with very modest reduction in blood pressure.[11] Cerebral blood flow falls when blood pressure is lowered with trimethaphan below 160/100 mm. Hg in men with pretreatment pressure averaging 206/132, but symptoms of cerebral ischemia occur only when pressure falls to about 110/50 mm. Hg.[12] These data plus rare anecdotal experience of hemiparesis or prolonged pain attributable to myocardial ischemia (Fig. 1) when systolic blood pressure is abruptly reduced below 130 mm. Hg suggest 150 to 160 mm. Hg as a reasonable goal for the first few days.

Are There Specific Antihypertensive Drugs to Avoid in Acute Management of Accelerated Hypertension?

The currently popular hypothesis of the pathogenesis of encephalopathy, that dilation of cerebral arteries unable to cope with very high intraluminal pressure allows leak of intravascular fluid into the brain, suggests avoidance of drugs whose major mechanism of antihypertensive action is arteriolar dilation. Extensive experience in managing encephalopathy with diazoxide,[9, 13] a drug whose sole antihypertensive action is

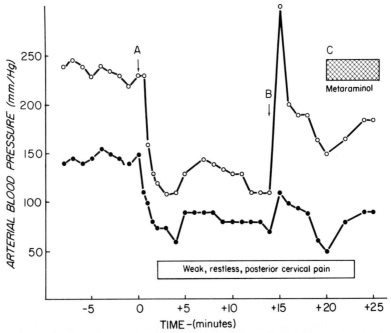

Figure 1. Unusual response to diazoxide. At A, diazoxide 300 mg. was injected intravenously in about 10 seconds. The patient developed neck pain similar to discomfort previously present during brisk walking. At B, she received epinephrine 0.3 mg. intravenously.

arteriolar dilation, effectively refutes the suggestion. Clearing of encephalopathy within one or two hours is the expected accompaniment of intravenous administration of diazoxide,[13] which remains the most convenient drug of great efficacy in the acute management of hypertensive encephalopathy. Nitroprusside, with which blood pressure can be gradually reduced (Fig. 2), also works by dilating peripheral arterioles.

Reserpine is best avoided. Response of blood pressure to a given dose varies widely in onset, magnitude and duration, and parenteral reserpine regularly clouds the sensorium. Parenteral hydralazine and methyldopa require several hours to achieve maximum reduction in blood pressure, and are probably less consistently effective in lowering pressure than diazoxide or nitroprusside.

Long-Term Management of Accelerated Hypertension

For patients who present in the accelerated phase of hypertension, a maintenance regimen including three drugs is usually required to maintain blood pressure below 160/95 mm. Hg. Hydralazine and a diuretic (thiazide if renal function is near normal; furosemide if BUN exceeds 50 or creatinine 5 mg. percent) are two usual components. Propranolol is first choice for the third drug because of a lower incidence of severe side effects. The reliability of propranolol, that is the proportion of patients with accelerated hypertension whose blood pressure it will control, is as yet uncertain. Methyldopa and guanethidine remain acceptable alternatives.

The maintenance regimen should be started as soon as the patient can take oral medications, to allow freedom from the encumbrance of intravenous infusions and to provide as much time as possible in the hospital for selection of the ideal dose of the drugs to be used for management. Methyldopa certainly, and hydralazine probably, interferes with measurement of urinary catecholamines, but not vanillylmandelic acid (VMA).

Diagnostic Management of Accelerated Hypertension

The presence of the accelerated phase indicates hypertensive disease severe enough to require a drug regimen which is complex, expensive, and usually unpleasant. Pro-

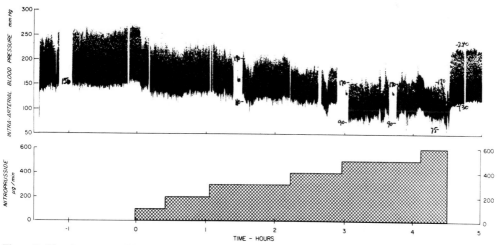

Figure 2. Usual response of blood pressure to nitroprusside. The upper record is intra-arterial blood pressure recorded at very slow paper speed. The top of the black band is systolic and the bottom of the band is diastolic pressure. Increases in the rate of nitroprusside infusion can be made as often as every five minutes to reduce blood pressure more rapidly.

231

longed adherence to such a regimen is difficult; therefore, discovery of a surgically correctable cause for the hypertension is especially valuable. Further, patients who have been in the accelerated phase are at increased risk for its recurrence; full evaluation including measurement of urinary catecholamines or VMA and arteriography to detect renal artery stenosis are a part of good management. Primary hyperaldosteronism very rarely produces fibrinoid necrosis; conversely in the accelerated phase of hypertension, hyperaldosteronism secondary to renal ischemia is common. Measurement of plasma or urinary aldosterone concentrations is usually not useful.

Prognosis in Treated Accelerated Hypertension

Drug treatment of accelerated hypertension clearly improves prognosis as compared to untreated patients, though the outlook is not perfect. Harrington, Kincaid-Smith, and McMichael[14] found one year mortality of 30 percent and five year mortality of 70 percent in patients with papilledema and normal renal function at the beginning of treatment. If renal function is abnormal when treatment begins, prognosis is even worse and chronic artificial dialysis is often required.[14, 15]

INTRACEREBRAL HEMORRHAGE

This devastating neurologic catastrophe is most common among hypertensive middle-aged males, and is among the most preventable of hypertensive complications.[6] Once the problem has developed enough for an accurate clinical diagnosis to be made (gross shift of intracranial structures, with or without bloody spinal fluid) serious neurological damage has already occurred. A complex clinical picture is present. Severe hypertension may have preceded the event, but the hypertension may also occur partly or wholly in reaction to ischemic brain tissue and/or raised intracranial pressure (it is possible that the raised arterial pressure serves as a "protective reflex").[16] Most disconcerting is the advancing neurological deficit, which will most likely worsen, whatever the management of the blood pressure.

Management of hypertension in this setting has not been systematically studied. Meyer[17] has reported a series of patients with intracerebral hemorrhage treated with antihypertensive agents; those whose hypertension was reduced fared better. However, his study is subject to criticism in regard to several matters of design and execution; firm conclusions are not warranted. The Clinical Management Study Group recommends a partial control of hypertension; 20 to 30 percent lowering of systolic pressure if >200 mm. Hg, with a goal of 160/100 mm. Hg if less severe.[16]

The question of the frequency and diagnosis of smaller (arrested) intracerebral hemorrhages with clear cerebrospinal fluid is unresolved. Pathological evidence suggests that such hemorrhages indeed occur, as small areas (lacunes) are found with walls containing hemosiderin-laden macrophages.[1] Diagnosis during life is tenuous, but can be suspected in the presence of a neurological deficit which could be explained by a small lesion, a lesion which does not shift the midline, or does not "show" on brain scan, EEG, or cerebral arteriogram. The CAT (Computerized Axial Tomography) scan of the brain can show small hematomas (1 cm.) in certain locations, and may help in the early diagnosis of some of these lesions. When such a lesion is diagnosed, immediate lowering of the blood pressure into the normal range should not be harmful, but clearcut evidence that this actually helps (by arresting the growth of the hemorrhage) is not available. Of course, the agent used should not be one that might itself cloud mental function, or cause unwanted hypotension (Table 2).

232

Table 2. Drugs for treatment of hypertensive emergencies

Drug	Dose and route	Mechanisms of action	Advantages	Disadvantages
Sodium Nitroprusside	100 μg./min. (or more) by IV titration	Direct vascular smooth muscle vasodilator	Always works, smooth, well tolerated	Requires intensive nursing and precise constant IV infusion
Trimethaphan	3 mg./min. (or more) by IV titration	Sympathetic and parasympathetic ganglionic blockade	Usually effective	Total ganglionic blockade (with GI and GU effects). Severe bradycardia (a few cases). Requires intensive nursing, constant IV infusion.
Diazoxide	300 mg. direct IV bolus in 30 sec.	Direct vascular smooth muscle vasodilator	Effective: After B.P. stabilizes (30 min.), patient does not require intensive care.	B.P. undershoot (sometimes with reactive tachycardia) occurs. May have to be repeated. Fluid retention, hyperglycemia can occur.
Methyldopa	500 mg. IV drip in 30 min.	Central action (on brain alpha receptors)	Smooth, gradual	Slow onset of action (2–5 hours). Drowsiness.
Reserpine	2–5 mg. IM q. 3–5 hours	Depletion of norepinephrine from nerve endings	IV not required	Slow onset (2 hours). Great drowsiness. Not suitable in neurological cases. Toxicity frequent if used for long. Erratic control.
Hydralazine	10–20 mg. (or more) IM q. 3–4 hours	Direct vascular smooth muscle vasodilator	IV not required	Erratic control. Cardiac stimulation.
Phentolamine	5 mg. (or more) IV intermittently as needed	Alpha blockade and direct vasodilator	Rapid. Specific for catecholamine excess.	Erratic duration of effect. Frequent IV dose by physician. Not widely applicable.

RUPTURED INTRACRANIAL ANEURYSM
WITH SUBARACHNOID HEMORRHAGE

To some degree this may also be a preventable hypertensive complication; it is theoretically reasonable that blood pressure, especially if raised, contributes to intracranial aneurysm formation and rupture. Clear data to prove that treatment of hypertension prevents this problem are unavailable. Once the subarachnoid hemorrhage has occurred, a complex pathophysiology is present. Raised intracranial pressure and blood-induced cerebral arterial spasm may each contribute to decreased cerebral blood flow; hypertension in this setting may be partially or wholly a protective mechanism, which restores blood flow. It is theoretically possible that lowering the blood pressure to normal in this setting may be counterproductive.[16] It is clear, however, and is generally agreed, that control of the hypertension will help to prevent the *second* hemorrhage, which also carries a high risk.[18] In the face of these conflicting clinical imperatives, various treatment schemes have been advanced, without a clear advantage proven for any. Indeed, a large cooperative study, which came to the conclusion that antihypertensive therapy helps in the acute phase, has been so severely criticized that its results have not been accepted.[19] A reasonable course would be partial control of severely elevated pressure during the first several days, then gradual lowering of blood pressure to normal, always being alert for further cerebral ischemia induced by lowering the blood pressure. Agents causing wide swings in blood pressure or an altered cerebral state must not be used (see Table 2).

AORTIC DISSECTION

Excruciating pain and very high mortality make aortic dissection a dreadful complication of hypertension. Rapid reduction of elevated arterial pressure is needed for most patients who reach a hospital, either to prevent further dissection until surgery can be accomplished or as the definitive, permanent measure to prevent extension of the dissection.

The mechanisms which underlie dissection remain vague.[20] Treatment of preexisting hypertension is the only measure considered valuable in preventing this catastrophe.

Recognition

Sudden severe pain in the anterior chest or back places aortic dissection among a list of diagnostic possibilities. A new murmur of aortic regurgitation, new absence of one or more major pulses, or new widening of the aortic shadow on chest x-ray makes the diagnosis quite likely, and should lead to prompt reduction of elevated arterial pressure to normal with trimethaphan (Arfonad) to reduce the danger of further dissection. Aortography will establish the diagnosis and the extent of dissection, and is remarkably safe even when the catheter is advanced in and dye injected into the false lumen.[21] Echocardiogram appears of little value because of the high prevalence of findings suggestive of dissection in normal people.[22]

Management

Chronic Dissection

Dissections present more than two weeks have better prognosis than very recent tears.[23] For patients who have survived two weeks, vigorous oral drug therapy to keep systolic blood pressure around 110 to 120 mm. Hg is indicated. Reduction of rate of rise of aortic pressure may also help prevent further dissection. Thus, drugs which reduce sympathetic discharge to the heart are specially indicated; propranolol, methyldopa, or guanethidine is suitable. Resting heart rate below 60 per minute is an encouraging occurrence, suggestive of adequate sympathetic blockade. Asymptomatic sinus bradycardia, no matter how slow, should not dissuade the physician from attaining normal blood pressure. For chronic dissection, surgical intervention is usually reserved for a specific problem, such as the appearance of a localized bulge on chest x-ray or severe leak of the aortic valve. Even with dissection of the ascending aorta, mortality after the first three weeks is at least as low in the medically treated (4 deaths/36 patients), as in those treated surgically (16 deaths/80 patients) for acute dissection.[24-31]

Acute Dissection

FIRST STEPS. With acute dissecting aneurysm, i.e., onset of symptoms within the past 48 hours, the first step in management is reduction in systolic blood pressure below 120 mm. Hg with a drug which does not increase the rapidity of cardiac contraction. Trimethaphan (Arfonad) is the first choice because it decreases the rate of rise of arterial pressure during each cardiac contraction,[32] in contrast to diazoxide and nitroprusside, and because surgeons are more comfortable and experienced with trimethaphan than with the other drugs. Reduction in blood pressure before aortography seems rational. Aortography, the second step, is done as soon as possible after reduction of blood pressure.

Once the extent of the dissection is defined aortographically, a decision about surgical or continued drug treatment can be based partly on experience available in the ten reported series[24-31, 33, 34] which compared medical against surgical treatment for acute dissection, plus the extensive surgical experience of Cooley's group.[35] These reports are summarized in Table 3.

ASCENDING AORTA. For acute dissection involving the ascending aorta, surgical repair resulted in significantly (Chi-square = 11, P < 0.001) lower three-week mortality than did medical management. Later mortality did not differ significantly. Most experienced authors recommend surgical repair of dissection involving the ascending aorta as soon as ideal operating personnel and equipment can be organized. Careful maintenance of normal blood pressure allows arrangements for surgery to be completed without panic, and allows a reasonably safe transfer from community physician to medical center.

DESCENDING AORTA. For dissections confined to the descending aorta, surgical repair has no clear advantage over medical management in immediate or later mortality (see Table 3). Treatment with antihypertensive drugs is the choice of most physicians; surgery is used for complications such as recurrent pain suggesting further dissection, a local bulge which threatens rupture through the outer wall, or symptomatic ischemia from obstruction of a major aortic branch. However, with medical therapy the mortality is 20 to 50 percent within three weeks in five series of patients published since 1974.[27-31] There are no new tools to suggest much improvement in the near future. Therefore, when very experienced vascular surgeons are available, surgical repair may prove preferable for dissection of descending as well as ascending aorta.

MEDICAL MANAGEMENT. Drug management of acute dissection begins with trimethaphan, infused intravenously. The initial rate is 1 mg. per minute with increases every 5 minutes to 2, 3, 4 mg./minute, until systolic blood pressure is below 120 mm. Hg or a maximal rate of 15 mg./minute is reached. Trimethaphan blocks parasympathetic as well as sympathetic ganglia. Unpleasant effects, including dry mouth and blurred vision, and the more serious difficulties of urinary retention and ileus preclude use of the drug for much more than 48 hours. Therefore, it is advisable to immediately begin drugs

Table 3. Comparison of medical with surgical management of acute dissection of aorta

Medical therapy		Surgery	
Deaths in 3 weeks	Later deaths	Deaths in 3 weeks	Later deaths
Type A — Ascending aorta involved			
43(52%)	4(11%)	39(30%)	20(19%)*
Type B — Descending aorta only			
34(29%)	2(3%)	42(30%)	6(8%)

*Number of deaths divided by number of patients with acute dissection. Several authors did not state extent of dissection in patients who died after 3 weeks; the total number of patients at risk as well as the number of deaths are different from those with immediate mortality. Data gathered from references 24–31 and 33–35.

which can be maintained permanently, including a diuretic and an agent which decreases sympathetic neural activation of arterioles and heart: either propranolol, methyldopa, or guanethidine. If oral drugs are impractical, intravenous methyldopa, 0.5 to 1.0 gm. every eight hours,[36] is convenient. When medicine can be swallowed, propranolol produces the least unpleasant effects, but is a drug with which American physicians have least experience and confidence. Large doses, 160 to 640 mg. daily, will be required. Daily administration of two doses is often enough for propranolol[37] as well as for methyldopa. Guanethidine can be given once daily. A loading dose of 100 to 150 mg. of guanethidine should be used because its onset of action is slow, the maximum effect of a given dose occurring 48 hours later.[38]

CORONARY ARTERY DISEASE

Hypertension raises the probability of developing symptomatic coronary disease. The annual incidence increased about 10 percent with each 20 mm. Hg increase in systolic pressure in Framingham men aged 55 to 64.[39] Myocardial infarction, angina pectoris, and intermediate syndromes are all common complications of hypertension. Reduction of blood pressure reduces cardiac work, wall tension, and oxygen demand, and is a logical tactic to decrease the frequency of angina, prevent myocardial necrosis in patients with bouts of prolonged pain, limit necrosis in the early hours of infarction, and relieve left ventricular failure resulting from myocardial ischemia. In practice, trials of reduction in blood pressure have produced convincing evidence of benefit for pulmonary edema complicating myocardial infarction,[40] and for relief of prolonged ischemic chest pain with or without myocardial infarction.[41] The conflicting evidence[42, 43, 48] about the value of reducing blood pressure to reduce infarct size in the absence of pulmonary congestion or recurrent pain is reviewed below in discussing the choice of antihypertensive drugs. Since aortic diastolic pressure is a major determinant of coronary blood flow, moderate reduction of 20 to 30 mm. Hg is the initial goal in management of coronary disease.[42]

Problems with this therapeutic approach are whether cardiac catheterization is needed to monitor pulmonary capillary pressure, and which drugs are most useful.

Is Monitoring of LV Filling Pressure Necessary?

Measurement of pulmonary pressure with a cardiac catheter is essential for management of pulmonary congestion with vasodilators when blood pressure is normal. The dose of the vasodilating drug is adjusted to reduce left heart filling pressure below 20 mm. Hg; this can usually be achieved with minor reduction in systemic arterial pressure.

With systemic hypertension, use of vasodilators *without* cardiac catheterization seems reasonable in the presence of pulmonary congestion. Reduction in blood pressure into high normal ranges has normalized the elevated left ventricular diastolic pressure in most patients with acute myocardial infarction.[40, 41, 44] Pulmonary rales, the loudness of the pulmonic component of the second heart sound, and the third heart sound can be used to monitor improvement.

In the absence of heart failure, where the goal is limitation of size of myocardial infarction, use of the Swan-Ganz catheter to monitor pulmonary capillary pressure is preferred because a reduction in arterial pressure has been accompanied by increase in ST segment elevation or in serum creatine phosphokinase concentrations in some [45, 46, 47] but not all[48] studies of patients with acute myocardial infarction and normal pulmonary capillary pressure.

When skilled personnel and adequate equipment are available, the ability to observe a decrease in left heart filling pressure and to document an increase in cardiac output reassures the physician considerably and probably outweighs the hazards and discomforts associated with the use of the cardiac catheter. In the absence of staff experienced in cardiac catheterization, thought, aided by auscultation of the heart, lungs, and Korotkov sounds will allow beneficial use of vasodilators in most hypertensive people with acute infarction.

Which Antihypertensive Drugs Are Most Useful?

Nitroglycerin may prove preferable to intravenous nitroprusside in acute myocardial infarction. Nitroglycerin decreases and nitroprusside increases ST segment elevation in man; in the dog nitroglycerin redistributes myocardial flow toward ischemic areas, in contrast to nitroprusside.[42] But ST segment mapping may not be a reliable measure of myocardial ischemia,[49, 50] and respected investigators have found opposite results, namely that nitroprusside consistently reduced ST segment elevation.[48] Current information is insufficient to be sure that nitroglycerin is preferable to nitroprusside, or to trimethaphan, in managing the patient with hypertension and myocardial ischemia.

Intravenous diazoxide given rapidly induced ST segment shifts suggesting myocardial ischemia in about half of 20 patients with acute myocardial infarction;[8] and, in combination with intravenous furosemide, produced substernal discomfort in 6, and ST or T changes in 7 of 14 patients without previous angina or myocardial infarction treated for severe elevation of blood pressure.[7] The abrupt large decrease in blood pressure, the marked reflex tachycardia, and these unattractive experiences preclude use of diazoxide, given as a bolus, to patients with manifest coronary disease. There is no experience with more slowly infused diazoxide in managing cardiac ischemia.

To summarize current belief about reduction of elevated blood pressure in the treatment of acute myocardial infarction, this maneuver will probably benefit patients with left ventricular pump failure as evidenced by pulmonary congestion or elevated left ventricular filling pressure. Because of controversy over the exactness of ST segment mapping or of serial blood creatine phosphokinase levels in predicting the extent of myocardial necrosis, the value of lowering blood pressure in the absence of heart failure is still uncertain.

CEREBRAL ATHEROSCLEROSIS

Transient ischemic attacks (TIAs) by definition resolve spontaneously within 24 hours.[16] They may be caused by narrowed cerebral arteries, or by "arterial-to-arterial" emboli from damaged arterial endothelium.[51] Theoretically, lowering blood pressure in the presence of narrowed cerebral arteries might be expected to cause a greater ischemia and worsened neurological deficit. This theoretical danger has given rise to pointed warnings about the danger of precipitating strokes by lowering of the blood pressure in the patient with recent onset of neurological findings suggesting ischemia.[52, 53, 54] However, no concrete data exist documenting such catastrophes.

The Clinical Management Study Group cites the known impairment of cerebral blood flow autoregulation in acute stroke (which may also occur in transient ischemia), and recommends avoidance of either extreme in blood pressure. Thus, hypotension may allow an unregulated drop in flow, with ischemic damage, while hypertension may allow an unregulated high flow, with damage by cerebral edema and further direct vascular deterioration.[16] They suggest that a systolic pressure of 160 mm. Hg might be a rational goal. Exact treatment goals in acute ischemic brain disease remain a clinical mystery, and would be a fruitful field for careful study. When blood pressure is to be lowered, it would seem prudent to affect a smooth change, without transient hypotension.

Regarding chronic outpatient therapy, the Hypertension-Stroke Study Group carefully followed the course of 452 post-stroke or post-TIA patients (randomized to treatment or no treatment).[55] Eighty-one of these patients had TIAs; treatment of the blood pressure on a chronic outpatient basis did not cause an increase or decrease in the number or severity of attacks. Thus, chronic treatment to lower blood pressure (to obtain benefits not related to stroke) is permissible without increased danger to the brain.

An unknown percent of patients with TIAs have their problems on an embolic rather than a stenotic basis. At times, certain clinical features (cholesterol embolus in retinal artery, ulcerated plaque on arteriogram) allow presumption of the embolic nature of the patient's problem, but precision is not possible. It is not to be expected that lowering the blood pressure would affect the basic disease in an important manner, though better knowledge about desirable blood pressure goals during the acute phase would be helpful.

Completed thrombotic strokes present a similar problem to that of TIAs, in that arterial disease is presumably already present. Lowering of blood pressure in the *acute* setting has not been well studied. However, an intriguing autopsy study of patients in whom cardiopulmonary resuscitation did not ultimately succeed suggests that acute hypotension does not often cause brain damage in those with cerebral atherosclerosis.[56] The Clinical Management Study Group recommends that the blood pressure of the severely hypertensive patient be smoothly controlled, without "undershoot," to a systolic pressure of 160 mm. Hg (for a choice of agents, see Table 2).

The chronic outpatient handling of the hypertensive post-stroke patient has been repeatedly studied. It has been demonstrated that acutely induced lowering of blood pressure (I.V. pentolinium and tilt-table) does not cause acute neurological deterioration in post-stroke patients.[57] Severely hypertensive post-stroke patients (diastolic > 120 mm. Hg) appear to suffer less recurrent strokes after blood pressure control.[58] Those with diastolic pressures greater than 110 mm. Hg also benefited in a similar fashion (those over 65 years old did not).[59] Thus at higher diastolic pressures, treatment of hypertension appears to prevent recurrent stroke (though some of these cases were doubtless intracerebral hemorrhage). The Hypertension-Stroke Study included 435 with completed strokes; untreated diastolic blood pressure averaged 100 mm. Hg; recurrent stroke was neither prevented nor precipitated by treatment, though other benefits were gained.[55] Thus, the ability to prevent stroke recurrence by treating hypertension appears related to the severity of the hypertension.

CONGESTIVE HEART FAILURE

Significant hypertension has emerged as an important etiology of chronic heart failure;[60] control of hypertension clearly prevents new episodes.[6] The effect of antihypertensive therapy upon established chronic heart failure is less well studied, as multiple interventions are usually thought to be in the patient's best interest. Mild hypertension can probably occur as a reaction to heart failure, and if this is the case, it should drop to normal with control of the heart failure. Severe or moderate hypertension deserves treatment per se in the presence of heart failure, as the energy requirements of the heart (related to heart rate and arterial pressure) can be thereby lowered.[61] Propranolol (a cardiac depressant) should be avoided in this situation; thiazide diuretics can have a desired effect both on the blood volume and arterial pressure. Other agents may also be used; the fluid retaining properties of guanethidine, methyldopa and certain vasodilators would require concomitant diuretic treatment. In acute heart failure, parenteral therapy may be quite helpful.

EXCESS CIRCULATING CATECHOLAMINES

The syndrome of headache, forceful and rapid pounding of the heart, tremulousness, sweating, hypertension and tachycardia suggests paroxysmal release of catecholamines into the blood. When alarming hypertension accompanies these symptoms, pheochromocytoma, withdrawal of clonidine (Catapres),[62] or ingestion of monamine oxidase inhibitors plus tyramine-containing foods[63] are frequent culprits.

Phentolamine (Regitine) and propranolol are the antagonists of choice. Phentolamine is given intravenously in doses of 5 mg. every 5 minutes until blood pressure is satisfactorily controlled. Propranolol, 1 or 2 mg. intravenously, is added as needed to control tachycardia.

ACKNOWLEDGMENT

We express great thanks to Mrs. Barbara Hendrick for expert typing and to Mrs. Hannah Overton for assistance in reviewing the literature.

REFERENCES

1. PICKERING, G.: *High Blood Pressure.* Grune and Stratton, New York, 1968.
2. FINNERTY, F.: *Hypertensive vascular disease: the long term effect of rapid repeated reductions of arterial pressure with diazoxide.* Am. J. Cardiol. 19:377, 1967.
3. WOODS, J. W., AND BLYTHE, W.: *Management of malignant hypertension complicated by renal insufficiency.* N. Engl. J. Med. 277:57, 1967.
4. GIFFORD, R. W., AND WESTBROOK, E.: *Hypertensive encephalopathy.* Prog. Cardiovasc. Dis. 17:115, 1974.
5. PICKERING, G. W., CRANSTON, W. I., AND PEARS, M. A.: *The Treatment of Hypertension.* Charles C Thomas, Springfield, Ill., 1961, p. 33.
6. VETERANS ADMINISTRATION COOPERATIVE STUDY GROUP ON ANTIHYPERTENSIVE AGENTS: *Effects of treatment on morbidity in hypertension.* JAMA 202:116, 1967 and 213:1143, 1970.

7. KANADA, S. A., KANADA, D. J., AND HUTCHINSON, R. A.: *Angina-like syndrome with diazoxide therapy for hypertensive crisis.* Ann. Intern. Med. 84:696, 1976.

8. O'BRIEN, K. P., GRIGOR, R. R., AND TAYLOR, P. M.: *Intravenous diazoxide in treatment of hypertension associated with recent myocardial infarction.* Br. Med. J. 4:74, 1975.

9. FINNERTY, F. A., JR.: *Hypertensive encephalopathy.* Cardiovasc. Clin. 1 (1):235, 1969.

10. MILLER, W. E., GIFFORD, R. W., HUMPHREY, D. C., ET AL.: *Management of severe hypertension with intravenous injections of diazoxide.* Am. J. Cardiol. 24:870, 1969.

11. KINCAID-SMITH, P. S.: *The treatment of resistant hypertension.* Drugs 11 (Suppl. 1): 78, 1976.

12. STRANDGAARD, S., OLESEN, J., SKINHOJ, E., ET AL.: *Autoregulation of brain circulation in severe arterial hypertension.* Br. Med. J. 1:507, 1973.

13. GIFFORD, R. W., JR.: *Management of hypertension complicated by cerebrovascular disease.* Drug Therapy 1:22, 1971.

14. HARRINGTON, M., KINCAID-SMITH, P. S., AND MCMICHAEL, J.: *Results of treatment in malignant hypertension: a seven-year experience in 94 cases.* Br. Med. J. 2:969, 1959.

15. WOODS, J. W., BLYTHE, W. B., AND HUFFINES, W. D.: *Management of malignant hypertension complicated by renal insufficiency.* N. Engl. J. Med. 291: 10, 1974.

16. CLINICAL MANAGEMENT STUDY GROUP: *Medical and surgical management of stroke.* Stroke 4:273, 1973.

17. MEYER, J., AND BAUER, R.: *Medical treatment of spontaneous intracranial hemorrhage by use of hypotensive drugs.* Neurology 12:36, 1962.

18. SLOSBERG, P.: *Nonoperative management of ruptured intracranial aneurysms.* Clin. Neurosurg. 21:99, 1974.

19. MILLIKAN, C.: *Summary of eighth Princeton conference on cerebrovascular disease.* Stroke 3:105, 1972.

20. HIRST, A. E., AND GORE, I.: *Is cystic medionecrosis the cause of dissecting aortic aneurysm?* Circulation 53:915, 1976.

21. HAYASHI, K., MEANEY, T. F., ZULCH, J. V., ET AL.: *Aortographic analysis of aortic dissection.* Am. J. Roentgenol. Radium Ther. Nucl. Med. 122:769, 1974.

22. BROWN, O. R., POPP, R. L., AND KLOSTER, F. E.: *Echocardiographic criteria for aortic root dissection.* Am. J. Cardiol. 36:17, 1975.

23. MCFARLAND, J., WILLERSON, J. T., DINSMORE, R. E., ET AL.: *The medical treatment of dissecting aortic aneurysms.* N. Engl. J. Med. 286:115, 1972.

24. AUSTEN, W. G., BUCKLEY, M. J., MCFARLAND, J., ET AL.: *Therapy of dissecting aneurysms.* Arch. Surg. 95:835, 1967.

25. DAILY, P. O., TRUEBLOOD, H. W., STINSON, E. B., ET AL.: *Management of acute aortic dissections.* Ann. Thorac. Surg. 10:237, 1970.

26. LIOTTA, D., HALLMAN, G. L., MILAM, J. D., ET AL.: *Surgical treatment of acute dissecting aneurysm of the ascending aorta.* Ann. Thorac. Surg. 12:582, 1971.

27. APPELBAUM, A., KARP, R. B., AND KIRKLIN, J. W.: *Ascending versus descending aortic dissections.* Ann. Surg. 183:296, 1976.

28. STRONG, W. W., MOGGIO, R. A., AND STANSEL, H. C.: *Acute aortic dissection.* J. Thorac. Cardiovasc. Surg. 68:815, 1974.

29. PARKER, F. B., NEVILLE, J. F., HANSON, E. L., ET AL.: *Management of acute aortic dissection.* Ann. Thorac. Surg. 19:436, 1975.

30. DALEN, J. E., ALPERT, J. S., COLIN, L. H., ET AL.: *Dissection of the thoracic aorta. Medical or surgical therapy?* Am. J. Cardiol. 34:803, 1974.

31. ANAGNOSTOPOULOS, C. E.: *Acute Aortic Dissections.* University Park Press, Baltimore, 1975, p. 3.

32. PALMER, R. F., AND LASSETER, K. C.: *Nitroprusside and aortic dissecting aneurysm* (letter to the editor). N. Engl. J. Med. 294:1403, 1976.

33. WHEAT, M. W., HARRIS, P. D. MALM, J. R., ET AL.: *Acute dissecting aneurysms of the aorta.* J. Thorac. Cardiovasc. Surg. 58:344, 1969.

34. ATTAR, S., FARDIN, R. HYELLZ, R., ET AL.: *Medical versus surgical treatment of acute dissecting aneurysms.* Arch. Surg. 103:568, 1971.

35. REUL, G. J., COOLEY, D. A., HALLMAN, G. L., ET AL.: *Dissecting aneurysm of the descending aorta.* Arch. Surg. 110:632, 1975.

36. KOCH-WESER, J.: *Hypertensive emergencies.* N. Engl. J. Med. 290:211, 1974.

240

37. BERGLUND, G., ANDERSSON, O., HANSSON, L., ET AL.: *Propranolol given twice daily for hypertension.* Acta Med. Scand. 194:513, 1974.

38. RICHARDSON, D. W., WYSO, E. M., MAGEE, J. H., ET AL.: *Circulatory effects of guanethidine.* Circulation 22: 184, 1960.

39. KANNEL, W. B., GORDON, T., AND SCHWARTZ, M. J.: *Systolic versus diastolic blood pressure and risk of coronary artery disease.* Am. J. Cardiol. 27: 335, 1971.

40. FRANCIOSA, J. A., ET AL.: *Improved left ventricular function during nitroprusside infusion in acute myocardial infarction.* Lancet 1:650, 1972.

41. VEITH, C. E., FELDMAN, M., AND HELFANT, R. H.: *Nitroprusside in patients with recurrent ischemia or ventricular arrhythmias associated with the intermediate syndrome of acute myocardial infarction.* Circulation 54:II-211, 1976.

42. SHELL, W. E., AND SOBEL, B. E.: *Protection of jeopardized ischemic myocardium by reduction of ventricular afterload.* N. Engl. J. Med. 291: 482, 1974.

43. CHIARIELLO, M., ET AL.: *Comparison between the effects of nitroprusside and nitroglycerin on ischemic injury during acute myocardial infarction.* Circulation 54:766, 1976.

44. KELLY, D. T., DELGADO, C. E., TAYLOR, D. R., ET AL.: *Use of phentolamine in acute myocardial infarction associated with hypertension and left ventricular failure.* Circulation 47: 729, 1973.

45. BORER, J. S., REDWOOD, D. R., LEVITT, B., ET AL.: *Reduction in myocardial ischemia with nitroglyerin or nitroglycerin plus phenylephrine administered during acute myocardial infarction.* N. Engl. J. Med. 293:1008, 1975.

46. ARMSTRONG, P. W., BOROOMAND, K., AND PARKER, J. O.: *Nitroprusside in acute myocardial infarction: correlative effects on hemodynamics and precordial mapping.* Circulation 54:II-76, 1976.

47. MAGNUSSON, P., ET AL.: *Increased creatine phosphokinase release following blood pressure reduction in patients with acute myocardial infarction.* Circulation 54:II-28, 1976.

48. AWAN, N. A., ET AL.: *Reduction of ST segment elevation with infusion of nitroprusside in acute myocardial infarction.* Am. J. Cardiol. 38:435, 1976.

49. FOZZARD, H. A., AND DAS GUPTA, D. S.: *ST segment potentials and mapping: theory and experiments.* Circulation 54:533, 1976.

50. IRVIN, R. G., AND COBB, F. R.: *Relationship between epicardial ST segment changes and extent of histologic myocardial infarction in awake dogs.* Circulation 54:II-15, 1976.

51. HASS, W.: *Medical management of cerebral vascular disease.* MCV/Q. 10:118, 1974.

52. WHITFIELD, A.: *Iatrogenic misadventure,* Br. Med. J. 1:733, 1972.

53. FOLKERTS, J.: *The treatment of hypertension and its possible risks for the cerebral circulation.* Psychiatr. Neurol. Neurochir. 75:459, 1972.

54. KOSTER, M.: *Hypertensive treatment and the risks for the cerebral blood flow.* Psychiatr. Neurol. Neurochir. 75:463, 1972.

55. HYPERTENSION-STROKE COOPERATIVE STUDY GROUP: *Effect of antihypertensive treatment on stroke recurrence.* JAMA 229:409, 1974.

56. TORVIK, A., AND SKULLERUD, K.: *How often are brain infarcts caused by hypotensive episodes?* Stroke 7:255, 1976.

57. HARMSEN, P., KJAERULFF, J., AND SKINHOJ, E.: *Acute controlled hypotension and EEG in patients with hypertension and cerebrovascular disease.* J. Neurol. Neurosurg. Psychiatry 34:300, 1971.

58. PIERSON, E., AND HOOBLER, S.: *Significance of transient encephalopathy in cases of benign hypertension.* Univ. Mich. Med. Bull. 23:446, 1957.

59. CARTER, A.: *Hypotensive therapy in stroke survivors.* Lancet 1:485, 1970.

60. McKEE, P., CASTELLI, W., McNAMARA, P., ET AL.: *The natural history of congestive heart failure: the Framingham study.* N. Engl. J. Med. 285:1441, 1971.

61. COHN, J.: *Vasodilator therapy for heart failure.* Circulation 48:5, 1973.

62. HANSSON, L., HUNYOR, S. N., JULIUS, S., ET AL.: *Blood pressure crisis following withdrawal of clonidine.* Am. Heart J. 85:605, 1973.

63. HORWITZ, D., LOVENBERG, W., ENGELMAN, K., ET AL.: *Monamine oxidase inhibitors, tyramine, and cheese.* JAMA 188:1108, 1964.

The Struggle for Drug Compliance in Hypertension

Donald G. Vidt, M.D.

Results of epidemiologic surveys have demonstrated that 10 to 15 percent of the adult American population have hypertension, making it the most common chronic disease seen by the practicing physician.[1-5] Hypertension is a major cause of death and disability in the United States and unquestionably represents a significant factor in rising health care costs to individuals, to society, and to government.[6-10]

It is now well recognized that effective treatment of hypertension can control high blood pressure and significantly reduce both morbidity and mortality from this insidious, often asymptomatic disease.[11, 12] Effective treatment is available not only for severe or complicated hypertension but also for a much larger majority of patients with mild or moderate, asymptomatic hypertension. Yet, the majority of Americans with hypertension are not receiving suitable long-term treatment. Despite the fact that hypertension is easy to detect, even when asymptomatic, many hypertensive patients have not been identified.

Progress has been made in detecting new hypertensive patients and improving treatment, with much of the impetus provided by the National High Blood Pressure Education Program introduced in 1973. Two reports from the Hypertension Detection and Followup Program (HDFP), involving 157,376 persons in 14 identified populations, showed that as many as 37.6 percent of all persons surveyed with high blood pressure had controlled hypertension.[13, 14] A recent report of the Community Hypertension Evaluation Clinic (CHEC) Program by Stamler and associates[15] has stated that 44.9 percent of persons with hypertension were under adequate control. The HDFP represented a systematic survey of hypertension in defined populations; the CHEC program represented intensive community screening efforts carried out in schools, shopping centers, and mobile vans. Despite the differences in populations screened, similar data were generated regarding the current effectiveness of treatment for hypertension, and both suggest that progress has been made since earlier surveys when hypertension was far less effectively treated and controlled. It should also be apparent that both surveys again confirm a vast population of persons with hypertension previously undetected, detected but untreated, or treated but still uncontrolled.

Data from the National Disease and Therapeutic Index[16] suggest that since 1971, there has been a 38 percent increase in initial patient visits to physicians for hypertension and hypertensive heart disease. Total patient visits for these conditions have increased 40 percent, considerably more than the increase of approximately 17 percent in initial and total patient visits for all other medical causes. It can also be shown that the number of prescriptions written for antihypertensive drugs has increased from 46 million in 1965 to 96 million in 1975.

Although these statistics suggest that progress has been made in detection and treatment of hypertension, they also point to the need for greatly increased efforts in expanded detection programs and increased physician and patient awareness of the benefits of long-term control of hypertension.

When considering a large population of recognized hypertensives who are either untreated or inadequately treated, patient compliance or adherence to the treatment regimen is always questioned. It is vital, however, that the medical community recognize that patient compliance is only one factor in our continued inability to provide appropriate, adequate long-term treatment. Physicians and other health professionals must shoulder a large share of the responsibility for inadequate long-term control of blood pressure. In assessing the responsibilities of the medical community, several problem areas can be identified.

THE PROBLEM OF BLOOD PRESSURE DETECTION

It is evident from currently available survey studies that more than 30 percent of patients with hypertension remain undetected, making it clear that population screening efforts must be increased. It is also apparent that opportunities for detecting hypertension among patients who have contacts with the health care system are not utilized. Simply stated, measurement of blood pressure is not routinely performed as a part of every physical examination. This is especially true for patients seen by physicians in nonmedical specialties and too often the case for patients seen in medical clinics and emergency rooms. A review of 800 randomly chosen charts from four hospitals (2 VA, 1 community, 1 private), by Frohlich and coworkers[17] revealed that 26 percent of patients never had their blood pressures recorded. Another 26 percent had blood pressures higher than 150/100 recorded, yet only one-fifth listed hypertension as a diagnosis. Similarly, the results of the much larger Chicago Heart Association detection project in industry reported by Schoenberger and associates[4] in 1972 revealed that 58.9 percent of patients denied a prior knowledge of hypertension, despite the fact that 90 percent of the women and 75 percent of the men screened had been examined by physicians in the preceding two years. It can be presumed that the physicians had never made the diagnosis of hypertension, or if they recognized elevated levels of blood pressure, had not informed their patients. It is apparent that we shall continue to experience a large, unresolved problem of control of hypertension until effective methods are implemented for the identification of previously unrecognized hypertensive persons.

THE PROBLEM OF NONTREATMENT OR INEFFECTIVE TREATMENT

There is general agreement on the benefits of therapy for accelerated or malignant hypertension, but it was not until the reports of the Veterans Administration Cooperative Study that benefits of treatment for mild to moderate, uncomplicated hypertension were recognized.[11, 12] Evidence that significant numbers of recognized hypertensives are not receiving therapy suggests that many physicians are not yet convinced of the efficacy of drug treatment, particularly for those patients with mild or moderate elevations of blood pressure.

Well intentioned detection programs are often poorly designed and do not provide adequate referral and followup mechanisms for individuals in whom initial screening indicates elevated blood pressure. Wilber and Barrow,[18, 19] and Finnerty and associates[20] have shown that prompt intensive referral mechanisms built into detection programs can assure that patients will get to a suitable source of patient education and care whether it be a clinic, hospital, or concerned physician. Following referral, patients must be provided persistent care to assure adequate treatment.

Another obstacle to physician followup and, for that matter, to patient compliance has been that pretreatment evaluation of a hypertensive patient is often too time-consuming and expensive. It is generally agreed that less than 10 percent of all hypertension is secondary or "potentially curable." Traditional teaching has emphasized intensive evaluation and elaborate diagnostic studies to identify those few patients with secondary hypertension. Limitations in manpower, facilities, and resources make a review of the traditional concepts of the hypertensive evaluation necessary, with efforts made to eliminate those examinations which are cumbersome, expensive and have a low yield in terms of objectives. For most asymptomatic patients, objectives of pretreatment evaluation should be to determine that hypertension is sustained, and to identify cardiovascular complications and other risk factors with a thorough history and physical examination plus a few economical, easily available laboratory studies. Physicians must be made aware of the value of a thorough history and physical examination and a few selected laboratory studies in providing clues to most patients with secondary hypertension. For the majority of asymptomatic patients, if this minimal evaluation is unrevealing, treatment should be instituted.[21]

THE PROBLEM OF PHYSICIAN COMPLIANCE

Discussions on compliance often focus on the failure of patients to comply with instructions given by the physician, failure to adhere to medication schedules, and failure to keep followup appointments. Insufficient attention has been paid to the responsibilities of the physician in terms of his adherence to optimum principles for the management of hypertension.

Medical education has traditionally focused on management of symptomatic disease with few efforts directed toward preventive medicine. Many physicians still have not accepted epidemiologic data pointing out the risks of asymptomatic hypertension, nor have they accepted data from the VA Cooperative Study showing that aggressive, continuous therapy for mild or moderate hypertension reduces cardiovascular morbidity and mortality. Efforts in continuing education must be aimed at convincing the practicing physician of the advantages of long-term treatment and adequate control of blood pressure.

Physician compliance entails earlier detection of hypertension through routine blood pressure measurements on every patient, thorough education of patients so they understand and respect the risks of untreated hypertension, and a system of routine followup on all patients to help insure adherence to treatment. The average busy practitioner does not have the time to provide the information needed to educate and motivate each new hypertensive patient; also, few practices are designed to assure adequate followup for missed appointments. These are areas where allied health professionals have an increasing role in providing the necessary education, followup, and patient motivation to assure improved adherence.

For the past two years, we have used a Certified Physician's Assistant to assist in the education and regular followup care of a large group of hypertensive patients at the Cleveland Clinic (Table 1). These health professionals have been well received by our patients, and patient compliance with prescribed drug regimens has improved. Patient visits with the physician's assistant are scheduled and performed at lower cost to the patient than regularly scheduled physician visits. A systematic appointment schedule is utilized for all patients. For a new hypertensive patient with previously untreated and uncomplicated essential hypertension, appointments are scheduled at 4-week intervals until diastolic blood pressures equal to or less than 90 mm. Hg for two visits are ob-

Table 1. Position description for certified physician assistant

Primary Function:

To assist the physician with the primary care of hypertensive patients under regular ongoing care at the Cleveland Clinic. To perform special duties and procedures under the medical staff's guidance and control.

Specific duties:

1. Assist in providing primary care to the patient while at the Cleveland Clinic for hypertension.
2. Schedule patients referred by staff physicians, to be seen at specified intervals.
3. Measure blood pressure in the supine and standing positions, question patients about side effects of medication, and adherence to regimen; encourage patients to be more compliant if they seem not to be following the regimen faithfully.
4. Participate in patient education regarding hypertension. Distribute literature obtained from the American Heart Association and other agencies, and discuss it with the patient.
5. Advise patients of changes in dosage of medication after consultation with the staff physician.
6. Call patients on behalf of the staff physician regarding changes in dosage and changes in scheduling.
7. Follow up patients who do not keep appointments; call them, if necessary, to make new appointments.
8. Assist in the training of patients for home blood pressure measurements.
9. Maintain an inventory of all patients undergoing active treatment for blood pressure and keep the hypertensive therapy sheet current.
10. Collect information by examination and grading of optic fundi, cardiac examination, arterial pulses, urinalysis, etc.
11. Assist in clinical studies of new antihypertensive drugs.

Level of responsibility:

To be directly responsible and act as an assistant to the medical staff with their various treatments and procedures.

Identity with staff physician will be maintained, because each patient will have an appointment to see his staff physician every 6 to 12 months at the discretion of the staff physician. The hypertensive therapy record will be reviewed by the staff physician after each visit.

tained. Visits are then scheduled at 6-week intervals, and finally at 12-week intervals when diastolic blood pressures are maintained below 90 mm. Hg. Appointment intervals will also be determined by individual patient evaluation and a determination of each patient's therapeutic and educational needs. Four-week appointment intervals are maintained as long as there are changes of dosages or medications. After each patient visit, the supervising physician reviews the patient's chart and blood pressure record. Any correspondence to the patient will be reviewed by the supervising physician before the letters are mailed. An important aspect of each patient visit is a review of all medications and dosages and an assessment of whether the patient is taking medication regularly or irregularly. A step-care plan of drug regulation for hypertension is utilized in our Clinic (Table 2).

The step-care plan for each patient must be approved and supervised by a physician present in the Clinic or immediately available by telephone. The physician's assistant using the step-care plan must be knowledgeable of the pharmacology of each medication, and particularly of the action of drugs, adverse effects, contraindications, recommended dosages, and the physical assessment of each individual patient. For each individual patient, the step-care plan is initiated by the physician responsible for that patient's care. The physician or the physician's assistant explains the plan and its purpose to the patient, stressing the importance of keeping appointments and taking medications regularly as prescribed. The patient is informed of the blood pressure goal and may keep a flow chart if he or she wishes.

Patients who express an interest in home blood pressure recordings are encouraged

246

Table 2. Stepped care plan for blood pressure control of the Department of Hypertension and Nephrology, Cleveland Clinic Foundation

Regular

Step

1. At least three sets of blood pressure readings on separate visits prior to starting therapy.
2. Thiazides*   q.d.
3. Thiazides   b.i.d. (not necessary for chlorthalidone or metolazone)
   Pathway determined in consultation with physician

4. Thiazides – b.i.d. methyldopa – 250 mg. b.i.d.*	Thiazides – b.i.d. clonidine – 0.2 mg. h.s.*	Thiazides – b.i.d. propranolol – 10 mg. q.i.d.*
5. Thiazides – b.i.d. methyldopa – 250 mg. t.i.d.	Thiazides – b.i.d. clonidine – 0.4 mg. h.s.	Thiazides – b.i.d. propranolol – 20 mg. q.i.d.
6. Thiazides – b.i.d. methyldopa – 250 mg. q.i.d.	Thiazides – b.i.d. clonidine – 0.2 mg. a.m. 0.4 mg. h.s.	Thiazides – b.i.d. propranolol – 40 mg. q.i.d.
7. Thiazides – b.i.d. methyldopa – 250 mg. q.i.d. hydralazine – 25 mg. b.i.d.	Thiazides – b.i.d. clonidine – 0.2 mg. a.m. 0.4 mg h.s. hydralazine – 25 mg. b.i.d.	Thiazides – b.i.d. propranolol – 40 mg. q.i.d. hydralazine – 25 mg. b.i.d.
8. Thiazides – b.i.d. methyldopa – 250 mg. q.i.d. hydralazine – 50 mg. b.i.d.	Thiazides – b.i.d. clonidine – 0.2 mg. a.m. 0.4 mg. h.s. hydralazine – 50 mg. b.i.d.	Thiazides – b.i.d. propranolol – 40 mg. b.i.d. hydralazine – 50 mg. b.i.d.
9. Thiazides – b.i.d. methyldopa – 250 mg. q.i.d. hydralazine – 100 mg. b.i.d.	Thiazides – b.i.d. clonidine – 0.2 mg. a.m. 0.4 mg. h.s. hydralazine – 100 mg. b.i.d.	Thiazides – b.i.d. propranolol – 40 mg. q.i.d. hydralazine – 100 mg. b.i.d.

10, 11, etc. Further increments in medication dosages, consideration of alternate drugs, and drug combinations are determined after consultation with the physician. The physician is consulted prior to proceeding to each additional step for blood pressures not controlled below 90 mm. Hg.

*Alternatives available: The physician may elect to prescribe spironolactone or furosemide as an alternative for thiazides for initial step therapy. A vasodilating agent (hydralazine, prazosin) may be prescribed instead of a sympathetic inhibitor in Step 4.

to purchase the apparatus and are trained in its use by the physician's assistant. We are of the impression that home blood pressure determinations which actively involve the patient in his ongoing care can be a positive factor in patient compliance. It serves as a daily reminder to the patient under a long-term treatment program, gives the patient a feeling of active participation in his own care, and the availability of serial blood pressure determinations which are reviewed at each office visit help overcome our concerns over the frequent inaccuracies and variations in random office determinations of blood pressure. Gibson and Sackett[22] have collected preliminary data suggesting that a behavioral intervention program including self-measurement of blood pressure, daily charting of blood pressure and pills taken, and the tailoring of medications to daily habits can improve compliance.

The physician's assistant follows the regular step-care plan unless it is contraindicated or adverse effects to medications necessitate a change in the plan. The physician must approve any alternates or deviations from the regular plan. In the event that an adverse effect of a medication develops, an alternate preparation may be recommended after consulting with the physician. In the event that the patient is not taking medication as prescribed and blood pressure is elevated at the time of an office visit, the same step is continued and the need for improved compliance is stressed to the patient. For elevations in blood pressure previously controlled on a given step, the same step is continued and the patient is re-evaluated after four weeks. If blood pressure remains elevated and the patient is compliant regarding medication, the physician's assistant proceeds to the next step. The physician is consulted before proceeding to the next step in the treatment plan. Unless otherwise specified by the supervising physician, the interval for each step is four weeks until blood pressure control is achieved.

We are also using a recently established Department of Patient Education to assist us with several well designed educational programs. These programs include a film strip with audio tape cassette, preprogram and postprogram testing questionnaires, review sheets for active participation by the patient at various stopping points during the program, and an illustrated booklet reviewing the program content and answering questions often asked by hypertensive patients, which the patient takes to read at home and share with the family.* Three educational programs are currently available: "An introduction to high blood pressure," "Self-measurement of blood pressure," and "Living with a low sodium diet." Additional educational programs are planned in this series.

Wilber and McCombs[23] have shown the effectiveness of the nurse or other allied health professionals on patient compliance with office visits and on the success of antihypertensive therapy. In their program, patients have accepted the nurses as therapists and, in turn, the nurses have accepted the increased responsibilities and feel comfortable functioning in an extended role. In their nurse-run clinics there have been fewer dropouts and better control of blood pressure compared to a survey of private patient records and hospital outpatient clinic records in the same community. In 18 months' experience with a nurse-managed clinic, 81 percent of patients returned regularly for followup visits and 52.5 percent achieved blood pressure control (Fig. 1).

THE PROBLEM OF PATIENT COMPLIANCE

Caldwell and coworkers[24] reported a pilot study of social and emotional factors influencing a patient's compliance with antihypertensive treatment. Patients who had experienced a hypertensive emergency following discontinuance of therapy were compared to a group of compliant patients. The dropouts were younger, had the disease for a shorter time, had less education, less income, and were most often black. They also reported that learned responses following personal experience of harmful effects of no treatment or inadequate treatment, and education of the patient about the disease and its treatment were also significant factors which influenced a patient's ability to follow an antihypertensive program. Contrary to these findings, an extensive literature review by Marsten[25] on compliance with medical regimens revealed no clear association between compliance behavior and sex, age, race, marital status, socioeconomic status, or education. Noncompliance with drug recommendations in a wide variety of illness situations ranged from 6 to 92 percent. The accuracy of such estimates is dependent upon the periods of observation and the measurement tools used. Objective measures such as pill counts and urine excretion tests can be expected to provide more accurate asessments of compliance than subjective measures such as patient reports or estimates of other observers. The severity of illness as perceived by the patient does not appear to result in increased compliance.

Noncompliance increases with the complexity of the treatment regimen and the degree with which a treatment regimen interferes with a patient's life style. This is true when multiple medications are prescribed and among patients for whom drug prescriptions and other therapeutic recommendations were made concurrently.[26-28] There is also some evidence to suggest that drugs with unpleasant side effects are likely to be

---

*Core Communications in Health, Inc., 1290 Avenue of the Americas, New York, NY 10019.

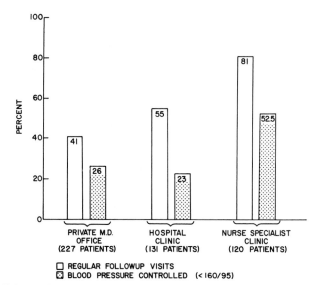

Figure 1. Relative efficiency of office, hospital clinic, and nurse specialist clinic on patient followup and blood pressure control. (Modified from Wilber and McCombs.[23])

omitted. Recommended restriction of behavior and changes in personal habits may be more difficult to comply with than prescriptions for medicine. Recommendations regarding diet have also been associated with decreasing compliance.[26, 29]

The types of interactions which occur between doctor and patient are predictive of patient behavior and, therefore, are an important determinant in the patient's response to medical advice. A few examples may serve to demonstrate the importance of the patient-physician relationship in promoting compliance. Davis[30] has reported that patient noncompliance could be correlated with the physician's disagreement with patient's opinions, and with requests by the physician for information without appropriate feedback to the patient. Korsch and colleagues[31] have shown that the extent to which a patient's expectations are met will influence satisfaction with a medical visit. The extent to which the patient's expectations of the medical visit are left unmet, lack of warmth in the doctor-patient relationship, and failure to receive an explanation of diagnosis and cause of illness are key factors in noncompliance. Charney and associates[32] have suggested that a long lasting relationship makes for increased compliance in private pediatric practices. This would indicate the importance of continuity of care by the same physician whenever possible. Finally, Williams and coworkers[33] have reported a significant correlation between patient preference for a strict or authoritarian attitude by the physician and subsequent control of their diabetes.

The efficacy of antihypertensive therapy in preventing complications has been demonstrated in random clinical trials reported by the VA Cooperative Study Group. It should be remembered, however, that these studies were properly limited to compliant patients. Frustrations in achieving similar benefits at the community level can be related in large part to the failure of hypertensive patients to comply with treatment. Finnerty and associates[20] have suggested that convenience in followup care is an important determinant of compliance. During screening and verification of sustained hypertension, high "no show" rates were reduced from 50 percent to fewer than 5 percent by early rescheduling, personal contact, or home visits by a paramedical member of the screening team. Further, they demonstrated that patients randomly assigned to an intensive personalized followup group were more compliant than patients left to followup in a general medical clinic, and that normal blood pressure was achieved in a significantly higher percentage of patients in the compliant group. Thus, they were able to demonstrate a direct relationship between patient compliance and ability to control blood pressure. A number of other randomized studies have shown that compliance in keeping appointments can be improved by the establishment of effective followup mechanisms.[34-37] Whether improved followup of patients with hypertension is indeed associated with improvement in medical care and blood pressure control has been left open to question by studies of Fletcher and coworkers.[38] Emergency room patients were chosen for this study because of recognized noncompliance of emergency room patients in returning for followup care. The use of a followup clerk improved compliance among patients directed to return for further evaluation and therapy, 84 percent compliance in the intervention group versus 63 percent of control patients. However, five months after the patient's emergency room visit, 51 percent of patients in the intervention group and 53 percent of control patients were normotensive. There were more diagnostic and therapeutic measures in the intervention group but long-term management was similar in both groups. Thus, improved followup care may not by itself lead to better blood pressure control among hypertensive patients.

Because convenience of followup care is believed to be an important determinant of compliance, and education of patients about their disease is considered a necessary factor in gaining their cooperation, Sackett and colleagues[39] tested these two strategies in a randomized clinical trial. One group saw their family physicians in their offices outside of working hours; the other group were afforded an augmented degree of convenience for hypertensive care and followup at their place of employment during working hours. The same patients were randomly assigned to receive an intensive educational program about hypertensive disease, benefits of therapy, and the need for compliance with medications. Surprisingly, compliance does not improve by attempts to make care and followup more convenient. Although an intensive educational program was highly effective in teaching these patients about hypertension and its management, it did not increase compliance. Further, individual compliance rates bore no relationship to knowledge about hypertension, either at entry into the study or at six months. Neither strategy affected the rates at which patients were designated both compliant and at goal blood pressure.

In contrast, more behaviorally-oriented strategies have shown some promising results. Meyer and Henderson,[40] in a randomized trial, achieved behavior changes affecting weight, smoking, diet, and physical activity, and changes in cholesterol and triglyceride levels. Behavior modification achieved greater initial change than individual counselling or physician consultation and maintained the changes longer.

It should be evident that the problem of patient compliance with medical regimens includes many variables. Compliance would seem to be affected by patient attitudes and beliefs, social-psychological factors including attitudes towards illness and attitudes towards the physician, complexity of medical regimens, and changes in patient life style, and may be influenced by followup mechanisms and educational processes. It is unlikely that changes in any one of these areas will have a significant impact on patient adherence to treatment. Rather, efforts must be undertaken to influence as many facets of the problem as possible.

When confronted with a noncompliant hypertensive patient, the clinician should first identify the patient's reasons for refusing to take medication and then determine whether the treatment approach should be changed. Some dependent patients may benefit from an increased frequency of office visits, medication charting, or training in home blood pressure determinations. Further tailoring of treatment to patient habits or life style can be assessed, and it may be worthwhile to see if behavior modification techniques can be adapted to larger scale behavioral changes. Further evaluation of medication dispensers seems warranted. The clinician must appreciate that compliance in hypertension is not merely a problem but rather represents a way of life for the patient.

To summarize, patients with hypertension, as a group, would seem to be at particularly high risk from noncompliance. Hypertension is a chronic illness requiring long-term maintenance with suppressive or preventive treatment. Ill effects after stopping medication are subtle and remote rather than dramatic or immediate. It is not the purpose of this review to point to the physician or to the patient as the major perpetrator in the failure to achieve long-term control of blood pressure in the hypertensive patient. Rather, it is my hope that the reader recognizes that compliance with the total antihypertensive regimen represents a complex mosaic of interacting factors between the patient, his physician, and the disease itself. It should be apparent that compliance will not be attained unless the regimen is designed and carried out in a manner that suitably addresses many or all of the variables discussed.

REFERENCES

1. HEALTH EXAMINATION SURVEY. *Health Statistics.* PHS Publication 1,000, Series 1, No. 4, U.S. Government Printing Office, Washington, D.C., 1966.

2. WILBER, J. A.: *Survey of hypertension in Baldwin County, Ga,* in STAMLER, J., STAMLER, R., AND PULLMAN, P. N. (EDS.): *Epidemiology of Hypertension.* Grude & Stratton, N.Y., 1967.

3. BORHANI, N. O., AND BORKMAN, T. S.: *Alamdea County blood pressure study.* State of California Department of Health, Berkeley, 1968.

4. SCHOENBERGER, J. A., STAMLER, J., SHEKELLE, R. B., ET AL.: *Current status of hypertension control in an industrial population.* JAMA 222:559, 1972.

5. NATIONAL CENTER FOR HEALTH STATISTICS: *Blood pressure of adults by age and sex, United States, 1960–62.* U.S. Department of Health, Education and Welfare, Vital and Health Statistics Series 11, No. 4, U.S. Government Printing Office, Washington, D.C., 1964.

6. STAMLER, J.: *Epidemiology of coronary heart disease.* Med. Clin. North Am. 57:5, 1973.

7. KANNEL, W. B., SCHWARTZ, M. J., AND McNAMARA, P. M.: *Blood pressure and risk of coronary heart disease: The Framingham study.* Dis. Chest 56:43, 1969.

8. *Build and Blood Pressure Study.* Society of Actuaries, Chicago, 1959.

9. KANNEL, W. B., CASTELLI, W. R., McNAMARA, R. M., ET AL.: *Role of blood pressure in the development of congestive heart failure.* N. Engl. J. Med. 287:781, 1972.

10. KANNEL, W. B., WOLFE, P. A., VERTER, J., ET AL.: *Epidemiologic assessment of the role of blood pressure in stroke: The Framingham study.* JAMA 214:301, 1970.

11. VETERANS ADMINISTRATION COOPERATIVE STUDY GROUP ON ANTIHYPERTENSIVE AGENTS: *Effects of treatment on morbidity in hypertension: I. Results in patients with diastolic blood pressures averaging 115–129 mm. Hg.* JAMA 202:1028, 1967.

12. VETERANS ADMINISTRATION COOPERATIVE STUDY GROUP ON ANTIHYPERTENSIVE AGENTS: *Effects of treatment on morbidity in hypertension. II. Results in patients with diastolic blood pressures averaging 90–114 mm. Hg.* JAMA 213:1143, 1970.

13. STEERING COMMITTEE: THE HYPERTENSION DETECTION AND FOLLOWUP PROGRAM. *Epidemiology and Control of Hypertension.* Symposia Specialists, Miami, 1975, p. 663.

14. HYPERTENSION DETECTION AND FOLLOWUP PROGRAM COOPERATIVE GROUP: *Results of two-stage screen.* Presented at the 47th Scientific Session of the American Heart Association, November 18–21, 1974, Dallas, Texas.

15. STAMLER, J., STAMLER, R., RIEDLINGER, W. F., ET AL.: *Hypertension screening of one million Americans. Community Hypertension Evaluation Clinic (CHEC) Program, 1973–1975.* JAMA 235:2299, 1976.

16. *National Disease and Therapeutic Index, 1965–1975,* IMS American Ltd., Ambler, Pennsylvania, 1975.

17. FROHLICH, E. D., CAMERON, E., HAMMARSTEN, J. E., ET AL.: *Evaluation of the initial care of hypertensive patients.* JAMA 218:1036, 1971.

18. WILBER, J. A., AND BARROW, J. G.: *Hypertension—a community problem.* Am. J. Med. 52:653, 1972.

19. WILBER, J. A., AND BARROW, J. G.: *Reducing elevated blood pressure.* Minn. Med. 52:1303, 1969.

20. FINNERTY, F. A., JR., MATTIE, E. C., AND FINNERTY, F. A., III: *Hypertension in the inner city. I. Analysis of clinic dropouts.* Circulation 47:73, 1973.

21. VIDT, D. G.: *The hypertensive evaluation: To what extent is it necessary?* Cardiovasc. Clin. 7(1):135, 1975.

22. GIBSON, E. S., AND SACKETT, B. L., Personal communication, February, 1976.

23. WILBER, J. A., AND McCOMBS, N. J.: *Hypertension 1975: The allied health professionals role.* Drug Therapy, May/June, 1975, p. 56.

24. CALDWELL, J. R., COBB, S., DOWLING, M. D., ET AL.: *The dropout problem in antihypertensive treatment. A pilot study of social and emotional factors influencing a patient's ability to follow antihypertensive treatment.* J. Chronic Dis. 22:579, 1970.

25. MARSTEN, M. V.: *Compliance with medical regimes: a review of the literature.* Nurs. Res. 19:312, 1970.

26. FRANCIS, V., KORSCH, B. M., AND MORRIS, M. J.: *Gaps in doctor-patient communication. Patient's response to medical advice.* N. Engl. J. Med. 280:535, 1969.

27. MADDOCK, R. K.: *Patient cooperation in taking medicines: a study involving isoniazid and aminosalicylic acid.* JAMA 199:169, 1967.

28. DAVIS, M. S., AND EICHHORN, R. L.: *Compliance with medical regimens: A panel study.* J. Health Soc. Behav. 4:240, 1963.

29. JOHNSON, W. L.: *Conformity to medical recommendations in coronary heart disease.* Presented at the meeting of the American Sociological Association, Chicago, Illinois, September, 1965.

30. DAVIS, M. S.: *Research in medical education: Attitudinal and behavioral aspects of the doctor-patient relationship as expressed and exhibited by medical students and their mentors.* J. Med. Educ. 43:337, 1968.

31. KORSCH, B. M., GOZZI, E. K., AND FRANCIS, V.: *Gaps in doctor-patient communication. I. Doctor-patient interaction and patient satisfaction.* Pediatrics 42:855, 1968.

32. CHARNEY, E., BYNUM, R., AND ELDREDGE, D.: *How well do patients take oral penicillin? Collaborative study in private practice.* Pediatrics 40:188, 1967.

33. WILLIAMS, T. F., MARTIN, D. A., AND HOGAN, M. D.: *The clinical picture of diabetic control—study in four settings.* Am. J. Public Health 57:441, 1967.

34. MARTIN, D. A.: *The disposition of patients from a consultant general medical clinic: Results of a controlled evaluation of an administrative procedure,* in WHITE, L. K. (ED.): *Medical Care Research.* Pergamon Press, London, 1965, pp. 113–120.

35. SCHROEDER, S. A.: *Lowering broken appointment rates at a medical clinic.* Med. Care 11:75, 1973.

36. LEWIS, C. E. AND RESNICK, B. A.: *Nurse clinics and progressive ambulatory patient care.* N. Engl. J. Med. 277:1236, 1967.

37. FINK, D., MALLOY, M. J., COHEN, M., ET AL.: *Effective patient care in the pediatric ambulatory setting: A study of the acute care clinic.* Pediatrics 43:927, 1969.

38. FLETCHER, S. W., APPLE, F. A., AND BOURGEOIS, M. A.: *Management of hypertension. Effect of improving patient compliance for follow-up care.* JAMA 233:242, 1975.

39. SACKETT, D. L., GIBSON, E. S., TAYLOR, D. W., ET AL.: *Randomized clinical trial of strategies for improving medication compliance in primary hypertension.* Lancet 1:1205, 1975.

40. MEYER, A. J., AND HENDERSON, J. B. *Multiple risk factor reduction in the prevention of cardiovascular disease.* Preventive Med. 3:225, 1974.

Beta-Blocking Drug Therapy in Hypertension

James Conway, M.D.

DISCOVERY OF THE ANTIHYPERTENSIVE EFFECT

The introduction of beta-blocking agents for the treatment of arrhythmias and angina[1] was followed in 1964 by the identification of the antihypertensive properties of propranolol.[2] Although in the early investigations there was some reservation regarding the significance of this effect,[3, 4] a clear antihypertensive action was abundantly confirmed by others in a large group of patients.[5, 6] Thus it has been established that beta-blockers are effective in a large proportion of hypertensive patients (Fig. 1). Side effects are few and it is important that lowering of blood pressure can be achieved without interfering with the patient's daily life. Subjects with both renal and essential hypertension respond, and a substantial fall in pressure is seen in severe or malignant hypertension as well as in the milder forms of the disease. Recumbent and standing pressures are both reduced equally, and postexercise hypotension, commonly experienced with the use of autonomic blocking agents, is not observed.[7] Moreover, a cutoff in the blood pressure response occurs at approximately normotensive levels. Thus, the symptoms of hypotension are unusual. Propranolol therefore appeared, like the diuretics, to be antihypertensive rather than hypotensive.

Thus, beta-adrenergic blocking drugs have emerged as new medicines in the armamentarium for the treatment of hypertension; and many studies have been devoted to an examination of their therapeutic potential.

DETAILS OF THE RESPONSE TO BETA-BLOCKERS IN HYPERTENSION

With any new treatment and particularly with one which was believed to act primarily on the heart, it was natural and prudent that a cautious approach was adopted to its investigation. As a consequence, while beta-blockers were thought initially to be of interest, they were not considered to be generally useful in the management of hypertension. The expansion of knowledge about these drugs has reversed this impression, and they have now been shown to be equal to the diuretics in the simplicity of their use in hypertension. Ideas have also begun to emerge on the possible modes of action of beta-blockers, although the precise mechanism responsible for the fall in pressure remains elusive.

The antihypertensive action of propranolol almost certainly resides in its beta-adrenoceptor blocking action since its inactive dextro-isomer does not lower blood pressure.[8]

Furthermore all the known beta-blockers lower pressure in spite of differences in physical and chemical properties.[9-11] It has also been shown that the dose response rela-

253

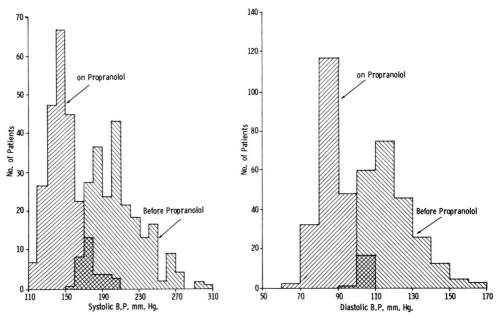

Figure 1. Distribution of systolic and diastolic pressure before and after treatment of hypertensive patients with propranolol. (From Zacharias and Cowen,[5] with permission.)

tionship for the antihypertensive effect generally follows that required for cardiac beta-blockade,[12, 13] although some have shown that cardiac blockade occurs at a lower dose than needed to produce an antihypertensive effect.[14] Much has been learned about the antihypertensive action of beta-blockers as newer ones have been developed, but a discussion of these will not be taken up here since only propranolol is presently available in the United States.

CHARACTERISTICS OF THE BLOOD PRESSURE RESPONSE

The response of blood pressure to beta-blockade has now been shown to persist for 24 hours and the elevation in pressure induced by stressful psychological stimuli is reduced.[15] During exercise, untreated hypertensive subjects are known to develop exceedingly high levels of systolic pressure.[16, 17] This stress to the vascular system is particularly well controlled by beta-blockade (Fig. 2). It has also been shown that whereas peripheral resistance rises with the fall in cardiac output after the acute administration of a beta-blocker, peripheral resistance returns to its initial level during chronic therapy, although cardiac output remains depressed.[13, 18]

Although it was originally thought that the full antihypertensive action of propranolol developed over many weeks, it has now been established that most, if not the entire, fall in pressure is seen within a matter of a few days or even hours (Fig. 3).[9, 12, 19-22]

Extended experience in the use of propranolol in hypertensive patients has led to a more precise estimate of the doses required to control blood pressure. These are much lower than was formerly believed. The maximal response to propranolol occurs with a dose which lies between 160 and 480 mg./day.[12, 19, 23] This, taken with the fact that cardiac side effects are very uncommon, has made it possible to simplify the dosage schedules. Thus, the starting dose of propranolol should be 80 mg. twice daily for all hypertensives.[24]

254

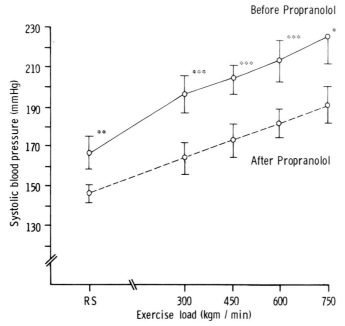

Figure 2. The effect of propranolol therapy on systolic blood pressure at rest (RS) and during exercise.

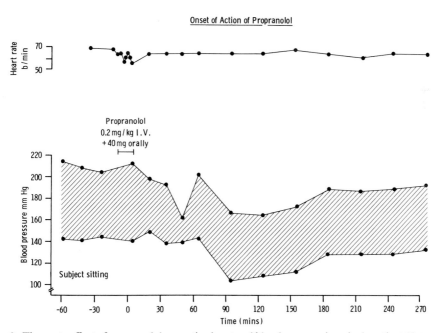

Figure 3. The acute effect of propranolol on resting heart and blood pressure in a single patient (data provided by Dr. P. Lauwers, Brussels).

The magnitude of the antihypertensive effect of propranolol appears to exceed that of the diuretics and to be equivalent to that of methyldopa (Fig. 4).[11] Furthermore it has been shown that an additive effect can be seen when beta-blocking agents are used in conjunction with many other antihypertensive drugs, e.g., diuretics,[25] methyldopa,[11] sympathetic neurone blockers and vasodilators. Reports attest to the value of combination therapy with any of these drugs in difficult cases. The use of vasodilators with beta-blockers is logical since the increase in heart rate and elevation of renin level induced by a vasodilator are controlled by beta-blockers.[29-31] The blood pressure response is enhanced when a vasodilator drug is added to propranolol therapy, but the total response is less than the sum of their individual effects.[27] More important, however, is the observation that a fall in blood pressure could be obtained in patients who had been refractory to other forms of treatment.[28, 32]

SIDE EFFECTS ATTRIBUTABLE TO BETA-BLOCKADE

The pharmacological actions of beta-blockers are seen primarily in their effects on the heart. Pulse rate and cardiac output are reduced, as is the force of cardiac contraction. On rare occasions, bradycardia may produce symptoms if the rate falls below 45 beats/min. If this occurs, the heart rate can be restored by the administration of atropine. If this is unsuccessful it is advisable to follow this with an isoprenaline infusion, recognizing that a very large dose will be needed in view of the prevailing beta-blockade.

The fall in cardiac output is followed by a reflex increase in alpha-sympathetic tone to blood vessels. This sometimes results in complaints of coldness of the hands and feet

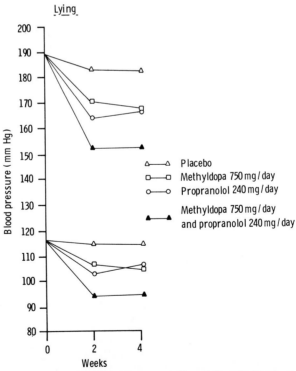

Figure 4. Comparison of propranolol and methyldopa on systolic and diastolic blood pressure. (Adapted from Petrie et al.,[11] with permission.)

and a syndrome similar to Raynaud's phenomenon. While this may be a nuisance, it is rarely so severe as to require the withdrawal of therapy. The fall in cardiac output and the reduced response to exercise may lead to complaints of tiredness on exercise, particularly in the legs. Again this is rarely of a sufficient degree to require withdrawal of treatment.

Stimulation of beta-adrenergic receptors in the lung produces bronchodilatation, consequently their blockade may lead to bronchoconstriction. This is of little consequence in normal subjects, but it can produce symptoms in patients who have asthma or a history of bronchospasm. Such a history is a contraindication to therapy with beta-blocking drugs. In Europe cardioselective agents, metoprolol and atenolol, have been developed to avoid this difficulty; but these drugs are not presently available in the United States.

The reduction in blood pressure and cardiac output can lead to fluid retention. Therefore, these drugs should not be used for the treatment of hypertension in subjects with a history of congestive heart failure or in those with evidence of cardiac dilatation when cardiac function is critically dependant on sympathetic drive. However, plasma volume is usually unchanged in the treatment of hypertension.[33, 34] Fluid retention is exceedingly uncommon, but, as has been shown with other antihypertensive drugs, when it does occur control of blood pressure is generally lost.[13, 35] In these circumstances, diuretics can be used to eliminate the accumulated fluid without interruption of antihypertensive therapy.

Renal function is well maintained as blood pressure is lowered with beta-blockers although glomerular filtration rate is reduced.[36] It must always be remembered that reduction in perfusion pressure with any antihypertensive agent can be harmful to subjects with severely compromised renal function.

Finally, it should be recognized that in diabetic subjects receiving insulin the physiological response to the hypoglycemia due to insulin overdosage includes the mobilization of hepatic glycogen. As this is a function of the beta-adrenergic system, hypoglycemia may therefore be more severe in patients on beta-blocking treatment.

SIDE EFFECTS UNRELATED TO BETA-BLOCKADE

The wide experience with the use of propranolol over the past 15 years has demonstrated a low incidence of adverse reactions. A full list of those seen during the treatment of hypertension has been published elsewhere.[38] Of the nonspecific adverse effects, vivid dreams, sleep disturbance and visual hallucinations are well documented. Another group of side effects are gastrointestinal disturbances. None of these are specific, but include heartburn, gastritis, nausea and "indigestion".

Overall, the freedom from adverse reactions has frequently been commented upon in the use of beta-blockers in hypertension, and there are no side effects which interfere with the daily life of the patient.[6, 39] In a recent survey of the treatment of hypertension in a Swedish community where beta-blockers are used extensively, the withdrawal rate from treatment in patients on these drugs was 8.1 percent as against 13.2 percent for diuretics.[40]

THEORIES FOR THE MODE OF ACTION OF BETA-BLOCKERS IN LOWERING BLOOD PRESSURE

As with most of the antihypertensive drugs, the mechanism responsible for the fall in pressure is unknown. This is not altogether surprising since the mechanism responsible for the increase in peripheral resistance in hypertension is itself unknown.

As indicated earlier, the fall in blood pressure can be attributed to beta-blockade since all the known drugs of this type lower blood pressure equally. It is also unlikely that the metabolites are responsible since hypotensive beta-blockers differ in the degree of metabolism and the type of metabolite.

The number of theories accounting for the reduction of pressure by beta-blockers increases with time. A list is given in Table 1. It would be premature to discuss these in detail since none fit all the known facts concerning their antihypertensive properties.

It is worthwhile, however, to consider the renin hypothesis, since this has been investigated more extensively than the others; and it offers, for the first time, the possibility of a rational approach to the choice of drugs for the treatment for hypertension. The theory is based on two related propositions which arose from observations by Bühler and coworkers in 1972.[41] First, patients who respond best to beta-blockers have an elevated plasma renin activity. Secondly, the fall in blood pressure results from the reduction in the level of the circulating vasoconstrictor substance angiotensin II, this fall being reflected by a decline in plasma renin activity.

Although there has been some disagreement over the evidence supporting the proposition that patients with elevated plasma renin respond well to beta-blockers,[42] on balance the evidence does appear to support this concept.[13, 43-45] The elevated plasma renin activity may, in fact, be a reflection of an increased sympathetic tone.[21] It must be pointed out, however, that the level of plasma renin activity has usually been measured after it has been raised by the stimulus of standing or by volume depletion, and this does not necessarily reflect the average level which persists throughout the day.

It has further been shown that all the presently available beta-blockers, with the possible exception of pindolol,[46] lower plasma renin activity.[21] However, there is considerable disagreement in the various reports as to whether the fall in blood pressure is related to the fall in renin. In several studies[44, 47, 48] the fall in blood pressure has correlated with the change in renin, and some have observed individual cases where the fall in blood pressure and renin activity occurred together.[20, 22] Others have been unable to relate the fall in renin to the fall in blood pressure;[9, 33, 49] and with one agent in particular, pindolol, it has been shown that the fall in blood pressure may not be accompanied by a fall in plasma renin activity.[45, 46]

Unfortunately, few of the reports provide adequate data on the levels of renin in their hypertensive patients compared with those seen in the normal population. This is of some importance since it is likely that when the level of plasma renin activity is grossly elevated the circulating angiotensin will be vasoconstrictor, and it is expected that its reduction would then lower blood pressure. This seems to apply most clearly in patients with renal failure.[22] At present, however, the precise levels of renin that result in plasma concentrations of angiotensin adequate to cause vasoconstriction have not been established.

On balance, therefore, it seems likely that a part of the antihypertensive action of beta-blockers can be accounted for by a fall in plasma renin activity. This may be seen in subjects with exceptionally high angiotensin levels. Conversely, subjects with an

Table 1. Theories for antihypertensive action of beta-blockers

1. Reduction in renin levels[41]
2. Cardiac output and heart rate depression with autoregulation in vasculature[12]
3. Reduction in the release of noradrenaline (presynaptic blockade)[52, 53]
4. Blockade of central beta-receptors[54]
5. Change in CNS control of BP resulting from the persistent cardiac effects[55, 56]
6. Control of surges in pressure leading to relaxation of vessels[15]
7. Restoration in the sensitivity of the beta-receptors[57]

abnormally low or "unresponsive" renin system respond poorly to beta-blocking drugs, but better to diuretics.[50, 51] Since subjects with normal renin levels also respond to beta-blockers, there must be an additional mechanism responsible for blood pressure reduction.[21, 44] The nature of this is unknown, and it cannot be determined which mechanism will predominate in a particular patient.

CONCLUSION

The introduction of beta-blocking drugs as antihypertensive agents seemed at first to be more of academic interest than of practical value. Further evaluation of their effectiveness in the treatment of large numbers of patients with hypertension has shown them to lower blood pressure in about 60 percent of patients. The overall effect has been to produce a fall in pressure of approximately 25/15 mm. Hg, which is greater than that seen with diuretics but equivalent to the effect of methyldopa. The fall in blood pressure occurs in the recumbent and upright positions and there is no postexercise hypotension. The dosage regimen for propranolol can be simplified to a recommendation of 80 mg. twice daily for most patients. Beta-blockers have thus emerged as drugs "of first choice" in the treatment of hypertension. Alone or in combination with diuretics, they can be used to manage the majority of uncomplicated hypertensives with a low incidence of side effects.

REFERENCES

1. DORNHORST, A. C., AND ROBINSON, B. F.: *Clinical pharmacology of a beta-adrenergic-blocking agent (Nethalide)*. Lancet 2:311, 1962.

2. PRICHARD, B. N. C., AND GILLAM, P. M. S.: *Use of propranolol in treatment of hypertension*. Br. Med. J. 2:725, 1964.

3. RICHARDSON, D. W., FREUND, J., GEAR, A. S., ET AL.: *Effect of propranolol on elevated arterial blood pressure*. Circulation 37:534, 1968.

4. PATERSON, J. W., AND DOLLERY, C. T.: *Effect of propranolol in mild hypertension*. Lancet 2:1148, 1966.

5. ZACHARIAS, F. J., COWEN, K. J., ET AL.: *Propranolol in hypertension: A study of longterm therapy, 1964–1970*. Am. Heart J. 83:755, 1972.

6. HANSSON, L., MALMCRONA, R., OLANDER, R., ET AL.: *Propranolol in hypertension. Report on 158 patients treated up to 1 year*. Klin. Wochenschr. 50:364, 1972.

7. PRICHARD, B. N. C. AND GILLAM, P. M. S. *Treatment of hypertension with propranolol*. Br. Med. J. 1:7, 1969.

8. RAHN, K. H., HAWLINA, A., KERSTING, F., ET AL.: *Studies on the antihypertensive action of the optical isomers of propranolol in man*. Nauyn Schmiedebergs Arch. Pharmacol. 286:319, 1974.

9. MORGAN, T. O., ROBERTS, R., CARNEY, S. L., ET AL.: *Beta-adrenergic receptor blocking drugs, hypertension and plasma renin*. Br. J. Clin. Pharmacol. 2:159, 1975.

10. DAVIDSON, C., THADANI, U., SINGLETON, W., ET AL.: *Comparison of antihypertensive activity of beta-blocking drugs during chronic treatment*. Br. Med. J. 2:7, 1976.

11. PETRIE, J. C., GALLOWAY, D. B., JEFFERS, T. A., ET AL.: *Methyldopa and propranolol or practolol in moderate hypertension*. Br. Med. J. 2:137, 1976.

12. CONWAY, J., AND AMERY A.: *The antihypertensive effect of propranolol and other beta-adrenoceptor antagonists*, in DAVIES, D. S. AND REID, J. L. (EDS.): *Central Action of Drugs in Blood Pressure Regulation*. Pitman, London, 1975, p. 277.

13. AMERY, A., BILLIER, L., BOEL, A., ET AL.: *Mechanism of hypotensive effect during beta-adrenergic blockade in hypertensive patients*. Am. Heart. J. 91:634, 1976.

14. LEONETTI, G., MAYER, G., MORGANTI, A., ET AL.: *Hypotensive and renin-suppressing activities of propranolol in hypertensive patients*. Clin. Sci. Mol. Med. 48:491, 1975.

15. LORIMOR, A. R., DUNN, F. G., JONES, J. V., ET AL.: *Beta-adrenoreceptor blockade in hypertension*. Am. J. Med. 60:877, 1976.

16. LUND-JOHANSEN, P.: *Hemodynamics in early essential hypertension*. Acta Med. Scand. (Suppl. 482), 1967.

17. AMERY, A., JULIUS, J., WHITLOCK, L. S., ET AL. *Influence of hypertension on the hemodynamic response to exercise.* Circulation 36:231, 1967.

18. TARAZI, R. C., AND DUSTAN, H. P.: *Beta-adrenergic blockade in hypertension.* Am. J. Cardiol. 29:633, 1972.

19. HANSSON, L.: *Beta-adrenergic blockade in essential hypertension.* Acta Med. Scand. (Suppl. 550), 1973.

20. STUMPE, K. O., VETTER, H., HESSENBRUCH, V., ET AL. *Einfluss einer chronischen beta-receptoren-blockade auf blutdruck renin, aldosteron und cortisolsekretion bei essentieller hypertension.* Klin. Wochenschr. 53:907, 1975.

21. BÜHLER, F. R., BURKART, F., LUTOLD, B. E., ET AL.: *Antihypertensive beta-blocking action as related to renin and age: a pharmacologic tool to identify pathogenetic mechanisms in essential hypertension.* Am. J. Cardiol. 36:653, 1975.

22. MOORE, S. B., AND GOODWIN, F. J.: *Effect of beta-adrenergic blockade on plasma renin activity and intractable hypertension in patients receiving regular dialysis treatment.* Lancet 2:67, 1976.

23. GALLOWAY, D. B., GLOVER, S. C., HENDRY, W. G., ET AL.: *Propranolol in hypertension: a dose response study.* Br. Med. J. 2:140, 1976.

24. BERGLUND, G., ANDERSSON, O., HANSSON, L., ET AL.: *Propranolol given twice daily in hypertension.* Acta Med. Scand. 194:513, 1973.

25. CHALMERS, J., HORVATH, J., TILLER, D., ET AL.: *Effects of timolol and hydrochlorothiazide on blood pressure and plasma renin activity.* Lancet 2:328, 1976.

26. PEARSON, R. M., BENDING, M. R., BULPITT, C. J., ET AL.: *Trial of combination of guanethidine and oxprenolol in hypertension.* Br. J. Med. 1:933, 1976.

27. ZACEST, R., GILMORE, E., AND KOCH-WESER, J.: *Treatment of essential hypertension with combined vasodilation and beta-adrenergic blockade.* N. Engl. J. Med. 286:1617, 1972.

28. KINCAID-SMITH, P.: *Management of severe hypertension.* Am. J. Cardiol. 32:575, 1973.

29. GILMORE, E., WEIL, J., AND CHIDSEY, C.: *Treatment of essential hypertension with a new vasodilator in combination with beta-adrenergic blockade.* N. Engl. J. Med. 282:521, 1970.

30. PETTINGER, W. A., AND MITCHELL, H. C.: *Renin release, saralasin and the vasodilator beta-blocker drug interaction in man.* N. Engl. J. Med. 292:1214, 1975.

31. PEDERSEN, E. B., AND KORNERUP, H. J.: *Effect of alprenolol and hydralazine on plasma renin concentration in patients with arterial hypertension.* Acta Med. Scand. 198:379, 1975.

32. SANNERSTEDT, R., STENBERG, J., VEDIN, A., ET AL.: *Chronic beta-adrenergic blockade in arterial hypertension.* Am. J. Cardiol. 29:718, 1972.

33. BRAVO, E. L., TARAZI, R. C., DUSTAN, H. P., ET AL.: *Dissociation between renin and arterial pressure responses to beta-adrenergic blockade in human essential hypertension.* Circ. Res. 36 & 37:I-241, 1975.

34. SEDENBERG-OLSEN, P., AND IBSEN, H.: *Plasma volume and extra-cellular fluid volume during long-term treatment with propranolol in essential hypertension.* Clin. Sci. 43:165, 1972.

35. FINNERTY, F. A.: *Relationship of extra-cellular fluid volume to the development of drug resistance in the hypertensive patient.* Am. Heart J. 81:563, 1971.

36. IBSEN, H., AND SEDENBERG-OLSEN, P.: *Changes in glomerular filtration rate during long-term treatment with propranolol in patients with arterial hypertension.* Clin. Sci., 41:129, 1973.

37. WARREN, D. J., SWAINSON, C. P., AND WRIGHT, N.: *Deterioration in renal function after beta-blockade in patients with chronic renal failure and hypertension.* Br. Med. J. 2:193, 1974.

38. CONWAY, J.: *Beta-adrenergic blockade and hypertension,* in OLIVER, M. F. (ED.): *Modern Trends in Cardiology,* 3. Butterworths, London, 1975, p. 376.

39. MATERSON, B. J., ULRICH, F. M., OSTER, J. R., ET AL.: *Antihypertensive effects of oxprenolol and propranolol.* Clin. Pharmacol. Ther. 20:142, 1976.

40. WILHELMSON, L.: *Treatment of hypertension in a Swedish community—the problem of borderline hypertension.* Acta Med. Scand. 197 (Suppl. 576):99, 1975.

41. BÜHLER, F. R., LARAGH, J. H., BAER, L., ET AL.: *Propranolol inhibition of renin secretion.* N. Engl. J. Med. 287:1209, 1972.

42. WOODS, J. W., PITTMAN, A. W., PULLIAM, C. C., ET AL.: *Renin profiling in hypertension and its use in treatment with propranolol and chlorthalidone.* N. Engl. J. Med. 294:1137, 1976.

43. STREETEN, D. H. P., ANDERSON, G. H., AND DALAKOS, T. G.: *Angiotensin blockade: its clinical significance.* Am. J. Med. 60:817, 1976.

44. HOLLIFIELD, J. W., SHERMAN, K., VANDER SWAGG, R. N. R., ET AL.: *Proposed mechanisms of propranolol's antihypertensive effect in essential hypertension.* N. Engl. J. Med. 295:68, 1976.

45. STUMPE, K. O., KOLLOCH, R., VETTER, H., ET AL.: *Acute and long-term studies of the mechanisms of action of beta-blocking drugs in lowering blood pressure.* Am. J. Med., 60:853, 1976.

46. STOKES, G. S., WEBER, M. A., AND THORNELL, I. R.: *Beta-blockers and plasma renin activity in hypertension.* Br. Med. J. 1:60, 1974.

47. CASTENFORS, J., JOHNSSON, H., AND ORO, L.: *Effect of alprenolol on blood pressure and plasma renin activity in hypertensive patients.* Acta Med. Scand. 193:189, 1973.

48. MENARD, J., BERTAGNA, X., N'GUYEN, P. T., ET AL.: *Rapid identification of patients with essential hypertension sensitive to acebutolol.* Am. J. Med. 60:886, 1976.

49. GEYSKES, G. G., BOER, P., VOS, J., ET AL.: *Effect of salt depletion and propranolol on blood pressure and plasma renin activity in various forms of hypertension.* Circ. Res. 36 & 37:I-248, 1975.

50. BÜHLER, F. R., AND GAVRAS, H.: *Antihypertensive action of propranolol. Specific antirenin responses in high and normal renin forms of essential, renal, renovascular and malignant hypertension.* Am. J. Cardiol. 32:511, 1973.

51. CAREY, R. M., DOUGLAS, J. G., SCHWEIKERT, J. R., ET AL.: *The syndrome of essential hypertension and suppressed plasma renin activity.* Arch. Intern. Med. 130:849, 1974.

52. DAHLÖF, C., ÅBLAD, B., BORG, K. O., ET AL.: *Prejunctional inhibition of adrenergic nervous vasomotor control due to beta-receptor blockade,* in ALMGREN, O., ET AL. (EDS.): *Chemical Books in Catecholamine Research,* II. North Holland Publishing Company, 1975.

53. ADLER-GRASCHINSKY, E., AND LANGER, S. Z.: *Possible role of a beta-adrenoceptor in the regulation of noradrenaline release by nerve stimulation through a positive feedback mechanism.* Br. J. Pharmacol. 53:43, 1975.

54. DAY, M. D., AND ROACH, A. G.: *Beta-adrenergic receptors in the central nervous system of the cat concerned with control of arterial blood pressure and heart rate.* Nature (New Biol.) 242:30, 1973.

55. LEWIS, P.: *The essential action of propranolol in hypertension.* Am. J. Med. 60:837, 1976.

56. RAINE, A. E. G., AND CHUBB, I. W.: *Long term β-adrenergic blockade reduces tyrosine hydroxylase and dopamine β-hydroxylase activities in sympathetic ganglia.* Nature 267:265, 1977.

57. AMER, M. S.: *Mechanism of action of beta-blockers in hypertension.* Biochem. Pharmacol. 26:171, 1977.

Management of Hypertension in the Patient with Chronic Renal Disease

Charles D. Swartz, M.D., and Kwan Eun Kim, M.D.

Hypertension is both a cause and a complication of chronic renal disease. In this chapter, we shall deal with the pathophysiology and management of patients with hypertension complicating the course of chronic renal disease.

An estimated 100,000 patients per year die of uremia. Over 20,000 are cared for by end-state renal disease programs which provide maintenance dialysis and renal transplantation. In all such programs, the major causes of death are the cardiovascular complications of myocardial infarction, congestive heart failure, and stroke. Therefore, it has become axiomatic that control of hypertension is mandatory for the long-term rehabilitation of all patients with chronic renal disease.

It has also been demonstrated that hypertension per se accelerates the deterioration of renal function by damaging renal arterioles. Therefore, to provide for the longest possible interval between the onset of renal parenchymal disease and the need for maintenance dialysis or transplantation, hypertension must be controlled.

HEMODYNAMICS OF HYPERTENSION IN CHRONIC RENAL DISEASE

Information regarding hemodynamic changes of hypertension in early chronic renal diseases suggests that the hypertension of chronic renal disease may start with an increased cardiac output.[1-3] With progression of hypertension, the cardiac output tends to decrease while peripheral resistance increases to sustain the hypertension. Finally, as the patient becomes progressively more azotemic and anemic, the cardiac output increases but the peripheral resistance fails to fall and hypertension persists.[4-7]

The pattern of hemodynamic changes in uremic patients has been extensively studied.[4-7] Cardiac output is significantly higher than in normal controls, whereas stroke volume is no different than that of normals. The higher cardiac output of uremic patients is accounted for by increased heart rate, and appears to be due to uremic anemia (Fig. 1). Cardiac output, heart rate, and stroke volume are similar in hypertensive and normotensive uremic patients, but total peripheral resistance is higher in the hypertensive patients. Therefore, the hypertension in end-stage renal disease is sustained mainly by high total peripheral resistance (Fig. 2).

PATHOPHYSIOLOGY OF BLOOD PRESSURE REGULATION IN PATIENTS WITH END-STAGE RENAL DISEASE

Salt and water balance and a vasopressor substance or substances from the diseased kidney are the two major factors that regulate blood pressure in patients with end-stage renal disease on maintenance hemodialysis.

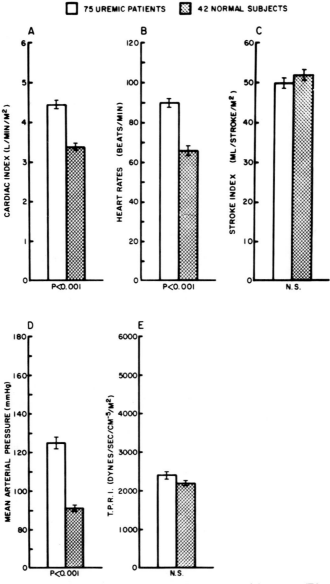

Figure 1. Cardiac index (A), heart rates (B), stroke index (C), mean arterial pressure (D), and total peripheral resistance index (E) of 75 patients with end-stage renal disease (hypertensives and normotensives, mean hematocrit 23 percent) compared with 42 normal controls (mean hematocrit 43 percent). Hemodynamic values are expressed as mean ± 1 SE; T.P.R.I. = total peripheral resistance index; N.S. = not statistically significant (from Kim, et al.,[4] with the permission of the American Heart Association, Inc.).

Ultrafiltration dialysis for the removal of salt and water controls hypertension in the majority of the patients. Bilateral nephrectomy in patients with severe and malignant hypertension on maintenance hemodialysis results in a significant reduction of blood pressure at equivalent levels of total exchangeable sodium and body weight.[4, 8]

The reduction of blood pressure after bilateral nephrectomy is associated with a decrease in total peripheral resistance without any change in cardiac output in severe but

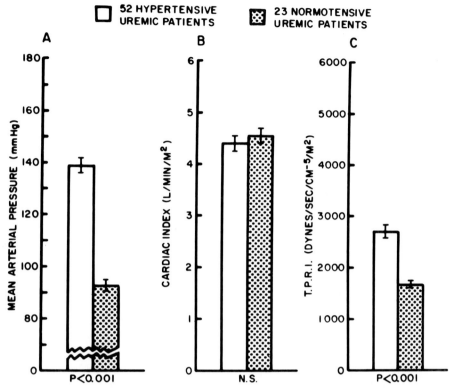

Figure 2. Comparison of mean arterial pressure (A), cardiac index (B), and total peripheral resistance index (C) of 52 hypertensive patients (mean hematocrit 23 percent) and 23 normotensive patients (mean hematocrit also 23 percent) with end-stage renal disease (from Kim, et al.,[4] with the permission of the American Heart Association, Inc.).

nonmalignant hypertensive uremic patients (Fig. 3).[4] In uremic patients with malignant hypertension, reduction of blood pressure after bilateral nephrectomy is associated with an actual increase in cardiac output and a more dramatic reduction in total peripheral resistance (Fig. 4).[4] These findings imply that a vasopressor substance or substances of renal origin increasing total peripheral resistance is a major factor in the pathophysiology of hypertension in end-stage renal disease.

RENAL EFFECTS OF ANTIHYPERTENSIVE AGENTS

Three categories of antihypertensive drugs are used in patients with chronic renal disease: diuretics, sympathetic nervous system inhibitors and vasodilators.

Diuretics

Acute administration of chlorothiazide reduces glomerular filtration. Heinemann and colleagues reported an average reduction of 16.9 percent with a range of 7.8 to 30 percent.[9] It also has been reported that the oral administration of chlorothiazide for 3 to 14 days reduces glomerular filtration rate; the mean reduction was 29 percent with a range of 16 to 50 percent.[10]

Acute administration of the loop blocking diuretics, furosemide and ethacrynic acid, ordinarily produces little or no change in glomerular filtration rate or renal plasma

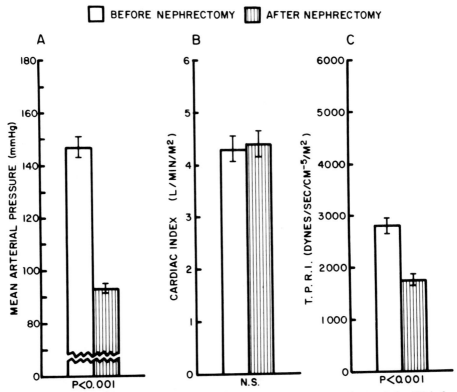

BEFORE NEPHRECTOMY ▦ AFTER NEPHRECTOMY

Figure 3. Mean arterial pressure (A), cardiac index (B), and total peripheral resistance index (C) before and after bilateral nephrectomy in 12 hypertensive patients (severe but nonmalignant) with end-stage renal disease. The hemodynamic values of each patient are compared at equivalent levels of exchangeable sodium and body weight. Exchangeable sodium ranged from 42 to 47 mEq./kg. before nephrectomy and 41 to 49 mEq./kg. after nephrectomy, indicating these patients were studied at dry weight (from Kim, et al.,[4] with the permission of the American Heart Association, Inc.).

flow.[11-17] Acute administration of large doses, however, may induce renal vasodilatation and increase renal blood flow.[18] It has been shown that acute administration of furosemide and ethacrynic acid redistributes renal blood flow; superficial renal cortical blood increases, while outer medullary blood flow and juxtamedullary blood flow decrease.[19]

Sympathetic Nervous System Inhibitors

Intravenous administration of guanethidine decreases glomerular filtration rate and renal blood flow.[20] It has been reported that short term oral administration of guanethidine also decreases glomerular filtration rate and renal plasma flow.[21] However, neither intravenous administration nor short term oral administration of alpha-methyldopa decreases glomerular filtration rate or renal plasma flow.[22, 23] Similarly, glomerular filtration rate and renal plasma flow do not decrease following acute or prolonged administration of clonidine.[24, 25]

It also has been reported that renal blood flow and glomerular filtration rate are not altered either after acute intravenous administration of reserpine or after oral administration of reserpine for three months.[26] However, glomerular filtration rate is reduced during long term administration of propranolol (mean reduction of 13 percent).[27] Treat-

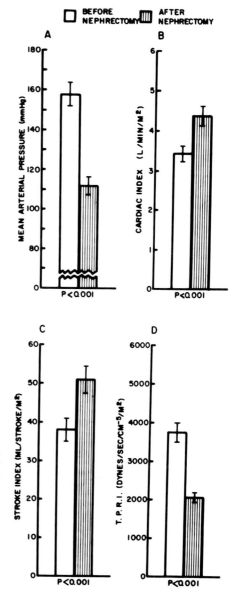

Figure 4. Mean arterial pressure (A), cardiac index (B), stroke index (C), and total peripheral resistance index (D) before and after bilateral nephrectomy in eight patients with end-stage renal disease and malignant hypertension. Hemodynamic values of each patient are compared at an equivalent level of total exchangeable sodium and body weight. Exchangeable sodium ranged from 43 to 49 mEq./kg. before nephrectomy and 45 to 48 mEq./kg. after nephrectomy (from Kim, et al.[4] with the permission of the American Heart Association, Inc.).

ment of hypertension with propranolol in patients with moderately severe renal failure may be followed by rapid deterioration of renal function.[28]

Vasodilators

A single subcutaneous or oral administration of hydralazine produces a significant increase in renal plasma flow without significant change in glomerular filtration rate.[29, 30] Direct injection of hydralazine into one renal artery produces an immediate decrease in renal blood flow on the injected side. When hydralazine reaches the systemic circulation, an increase in renal blood flow occurs contralaterally.[31] These findings indicate that hydralazine increases renal blood flow secondary to an increase in cardiac output.

However, the percentage increase in cardiac output exceeds the percentage increase in renal blood flow.[32] It has been reported further that prolonged administration of hydralazine (at the end of the 11 to 15 weeks of treatment) does not significantly increase renal plasma flow.[30]

MANAGEMENT OF PATIENTS WITH CHRONIC RENAL DISEASE NOT YET ON DIALYSIS

During severe salt restriction, a normal person can lower urinary sodium excretion nearly to zero. However, patients with chronic renal disease sometimes have an impaired ability to conserve sodium. In addition, patients with chronic renal insufficiency often cannot excrete a high salt intake. Such patients are vulnerable to salt and water retention, and circulatory congestion. On the other hand, severe salt restriction may cause salt depletion, dehydration and further deterioration of renal function. There is a small group of patients with chronic renal disease in whom massive salt wasting occurs. Thus, severe salt restriction should be avoided in patients with chronic renal disease unless they are fluid overloaded or have nephrotic syndrome.

Table 1 outlines the drug therapy of the patient with chronic renal disease who is not yet on dialysis.

Thiazide diuretics should be avoided in hypertensive patients with renal insufficiency because these agents decrease glomerular filtration rate[9, 10] and diuretic action (and probably antihypertensive action as well) is lost when the glomerular filtration rate is reduced below 20 ml. per minute. Furosemide and ethacrynic acid, however, continue to exhibit natriuretic and diuretic effects, even at low glomerular filtration rates.[33, 34] Therefore, if the patient is not a renal salt waster, furosemide or ethacrynic acid should be the starting therapeutic agent for the treatment of hypertension.

The dosage of furosemide varies, depending on the severity of the hypertension and the degree of impairment of the glomerular filtration rate. Forty milligrams may be given twice daily in the patient with mild to moderate hypertension and mild reduction of the glomerular filtration rate. Patients with severe reduction of the glomerular filtration rate may require 120 mg. four times per day or more.

Potassium-sparing diuretic agents, such as spironolactone or triamterene, are contraindicated when azotemia is present, because of the danger of hyperkalemia.

Table 1. Management of the patient with chronic renal disease not yet on dialysis

Start with diuretics unless patient is proven salt waster		
Loop Blocking Diuretics	*Starting Dose*	*Maximum Dose*
Furosemide	40 mg. b.i.d.	120 mg. q.i.d.
Ethacrynic Acid	50 mg. b.i.d.	150 mg. q.i.d.
AVOID thiazides and potassium sparing diuretics		
Sympathetic Blocking Drugs	*Starting Dose*	*Maximum Dose*
Alpha-methyldopa	250 mg. b.i.d.	500 mg. q.i.d.
Clonidine	0.1 mg. b.i.d.	0.6 mg. q.i.d.
AVOID guanethidine and propranolol as both may worsen azotemia		
Peripheral Vasodilators	*Starting Dose*	*Maximum Dose*
Hydralazine	10 mg. q.i.d.	100 mg. t.i.d.
Prazosin*	1 mg. b.i.d.	10 mg. b.i.d.
Minoxidil†	5 mg. o.d.	70 mg. o.d.

*Prazosin may be used without sympathetic blocking drug.
†Minoxidil—investigational drug.

If blood pressure is not controlled with a diuretic alone, the second drug to be added is alpha-methyldopa or clonidine. Both of these agents preserve glomerular filtration rate and renal blood flow.[22-25] Titration of drug dosage is essential with these agents.

The starting dosage of alpha-methyldopa is 250 mg. twice daily. If a satisfactory decrease in blood pressure is not obtained, the dosage should be increased by increments of 250 to 500 mg. depending on the severity of hypertension, until a satisfactory response is obtained or side effects become prohibitive. The maximum dosage of alpha-methyldopa is 2 to 3 grams per day. Drowsiness, fatigue, dry mouth, orthostatic hypotension, Coombs positive erythrocytes, rare hepatotoxicity and bone marrow suppression are potential untoward effects.

The initial dose of clonidine is 0.1 mg. twice per day. If an adequate response is not obtained, the dosage of clonidine should be increased by increments of 0.2 to 0.3 mg. until a satisfactory decrease in blood pressure is obtained or side effects become prohibitive. The maximum dosage of clonidine is 1.8 to 2.4 mg. per day, administered in three divided doses. Drowsiness and dry mouth are common side effects. A marked blood pressure rise with restlessness, insomnia and tremor following withdrawal of clonidine has been reported.[35] However, extensive experience with clonidine reveals the latter to be a rare complication.

If blood pressure is not controlled with furosemide (or ethacrynic acid) and alpha-methyldopa (or clonidine), hydralazine is the third drug to be added. The initial dosage of hydralazine is 10 mg. four times daily (or 25 mg. twice daily). If an adequate response is not obtained, the dosage of hydralazine should be increased by increments of 25 to 50 mg. until an adequate blood pressure reduction is achieved. Maximum dosage of hydralazine is 100 mg. three to four times per day. With the addition of hydralazine, the dosage of alpha-methyldopa (or clonidine) sometimes can be reduced, with satisfactory control of supine pressure and a reversal of any accompanying orthostatic hypotension. The concomitant administration of alpha-methyldopa (or clonidine) usually prevents the reflex tachycardia produced by hydralazine.

Prazosin is a newly released vasodilator which also may be used either with a diuretic alone or in combination with a diuretic and a sympathetic blocking agent.

If adequate control of blood pressure is not achieved with standard therapy, the combination of minoxidil, propranolol and furosemide may be effective. Minoxidil is the most potent oral vasodilator available, but currently is available only as an investigational drug. Fluid retention and hirsutism are common side effects induced by minoxidil. The drug should be administered with propranolol to prevent reflex tachycardia and with furosemide to prevent fluid retention. Minoxidil and propranolol administration should be undertaken with frequent monitoring of blood pressure and pulse rate.

Guanethidine should be avoided because this drug frequently causes severe orthostatic hypotension and decreases glomerular filtration rate and renal blood flow. Reserpine is rarely used because it lacks adequate potency and because of its side effects, e.g., mental depression and nasal congestion.

MANAGEMENT OF THE HYPERTENSIVE PATIENT WITH END-STAGE RENAL DISEASE ON MAINTENANCE HEMODIALYSIS

In most patients with end-stage renal disease on maintenance hemodialysis, hypertension can be controlled by removal of sodium and water by ultrafiltration dialysis and by restriction of salt and water intake. These patients have virtually no renal excretory function, and their body fluids are controlled by their salt and fluid intake and by the amounts of salt and water removed by the artificial kidney. Therefore, the initial treatment of hypertension consists of ultrafiltration dialysis for removal of excess body fluid plus dietary restriction of salt and water intake.

Table 2. Management of the patient with end-stage renal disease
on maintenance dialysis

Step 1 — Dehydration by ultrafiltration dialysis. Diuretics are not effective when glomerular filtration falls below 3 to 5 ml./min.

Step 2 — If dehydration fails to control blood pressure, add sympathetic blocking drugs

	Starting Dose	*Maximum Dose*
Propranolol	40 mg. t.i.d.	120 mg. q.i.d.
Alpha-methyldopa	250 mg. b.i.d.	500 mg. q.i.d.
Clonidine	0.1 mg. b.i.d.	0.6 mg. q.i.d.

Step 3 — Add vasodilator

	Starting Dose	*Maximum Dose*
Hydralazine	10 mg. q.i.d.	100 mg. t.i.d.
Minoxidil	5 mg. o.d.	70 mg. o.d.

Step 4 — Bilateral nephrectomy, if preceding regimen fails to control the blood pressure

Table 2 outlines the management of hypertension in these patients.

When hypertension is not controlled by ultrafiltration dialysis and dietary restriction of salt and water, antihypertensive drug therapy should be administered. Alpha-methyldopa or clonidine is usually the first antihypertensive drug employed for the treatment of hypertension in these patients. If blood pressure is not controlled with alpha-methyldopa or clonidine alone or if the side effects become prohibitive, the next drug to be added is hydralazine. An alternative therapeutic regimen is the combined use of hydralazine and propranolol.

If adequate control of the hypertension is not achieved with ultrafiltration dialysis, dietary restriction of salt and water, and the use of antihypertensive drugs as outlined, the combination of minoxidil and propranolol may be effective in controlling the refractory hypertension.[36]

Bilateral nephrectomy is recommended for the control of hypertension when uremic patients with severe and malignant hypertension are refractory to ultrafiltration dialysis and antihypertensive drug therapy. Bilateral nephrectomy in these patients results in a significant reduction of blood pressure, and a marked general clinical improvement usually follows.

In the anephric state, blood pressure is normal or only mildly elevated when the patient is at clinically dry weight. There is a positive correlation between blood pressure and total exchangeable sodium or body fluid. A very small percentage of anephric patients may exhibit severe hypertension even at dry weight. Their blood pressure is usually controlled by ultrafiltration dialysis and dietary restriction, but antihypertensive drugs as outlined above should be added if dehydration fails to control the blood pressure.

REFERENCES

1. BROD, J.: *Chronic renal parenchymal disease and hypertension.* Kidney Int. 8 (Suppl. 5):235, 1975.

2. KIM, K. E., ONESTI, G., FERNANDES, M., ET AL.: *Hemodynamics of hypertension,* in ONESTI, G., FERNANDES, M., AND KIM, K. E. (EDS.): *Regulation of Blood Pressure by the Central Nervous System.* Grune & Stratton, New York, 1976, pp. 337–353.

3. ONESTI, G., KIM, K. E., FERNANDES, M., ET AL.: *Hypertension of renal parenchymal disease. Hemodynamic patterns and mechanisms,* in GIOVANETTI, S., BONOMINI, V., AND D'AMICO, G. (EDS.): *Proceedings of the Sixth International Congress of Nephrology.* S. Karger, Basel, 1976, pp. 284–304.

4. KIM, K. E., ONESTI, G., SCHWARTZ, A. B., ET AL.: *Hemodynamics of hypertension in chronic end-stage renal disease.* Circulation 46:456, 1972.

5. NEFF, M. S., KIM, K. E., PERSOFF, M., ET AL.: *Hemodynamics of uremic anemia.* Circulation 43:876, 1971.

6. KIM, K. E., ONESTI, G., NEFF, M. S., ET AL.: *Hemodynamic alterations in hypertension of chronic end-stage renal disease,* in ONESTI, G., KIM, K. E., AND MOYER, J. H. (EDS.): *Hypertension: Mechanisms and Management.* Grune & Stratton, New York, 1973, pp. 609–616.

7. KIM, K. E., ONESTI, G., AND SWARTZ, C.: *Hemodynamics of hypertension in uremia.* Kidney Int. 7 (Suppl. 2):155, 1975.

8. ONESTI, G., KIM, K. E., GRECO, J. A., ET AL.: *Blood pressure regulation in end-stage renal disease and anephric man.* Circ. Res. 36 & 37 (Suppl. 1): 145, 1975.

9. HEINEMANN, H. O., DIMARTINI, F. E., AND LARAGH, J. H.: *The effect of chlorothiazide on renal excretion of electrolytes and free water.* Am. J. Med. 26:853, 1959.

10. CORCORAN, A. C., MACLEOD, C., DUSTAN, H. P., ET AL.: *Effects of chlorothiazide on specific renal functions in hypertension.* Circulation 19:355, 1959.

11. KIM, K. E., ONESTI, G., MOYER, J. H., ET AL.: *Ethacrynic acid and furosemide. Diuretic and hemodynamic effects and clinical uses.* Am. J. Cardiol 27:407, 1971.

12. CANNON, P. J., HEINEMANN, H. O., STASON, W. B., ET AL.: *Effectiveness and mode of diuretic action in man.* Circulation 31:5, 1965.

13. STASON, W. B., CANNON, P. J., AND HEINEMANN, H. O.: *Furosemide, a clinical evaluation of its diuretic action.* Circulation 34:910, 1966.

14. STEIN, J. H., WILSON, C. B., AND KIRKENDALL, W. M.: *Differences in the acute effects of furosemide and ethacrynic acid in man.* J. Lab. Clin. Med. 71:654, 1968.

15. BREST, A. N., ONESTI, G., SELLER, R., ET AL.: *Pharmacodynamic effects of a new diuretic drug, ethacrynic acid.* Am. J. Cardiol. 16:99, 1965.

16. REUBI, F. C.: *Clinical use of furosemide.* Ann. N. Y. Acad. Sci. 139:433, 1966.

17. NASH, H. L., FITZ, A. E., WILSON, W. R., ET AL.: *Cardiorenal hemodynamic effects of ethacrynic acid.* Am. Heart J. 71:153, 1966.

18. HOOK, J. B., BLATT, A. H., BRODY, M. J., ET AL.: *Effects of several saluretic agents on renal hemodynamics.* J. Pharmacol. Exp. Ther. 154:667, 1966.

19. BIRTCH, A. G., ZAKHEIM, R. M., JONES L. G., ET AL.: *Redistribution of renal blood flow produced by furosemide and ethacrynic acid.* Circ. Res. 21:869, 1967.

20. ONESTI, G., KIM, K. E., SWARTZ, C., ET AL.: *Hemodynamic effects of antihypertensive agents,* in ONESTI, G., KIM, K. E., AND MOYER, J. H. (EDS.): *Hypertension: Mechanisms and Management.* Grune & Stratton, New York, 1973, pp. 227–240.

21. RICHARDSON, D. W., WYSO, E. M., MAGEE, J. H., ET AL.: *Circulatory effects of guanethidine. Clinical, renal, and cardiac responses to treatment with a novel antihypertensive drug.* Circulation 22:184, 1960.

22. ONESTI, G., BREST, A. N., NOVACK, P., ET AL.: *Pharmacodynamic effects of alpha-methyldopa in hypertensive subjects.* Am. Heart J. 67:32, 1964.

23. SANNERSTEDT, R., BOJS, G., AND VARNAUSKAS, E.: *Alpha-methldopa in arterial hypertension. Clinical, renal, and hemodynamic studies.* Acta Med. Scand. 174:53, 1963.

24. ONESTI, G., SCHWARTZ, A. B., KIM, K. E., ET AL.: *Pharmacodynamic effects of a new antihypertensive drug, Catapres (ST-155).* Circulation 39:219, 1969.

25. BOCK, K. D., HEIMSOTH, V., MERGUET, P., ET AL.: *Klinische und klinische-experimentelle untersuchungen mit einer neuen blutdrucksenkenden substanz: Dichlorphenylaminoimidazolin.* Deutsch Med. Wschr. 91:1761, 1966.

26. MOYER, J. H., HUGHES, W., HUGGINS, R., ET AL.: *The cardiovascular and renal hemodynamic response to the administration of reserpine (Serpasil).* Am. J. Med. Sci. 227:640, 1954.

27. IBSEN, H., AND SEDERBERG-OLSEN, P.: *Changes in glomerular filtration rate during long-term treatment with propranolol in patients with arterial hypertension.* Clin. Sci. 44:129, 1973.

28. WARREN, D. J., SWAINSON, C. P., AND WRIGHT, N.: *Deterioration in renal function after beta-blockade in patients with chronic renal failure and hypertension.* Br. Med. J. 2:193, 1974.

29. REUBI, F. C.: *Renal hyperemia induced in man by a new phthalazine derivative (17591).* Proc. Soc. Exper. Biol. Med. 73:102, 1950.

30. VANDERKOLK, K., DONTAS, A. S., AND HOOBLER, S. W.: *Renal and hypotensive effects of acute and chronic oral treatment with 1-hydrazinophthalazine (Apresoline) in hypertension.* Am. Heart J. 48:95, 1954.

31. MOYER, J. H.: *Discussion* in BREST, A. N. AND MOYER, J. H. (EDS.): *Hypertension: Recent Advances.* Lea and Febiger, Philadelphia, 1961, p. 309.

32. WILKINSON, E. L., BACKMAN, H., AND HECHT, H. H.: *Cardiovascular and renal adjustments to a hypotensive agent (1-hydrazinophthalazine: CIBA BA-5968: Apresoline).* J. Clin. Invest. 31:872, 1952.

33. MUTH, R. G.: *Diuretic response to furosemide in the presence of renal insufficiency.* JAMA 195:1066, 1966.

34. MAHER, J. F., AND SCHREINER, G. E.: *Studies on ethacrynic acid in patients with refractory edema.* Ann. Intern. Med. 62:15, 1965.

35. HANSSON, L., HUNYOR, S. N., JULIUS, S., ET AL.: *Blood pressure crisis following withdrawal of clonidine (Catapres, Catapresan), with special reference to arterial and urinary catecholamine levels, and suggestions for acute management.* Am. Heart J. 85:605, 1973.

36. PETTINGER, W. A., AND MITCHELL, H. C.: *Minixodil — an alternative to nephrectomy for refractory hypertension.* N. Engl. J. Med. 289:167, 1973.

Recent Acquisitions in Antihypertensive Therapy: Clonidine, Minoxidil and Prazosin

Gaddo Onesti, M.D., and Michael Fernandes, M.D.

Progress in cardiovascular pharmacology has recently provided the clinician with antihypertensive agents that are more potent and clinically acceptable than conventional drugs. Since the physiology of hypertension remains uncertain, the pharmacologic approach has been empirical. The development of new compounds has been directed toward the central neurogenic mechanisms regulating the blood pressure and also the peripheral vascular smooth muscle.

Clonidine is the prototype antihypertensive agent acting on the vasomotor centers of the brain. Its development has significantly stimulated the study of the mechanisms regulating blood pressure by the central nervous system.[1] Its introduction into clinical medicine represents a useful innovation in therapeutic strategy. Minoxidil represents the most potent oral vasodilator synthesized and is probably the best hope for severely hypertensive patients refractory to standard therapy. Prazosin is also a vasodilator and is notable for the lack of reflex cardiac stimulatory effects.

It is the purpose of this chapter to describe the pharmacology, hemodynamic effects, and clinical use of these three agents.

CLONIDINE

It is now well accepted that the central nervous system directly regulates cardiovascular functions in general and blood pressure in particular. Cortical, limbic, hypothalamic, and bulbospinal autonomic mechanisms normally participate in a highly integrated manner in circulatory control.[2] Before reaching the cardiovascular system, their effects are integrated at the level of the medulla oblongata. This area contains the nucleus tractus solitarius, the vasomotor centers, and the vagal nuclei (Fig. 1).[2, 3] Afferent nerves from the arterial baroreceptors (in the carotid sinus and aortic arch) have their primary synapse in the nucleus tractus solitarius. Inhibitory neurons from the nucleus tractus solitarius control the vasomotor centers from which sympathetic preganglionic fibers originate. Connections from the nucleus tractus solitarius to the vagal nuclei control vagal activity. Thus, heart rate, cardiac output, arteriolar and venous tone are ultimately regulated. Cardiovascular stimulatory effects integrated at this level include a combination of sympathetic stimulation and vagal inhibition resulting in increased cardiac output, heart rate, peripheral vascular resistance, and blood pressure. The cardiovascular inhibitory actions of the central nervous system—predominantly the result of vagal stimulation and sympathetic inhibition—include decreased cardiac output, heart rate, total peripheral vascular resistance and blood pressure.

MEDULLA OBLONGATA

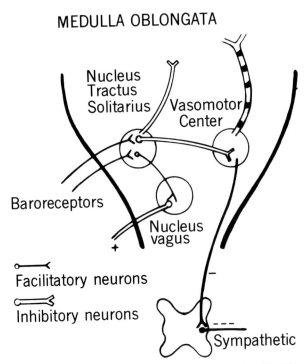

Figure 1. Central neurogenic mechanism regulating the blood pressure (modified from Chalmers[3]).

The modulation of such integrated cardiovascular responses is effected by the central adrenergic neurons with their cell bodies primarily located in the hypothalamic area and in the lower brain stem. It is now becoming apparent that these central adrenergic neurons are provided with alpha- and beta-adrenergic receptors similar to the receptors located in the peripheral organs. It is also evident that the most important central neurotransmitter is norepinephrine.[4] Recent evidence indicates that *stimulation* of central alpha-adrenergic receptors by norepinephrine results in the cardiovascular *inhibitory* effects previously described. Thus, in a seemingly paradoxical manner, a *central* norepinephrine effect results in a decreased peripheral adrenergic tone.

Clonidine hydrochloride is the prototype pharmacologic agent acting on central adrenergic neurons, lowering blood pressure through a decrease in peripheral adrenergic activity associated with an increase in vagal tone.[5, 6] When Kobinger injected a small dose (1 μg./kg.) of clonidine into the cisterna magna of the anesthesized dog, a significant decrease in blood pressure associated with bradycardia resulted. It was concluded that the blood pressure lowering effect and the bradycardia were due to a direct effect of clonidine within the central nervous system.[6] The cardiovascular effect of clonidine mediated by central adrenergic neurons may be prevented by pretreatment with the alpha-adrenergic blocker, phenoxybenzamine.[6] Thus, it is now accepted that the mode of action of clonidine involves interaction with the alpha-adrenergic receptors of the central adrenergic neurons. Additional studies by Sattler and van Zwieten,[7] Sherman and coworkers,[8] and Schmitt and associates[9] support these conclusions.

Systemic Hemodynamic Effects in Essential Hypertension

The acute cardiovascular effect resulting from the oral administration of clonidine to patients with essential hypertension includes a decrease in blood pressure, a modest reduction in cardiac output and an unchanged total peripheral vascular resistance. In the erect position, however, a marked decrease in the peripheral vascular resistance becomes evident, while cardiac output is minimally reduced. The decline in cardiac output is due to a decrease in blood pressure and heart rate (Fig. 2).[10] Prolonged oral administration is associated with a decrease in heart rate, minor reduction in cardiac output and a decrease in total peripheral vascular resistance.[11, 12] These latter studies were conducted at rest in the sitting position. During exercise the physiologic increase in cardiac output is preserved during clonidine therapy.[12]

Acute and chronic administration of clonidine to patients with essential hypertension preserves renal blood flow and decreases renal vascular resistance.[10, 13] Muscular blood flow is unchanged during the hypotensive response to clonidine.[14]

The effect of clonidine on cardiac output is predominantly due to the centrally mediated increase in vagal tone. The mild decrease in cardiac output is not due to any myocardial suppressive effect.[15] Thus, the final effect of clonidine on the cardiovascular system appears to be a combined vagal stimulation and decrease in adrenergic tone. This latter effect appears to be directed predominantly to the resistance vessels.[10, 16]

Effect on Renin

Administration of clonidine directly into the central nervous system (via the cisterna magna or cerebral ventricle) significantly reduces the release of renin by the kidney in the experimental animal. This effect is mediated by a decrease in adrenergic tone to the juxtaglomerular apparatus via the renal nerves.[17]

In hypertensive patients clonidine significantly decreases peripheral plasma renin activity (Fig. 3).[10] This observation has raised the possibility that suppression of renin may contribute to the antihypertensive effectiveness of the drug. Indeed, Weber and coworkers have shown that the antihypertensive effect of clonidine in hypertensive patients with normal or high renin is greater than in patients with low renin, and that the decrease in blood pressure is proportional to the concomitant decline in renin.[18]

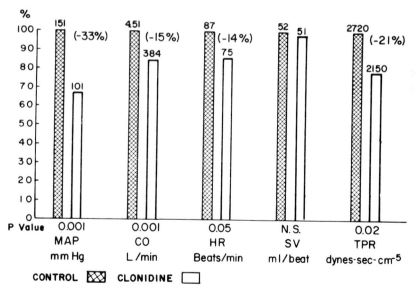

Figure 2. Acute effect of orally administered clonidine on mean arterial pressure (MAP), cardiac output (CO), heart rate (HR), stroke volume (SV), and total peripheral vascular resistance (TPR) in seven hypertensive patients (from Onesti et al.,[10] with permission).

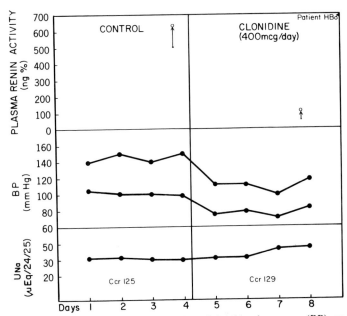

Figure 3. Effect of clonidine on peripheral plasma renin activity, blood pressure (BP), and urinary sodium (UNa) in a patient with essential hypertension (erect posture). Ccr = endogenous creatinine clearance. The arrow indicates the increase in plasma renin activity from the supine position (dot) to upright position (open circle) after passive tilt (from Onesti et al.,[10] with permission).

Clinical Use

Our experience with clonidine in the treatment of hypertension started in 1966.[10] It was demonstrated that daily doses of 0.15 to 0.9 mg. resulted in significant blood pressure reduction. Subsequently, it became apparent that the concomitant administration of a diuretic (chlorthalidone) enhanced the antihypertensive effectiveness of the drug.[13] In a third investigation it was determined that higher doses of clonidine, alone or in combination with chlorthalidone, were effective in the great majority of the patients treated.[19] It is noteworthy that the combination of clonidine and chlorthalidone produced "significant blood pressure reduction" in 95 percent of the patients treated. It is of particular importance that a satisfactory response was obtained in both the supine (89 percent) and standing (95 percent) positions. There is, in fact, no significant orthostatic effect exhibited in patients on long-term therapy.

A comparative analysis of the effects of clonidine revealed that this drug resulted in greater effectiveness than alpha-methyldopa, guanethidine, or pargyline.[20] The advantage was particularly evident on the supine blood pressure. An important clinical attribute of clonidine is its similar effect in supine and standing positions.

Hoobler and Sagastume[21] described a large series studied at the University of Michigan Medical Center, including 57 hypertensive patients treated with clonidine plus a diuretic. After evaluating their cumulative experience of clonidine in combination with a diuretic, the following conclusions were reached. There was no loss of drug effectiveness with the passage of time, since the average reduction in blood pressure and dose of drug remained about the same in the sixth and in the final months of treatment. Furthermore, the severity of the original hypertension did not alter the overall success rate (about 66 percent). Of the 25 patients with hypertension severe enough to require guanethidine originally, 15 showed improvement on a clonidine regimen (overall 60 percent favorable effect). Orthostatic hypotension was rarely a problem with clonidine, and 7 out of 12 patients (58 percent) previously taking alpha-methyldopa (1000 mg./24 hr. or more) were more successfully managed with clonidine administration. Clonidine showed a slight additive effect with hydralazine and reserpine but not with alpha-methyldopa. Clonidine added to guanethidine decreased both standing and recumbent blood pressure with a slight increase of the orthostatic gradient. After guanethidine had been replaced by clonidine in these patients, the recumbent blood pressure was lower than during the administration of guanethidine and there was a lesser orthostatic gradient.[21]

Side Effects

Unquestionably, the most common and important side effects are drowsiness and dryness of the mouth. In our experience,[10, 13] and in the experience of other investigators, these symptoms tend to decrease in severity and frequently subside.[19] Adverse reactions that have been inconsistently reported include nausea, vomiting, dryness of the nasal mucosa, parotid gland pain, and Raynaud's phenomenon. Table 1 provides a summary of the most consistently reported side effects based on an appraisal of their incidence reported in the literature.

One of the reported adverse reactions requires some detailed comment. In 1970 Hökfelt, Hedeland and Dymling reported that interruption of clonidine administration resulted in a rapid return of blood pressure to pretreatment levels.[22] Clonidine was shown to markedly decrease urinary catecholamines. When clonidine was discontinued, the investigators recorded a significant increase in urinary catecholamines above pretreatment levels, accompanied by symptoms of anxiety, nervousness, and restlessness. Subsequently, Hansson and coworkers[23] again reported a rapid increase of the blood pressure to pretreatment levels or possibly higher when clonidine was abruptly discontinued in 5 patients. These 5 patients had severe essential hypertension and had been treated for 24 to 48 months with clonidine. Pretreatment blood pressures were not recorded. Plasma and urinary catecholamines increased significantly. The same 5 patients were described three times in three different publications.[23, 24, 25] Similarly, Conolly and colleagues[26] reported severe hypertension after discontinuation of clonidine in 3 patients. In at least 1 patient, the blood pressure exceeded the pretreatment level.

Although other instances of rapid rise in blood pressure upon discontinuation of clonidine have been described,[27-30] most of the authors have failed to report pretreatment blood presure levels. Thus, the existence of a true "rebound" of blood pressure is difficult to document.[31, 32] The published reports of clonidine reversal or the "rebound" phenomenon are listed in Table 2. We have defined *reversal* as the return of the blood pressure to pretreatment levels and *rebound* as the documented increase in blood pressure above pretreatment levels.

Of significant practical importance are the instances of severe blood pressure elevation after discontinuation of clonidine in patients undergoing surgery.[26, 33] These eleva-

Table 1. Side effects of clonidine[13, 21, 26]

Side effect	Incidence (%)
Drowsiness	50–80 (Transient in about 50% of affected patients)
Dry mouth	30–80 (Transient in about 50% of affected patients)
Parotid gland pain	0–10
Impotence	0–24

Table 2. Clonidine reversal or rebound

Investigator	Cases reported
Hökfelt et al.[22]	5 (reversal)
Conolly et al.[26]	5 (1 rebound; 4?)
Hansson et al.[25]	5 (2?, probably rebound; 3?)
Hunyor et al.[24]	5*
Hansson et al.[23]	5*
Webster et al.[27]	1 (?, probably rebound; clonidine given with bethanidine)
Bailey[28]	6 (2?, probably rebound; 4?)
Wilkinson et al.[29]	9 (?)
Stelzer et al.[30]	1 (?)

Key: Question mark (?) indicates that pretreatment baseline blood pressure was not reported.
*Same patients as those reported by Hansson et al.[25]

tions have been reported to occur on induction of anesthesia, during anesthesia, and immediately after surgery. This problem may indicate a potential interaction with anesthetic agents—but again, our analysis indicates that although a true "rebound" may occur, clear documentation of blood pressure above pretreatment levels is not available. The rebound phenomenon was not observed in the most extensive clinical trials[13] and the only prospective study designed to reproduce it failed to do so.[34]

It is obvious that physicians and patients should not discontinue any antihypertensive drug abruptly. Since true "rebound" has been documented in only a few instances, it must, therefore, be an uncommon event and should not discourage the widespread application of a most useful and effective antihypertensive agent.

MINOXIDIL

Pharmacology and Hemodynamic Effects

Minoxidil is a potent oral vasodilator currently undergoing clinical trials in the United States. The vasodilator effect results from direct smooth muscle relaxation without inhibition of adrenergic tone or interference with cardiovascular reflexes.[35, 36]

Parenteral administration of minoxidil in experimental animals resulted in an immediate decrease in blood pressure which was sustained for at least 24 hours. Interestingly, during this period, rapid clearance of drug from the blood was noted.[36] Pluss, Orcutt and Chidsey studied the blood pressure response to the intraperitoneal injection of minoxidil in normotensive rats.[37] Plasma levels of minoxidil declined rapidly and concomitantly with the prompt decrease in blood pressure. Twelve hours later, a significant reduction in blood pressure persisted in the presence of low plasma levels of minoxidil (less than 1 percent peak level). Analysis of tissue distribution of the drug revealed its high concentration in arterial tissue. It appears, therefore, that persistent concentration of minoxidil in arterial smooth muscle is responsible for the prolonged hypotensive effect.[37]

The hemodynamic response to the administration of minoxidil includes a reduction in the systemic blood pressure associated with a decrease in the peripheral vascular resistance, whereas the cardiac output increases. The increase in the cardiac output is due predominantly to an increase in the heart rate.[36] This hemodynamic response is consistent with a drug effect limited to arteriolar dilatation; interference with adrenergic trans-mission or venous capacitance does not appear to be present.

Systemic vasodilatation by minoxidil (as with other vasodilators) increases cardiac output, induces sodium retention, disturbs transcapillary fluid exchange promoting the development of edema, and increases plasma renin activity.[38, 39] In addition to these effects, pulmonary hypertension has been noted to result from administration of minox-idil.[40-42]

Effect on Body Fluid and Renin

Treatment with minoxidil in combination with propranolol results in a markedly posi-tive sodium balance leading to fluid retention, hypervolemia and edema.[43, 44] Thus, con-comitant administration of relatively large doses of diuretics appears to be mandatory.

In contrast with other antihypertensive agents, the fluid retention and the hypervol-emia do not interfere with the antihypertensive efficacy of the drug.[44] A likely explana-tion for this fluid retention is the dramatic decrease in renal perfusion pressure resulting from the antihypertensive potency of the drug. In our experience, however, the magni-tude of edema has suggested the possibility that marked arteriolar dilatation might al-low transmission of a higher hydrostatic pressure distally into the capillary bed. In-crease in intracapillary pressure might disturb transcapillary fluid exchange resulting in a shift of fluid outside the capillary wall and resultant edema formation.

Administration of minoxidil, as other vasodilators, results in a marked rise in plasma renin.[38, 39] This is probably due to both an increased reflex activity and a reduction in renal perfusion pressure.[39] Concomitant administration of the beta-adrenergic blocker propranolol minimizes but does not abolish the increase in renin.[38] Whether the sup-pression of renin induced by propranolol contributes to the antihypertensive effect is open to speculation.

Clinical Use

Until recently, the only oral peripheral vasodilator available for the treatment of hy-pertension had been hydralazine. The effectiveness of hydralazine was limited by its modest potency, by immunologic disturbances and by the development of lupus erythe-matosus-like syndrome.[36] Minoxidil represents an oral peripheral vasodilator of un-usually high potency and long duration of action. Furthermore, its use has not been accompanied by the development of antinuclear antibodies nor the lupus erythemato-sus-like syndrome.[40, 44]

Minoxidil in combination with propranolol and a diuretic has been extensively em-ployed for the treatment of severe hypertension refractory to standard antihypertensive agents.[40, 45, 46] At the time of this writing its use remains limited to investigational proto-cols. However, a cumulative report of 510 patients with refractory hypertension treated with minoxidil has appeared.[47] The drug may be administered once or twice a day, from a starting dose of 10 mg. to a maximum of 100 mg. per day. Concomitant administration of propranolol is mandatory in order to prevent the severe reflex tachy-cardia (Fig. 4). A diuretic agent in large doses (generally a loop diuretic) is also neces-sary.

Dormois and coworkers have published extensive data on the effectiveness of mi-noxidil in combination with propranolol and other agents (methyldopa and guanethi-dine) in severe refractory hypertension. Furosemide was the diuretic employed.[40] Simi-lar effectiveness has been described by Pettinger and Mitchell.[46]

The safety and efficacy of minoxidil in the treatment of malignant hypertension in

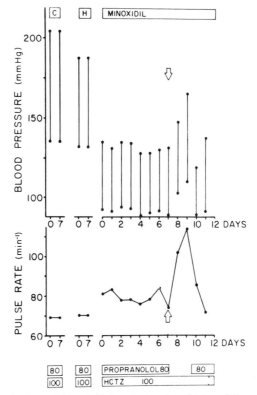

Figure 4. Blood pressure and pulse rate in an initial control period of 7 days followed by 7 days of hydralazine and 11 days of minoxidil therapy. Hydrochlorothiazide and propranolol were given continuously except for a temporary discontinuation of propranolol during days 7, 8, and 9 (from Chidsey et al.,[36] with permission).

chronic renal failure has been demonstrated and reported in detail.[48] Minoxidil in combination with propranolol has also been used successfully in hypertensive patients on hemodialysis[45] and has been considered a pharmacologic alternative to bilateral nephrectomy.[46]

In addition to marked potency, the combination of minoxidil and propranolol is not accompanied by orthostatic hypotension. This is a significant advantage, particularly in hemodialysis patients undergoing ultrafiltration.[45] Hemodialysis patients treated with sympathetic inhibitors are prone to severe hypotensive episodes during ultrafiltration dialysis.

The most important side effect of minoxidil is hypertrichosis which occurs even at relatively small doses. The excessive hair growth is particularly evident over the malar area, the temples, the shoulders, the dorsal area, and the forearms. This effect can be very severe.

The aforementioned fluid retention is a direct consequence of the pharmacologic effect of minoxidil and is generally corrected with the addition of high doses of potent diuretics.

Pulmonary hypertension has been reported with minoxidil.[40-42] Subsequent studies, however, have failed to reproduce these data when minoxidil was used in combination with propranolol and a diuretic in patients with previously normal pulmonary hemodynamics.[49]

280

PRAZOSIN

Mechanism of Action

Prazosin, a quinazoline derivative, has been shown to lower blood pressure in the experimental animal.[50] When prazosin is administered to renal hypertensive dogs the decrease in blood pressure lasts approximately 24 hours. Changes in heart rate are minimal and transient and limited to the period of maximum blood pressure decrease. This effect is different from that observed in the same dogs treated with hydralazine, in which equivalent decreases in blood pressure were accompanied by significant tachycardia.[51] Thus, reflex tachycardia is not a predominant feature of prazosin effect. Similarly, the profound decrease in blood pressure which follows intravenous administration of prazosin to genetic hypertensive rats (Okamoto-Aoki strain) is accompanied by some actual decrease in heart rate (Fig. 5).[52]

The lack of significant reflex tachycardia could be explained by an additional effect of the drug on venous tone, the baroreceptor mechanism or the central nervous system mechanisms governing cardiovascular function. Administration of prazosin directly into the cerebral ventricles of the genetic hypertensive rat (New Zealand strain) gave the same decrease in blood pressure as systemic administration.[53] Furthermore, the perfusion of an innervated hind limb preparation with circulation separate from the donor animal did not change when prazosin was injected into the circulation of the donor.[51] These studies represent strong evidence against a significant effect of prazosin on the central nervous system.

The studies of Constantine and coworkers established that prazosin exerts a vasodilatory effect by direct action upon the vascular smooth muscle.[51] In the hind limb preparation, intra-arterial administration of prazosin caused a dose related increase in blood

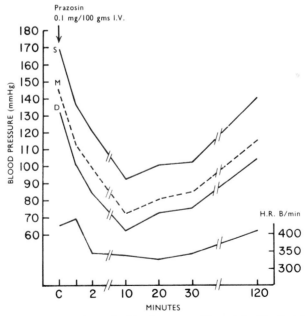

Figure 5. Effect of intravenous prazosin on the blood pressure (S: systolic, D: diastolic, M: mean arterial pressure) and heart rate (HR) in the conscious spontaneously hypertensive rat.

281

flow. In the same preparation prazosin caused seventeen times less vasodilation after ganglionic blockade with hexamethonium. In contrast the increase in blood flow caused by pure direct smooth muscle relaxants (papaverine and diazoxide) were minimally affected by ganglionic blockade. The increase in blood flow with alpha-adrenergic blockade (phentolamine) was completely abolished by ganglionic blockade. It is well accepted that the decrease in vasodilator activity of a drug after ganglionic blockade represents that component of drug action secondary to interference with adrenergic function. Thus, the residual vasodilation response elicited by prazosin (after ganglionic blockade) represents that component of drug action secondary to direct vascular smooth muscle effect (Fig. 6).[51]

The pharmacologic evaluation by Constantine and coworkers demonstrated that prazosin also interfered with peripheral adrenergic neurotransmission. Interference with perpheral adrenergic function is confined to the alpha-adrenergic receptors and represents a unique mechanism of action. Conventional alpha-adrenergic blockade involves occupancy of receptor site (e.g., with phentolamine). A functional disruption of the alpha-receptor mechanism without receptor occupancy (distal alpha-adrenergic blockade) results from the administration of prazosin.[54]

This unique action of prazosin has been tentatively linked to the biochemical correlates of muscle contraction.[54] Stimulation of beta-adrenergic receptors increases the production of cyclic adenosine monophosphate (AMP) and results in vasodilation. In contrast, stimulation of the alpha-adrenergic receptors decreases the production of cyclic AMP and results in vasoconstriction. Tissue levels of cyclic AMP are regulated by two enzymes: (a) adenyl cyclase which increases its synthesis from adenosine triphosphate (ATP), and (b) phosphodiesterase which causes its degradation to inactive 5'-AMP. Activation of adenyl cyclase may be accomplished by beta-adrenergic receptor stimulation (e.g., with isoproterenol). This will increase smooth muscle levels of AMP with consequent vasodilation. Also, inhibition of phosphodiesterase will impair the degradation of AMP and increase its smooth muscle levels with consequent vaso-

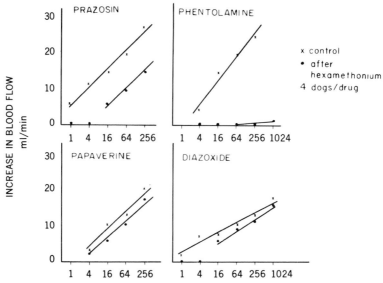

Figure 6. Effect of intravenously administered hexamethonium (2 mg./kg. body weight) on vasodilator responses in the hind limb of dogs anesthetized with intravenously administered sodium pentobarbital (30 mg./kg. body weight). Effect of each drug was studied in four dogs (from Constantine et al.,[51] with permission).

dilation. It is now apparent that prazosin is a potent inhibitor of phosphodiesterase.[54] Thus, increased levels of cyclic AMP by this mechanism may explain both the direct vasodilation and the inhibition of peripheral adrenergic neurotransmission exerted by prazosin (Fig. 7).

Systemic Hemodynamic Effects

Systemic hemodynamic studies in patients with essential hypertension have been performed after acute intravenous administration,[52, 55] short term oral administration[55, 56] and after long term treatment.[57] In general, the decrease in blood pressure was associated with a decrease in total peripheral vascular resistance without significant changes in cardiac output and heart rate.

Systemic hemodynamic studies, at rest and during exercise, were conducted by Lund-Johansen in ten hypertensive subjects treated with prazosin (3 to 7.5 mg./day) for one year (Fig. 8).[57] At rest, the decrease in mean arterial pressure was associated with a decrease in the vascular resistance; cardiac output remained unchanged. A similar cardiovascular response was obtained after acute drug administration in the supine position in our laboratory.[52] During exercise, at three work loads, the blood pressure and resistance remained below control values while cardiac output actually increased. This increase in cardiac output was primarily due to an increase in stroke volume. Changes in heart rate were not noted.[57]

Reduction in blood pressure associated with a decrease in vascular resistance, minimal changes in cardiac output and heart rate at rest, lack of postural hypotension, and the ability of the cardiac output and stroke volume to increase during exercise represent favorable effects on the cardiovascular system. It is our opinion, however, that the present knowledge of the pharmacology of prazosin does not fully explain the absence of reflex tachycardia. Beta-adrenergic blockade has been excluded.[51]

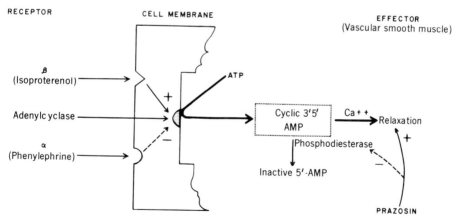

Figure 7. Proposed biochemical rationale for the action of prazosin. Beta-adrenergic stimulation increases and alpha-adrenergic stimulation decreases the production of 3'5'-cyclic adenosine monophosphate (cyclic AMP) from cellular adenosine triphosphate (ATP). This effect is modulated via the membrane-bound enzyme, adenylcyclase. Alpha-adrenergic blockade (as with phentolamine) results in increased cyclic AMP by inhibition of an inhibitory pathway. Cyclic AMP is degraded to inactive 5'-AMP by the enzyme, phosphodiesterase. Phosphodiesterase inhibition, as with prazosin, results in increased levels of cyclic AMP. Increased levels of cyclic AMP at the level of the effector (in this case, vascular smooth muscle) elicit a specific response (relaxation) (reprinted from Fernandes and Fiorentini, with permission).

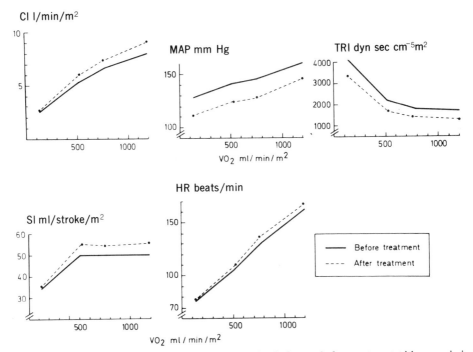

Figure 8. Hemodynamic changes at rest and during exercise before and after treatment with prazosin in ten hypertensive patients, CI: cardiac index; MAP: mean arterial pressure; TRI: total peripheral resistance index; SI: stroke index; HR: heart rate; VO_2: oxygen consumption (from Lund-Johansen,[57] with permission).

Effect of Renal Function, Body Fluid and Renin

Acute and chronic administration of prazosin resulted in no decrease in renal blood flow or glomerular filtration rate.[58] In fact, an actual improvement in renal function has been clearly demonstrated.[56] In a large clinical study (806 patients) 16.5 percent of patients had impaired renal function. Chronic administration of prazosin resulted in blood pressure reduction; further deterioration in renal function was not observed.[59] Chronic oral administration of prazosin in patients with essential hypertension does not result in plasma volume expansion.[55] Stokes and Weber recorded no significant short term effects of prazosin on plasma renin activity in patients with essential hypertension,[60] whereas Bolli and coworkers described an actual decrease in plasma renin activity.[61]

Clinical Trials

At Hahnemann Medical College and Hospital 48 patients with essential hypertension received prazosin, 6 to 20 mg./day, for 4 to 6 months. Prazosin was given after a period of 4 to 10 weeks' administration of placebo. All patients returned at two week intervals. Dosage was increased until a standing pressure of 140/90 mm. Hg was attained or maximum dose was reached.[52]

In the supine position, the average diastolic pressure at the end of the placebo period was 116 ± 12.3 mm. Hg. At the end of prazosin therapy the average diastolic pressure was 104 ± 13.6 mm. Hg (10 percent decrease, $p < 0.001$).

In the standing position, the average diastolic blood pressure at the end of the placebo period was 117 ± 11.3 mm. Hg. At the end of the prazosin treatment period, the average diastolic pressure was 101 ± 14 mm. Hg (11 percent decrease, $p < 0.005$). Heart

284

rate did not change significantly in the supine position. In the standing position, heart rate increased from a control value of 86 ± 8.2 beats per min. to 94 ± 11.7 beats per min. (9 percent increase, $p < 0.001$).

Twenty-eight of the 48 patients who did not achieve a standing blood pressure of 140/90 mm. Hg or less on maximum dosages (20 mg./day) of prazosin alone, were treated with the combination of prazosin and polythiazide. Polythiazide dosage was 1 mg. twice a day. Prazosin alone was continued for four months; combination therapy was continued for 3 to 8 months.

In the supine position, the average diastolic blood pressure of these twenty-eight patients at the end of the placebo period was 118 ± 13.2 mm. Hg. At the end of therapy with prazosin alone, the average diastolic pressure was 109 ± 11.3 mm. Hg (8 percent decrease, $p < 0.005$). At the end of the period of combination therapy, the average diastolic pressure was 92 ± 8.3 mm. Hg (22 percent decrease, $p < 0.001$). Heart rate did not change significantly during the prazosin treatment period. During the period of combination therapy, heart rate increased from a placebo control of 80 ± 7 beats per min. to 84 ± 8 beats per min. (5 percent increase, $p < 0.001$).

In the standing position, the average diastolic blood pressure at the end of the placebo period was 120 ± 12 mm. Hg. At the end of therapy with prazosin alone the diastolic pressure was 106 ± 11.3 mm. Hg (11 percent decrease, $p < 0.005$). At the end of combination therapy the average diastolic pressure was 91 ± 8.2 mm. Hg (24 percent decrease, $p < 0.001$). Heart rate did not change significantly during therapy with prazosin alone. At the end of combination therapy, heart rate increased from 87 ± 8.5 beats per min. to 102 ± 9.9 beats per min (17 percent increase, $p < 0.001$).

Side effects during the initial 2 to 4 weeks were palpitation (15 percent), headache (8 percent) and dizziness. Initially, prazosin may cause syncope with a sudden loss of consciousness;[62] in the majority of patients, it is believed to result from an excessive postural hypotensive effect, although occasionally the episode has been preceded by a bout of tachycardia. The incidence of syncopal episodes has been reported to be approximately 1 percent in patients given an initial dose of 2 mg. or greater.

In addition, a comparative study of the antihypertensive efficacy of prazosin versus alpha-methyldopa was performed with double blind technique in 53 ambulatory patients with essential hypertension.[52] Daily doses of 3 mg., 6 mg., 10 mg., 15 mg., and 20 mg. of prazosin were compared with doses of alpha-methyldopa of 750 mg., 1000 mg., 1500 mg., and 2000 mg. respectively. With each drug the dosage was increased until a standing pressure of 140/90 mm. Hg was obtained or the maximum dosage was reached. In the group treated with alpha-methyldopa the average control supine mean arterial pressure was 137 ± 12.7 mm. Hg; at the end of the treatment period it was 115 ± 17.8 (16 percent decrease, $p < 0.001$). In the prazosin treated group the average control mean arterial pressure was 137 ± 12.7 mm. Hg; in the alpha-methyldopa treated group, after therapy, it was 109 ± 14.7 mm. Hg (20 percent decrease, $p < 0.001$). Thus, at the arbitrary doses employed prazosin and alpha-methyldopa exhibited similar antihypertensive efficacy on the supine pressure. Standing pressure, however, was lower with alpha-methyldopa. The predominantly orthostatic antihypertensive effect of alpha-methyldopa is well established. At present, prazosin emerges as an antihypertensive agent with similar effectiveness in the standing and supine position.

These results confirm the clinical experience of prazosin reported in the literature.[59, 60, 63-69]

Role of Prazosin in the Treatment of Hypertension

Prazosin appears to be an effective and safe antihypertensive agent characterized by a favorable hemodynamic effect and preservation of cardiac performance. Its useful-

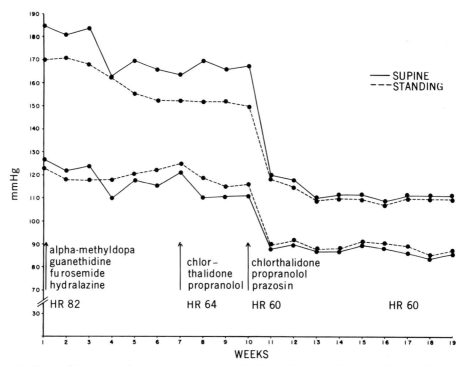

Figure 9. Successful control of severe hypertension with the combination of chlorthalidone 100 mg. o.d., propranolol 40 mg. t.i.d. and prazosin 5 mg. t.i.d. This patient was previously refractory to a four drug regimen. Note the similar effect in the supine and standing positions.

ness as a safe antihypertensive agent is limited to mild hypertension. It is still our approach to implement an oral diuretic as a first drug in these patients. Prazosin, added to an oral diuretic, however, has an important role in the management of hypertension. The effect is the same regardless of body position. The increase in heart rate is mild and well tolerated. Furthermore, in moderate and severe hypertension, prazosin may be successfully used in combination with a diuretic and propranolol (Fig 9). Clinical experience indicates that this regimen is effective and well tolerated.[70]

REFERENCES

1. ONESTI, G., FERNANDES, M., AND KIM, K. E. (EDS.): *Regulation of the Blood Pressure by the Central Nervous System.* Grune & Stratton, New York, 1976.

2. KORNER, P. I.: *Central control of blood pressure: Implications in the pathophysiology of hypertension,* in ONESTI, G., FERNANDES, M., AND KIM, K. E. (EDS.): *Regulation of the Blood Pressure by the Central Nervous System.* Grune & Stratton, New York, 1976, p. 3.

3. CHALMERS, J. P.: *Brain amines and models of experimental hypertension.* Circ. Res. 36:469, 1975.

4. STARKE, K., TAKAHIKO, E., AND TAUBE, H. D.: *Central noradrenergic mechanisms of neurotransmission,* in ONESTI, G., FERNANDES, M., AND KIM, K. E. (EDS.): *Regulation of the Blood Pressure by the Central Nervous System.* Grune and Stratton, New York, 1976, p. 21.

5. KOBINGER, W., AND WALLAND, A.: *Investigations into the mechanism of the hypotensive effect of 2-(2, 6-dichlorphenylamino)-2-imidazoline HCl.* Eur. J. Pharmacol. 2:155, 1967.

6. KOBINGER, W.: *Central modulation of cardiovascular activity by clonidine and other adrenal substances,* in ONESTI, G., FERNANDES, M., AND KIM, K. E. (EDS.): *Regulation of the Blood Pressure by the Central Nervous System,* Grune & Stratton, New York, 1976, p. 283.

7. SATTLER, R. W., AND VAN ZWIETEN, P. A.: *Acute hypotensive action of 2-(2,6-dichlorophenylamino)-2-imidazoline hydrochloride (ST-155) after infusion into the cat's vertebral artery.* Eur. J. Pharmacol. 2: 9, 1967.

286

8. SHERMAN, G. P., GREGA, G. J., WOODS, R. J., ET AL.: *Evidence for a central hypotensive mechanism of 2-(2,6-dichlorophenylamino)-2-imidazoline (Catapresan ST 155)*. Eur. J. Pharmacol. 2:326, 1968.

9. SCHMITT, H., SCHMITT, H., BOISSIER, J. R., ET AL.: *Cardiovascular effect of 2-(2,6-dichlorophenyl-amino)-2-imidazoline hydrochloride (ST-155): II. Central sympathetic structures*. Eur. J. Pharmacol. 2: 340, 1968.

10. ONESTI, G., SCHWARTZ, A. B., KIM, E., ET AL.: *Antihypertensive effect of clonidine*. Circ. Res. 29 (Suppl. II):53, 1971.

11. SCHNEIDER, K. W.: *Cardiane hamodynamik im akuten versuch, nach chronischer behandlung und im belastungstest mit St 155*, in HEILMEYER, L., HOLTMEIER, H. J., AND PFEIFFER, E. T. (EDS.): *Hoch-drucktherapie: Symposion uber 2-2(2,6-dichlorophenylamino)-2-imidazolin hydrochlorid*. Thieme, Stuttgart, 1968, p. 78.

12. STENBERG, J., HOLMBERG, S., NAETS, E., ET AL.: *Hemodynamic effects of Catapresan: Central circulation at rest; circulation at rest and under exercise*, in HEILMEYER, L., HOLTMEIER, H. J., AND PFEIFFER, E. F. (EDS.): *Hochdrucktherapie: Symposion uber 2-(2,6-dichlorphenylamino)-2-imidazolin hydrochlorid*. Thieme, Stuttgart, 1968, p. 68.

13. ONESTI, G., BOCK, K. D., HEIMSOTH, V., ET AL.: *Clonidine, a new antihypertensive agent*. Am. J. Cardiol. 28:74, 1971.

14. BOCK, K. D., MERGUET, P., BRANDT, T., ET AL.: *Experimental studies with clonidine hydrochloride in normotensive and hypertensive subjects*, in CONOLLY, M. F. (ED.): *Catapres in Hypertension, A Symposium held at the Royal College of Surgeons of England*. March, 1969. Butterworth, London, 1970, p. 101.

15. CONSTANTINE, J. W., AND MCSHANE, W. K.: *Analysis of the cardiovascular effects of 2-(2,6-dichlor-phenylamino)-2-imidazoline hydrochloride (Catapres)*. Eur. J. Pharmacol. 4:109, 1968.

16. LUND-JOHANSEN, P.: *Hemodynamic changes at rest and during exercise in long-term clonidine therapy of essential hypertension*. Acta Med. Scand. 195:111, 1974.

17. ONESTI, G., SCHWARTZ, A. B., KIM, K. E., ET AL.: *Antihypertensive effect of clonidine*. Circ. Res. 28–29 (Suppl. II):53, 1971.

18. WEBER, M. A., CASE, D. B., BAER, L., ET AL.: *Renin and aldosterone suppression in the antihypertensive action of clonidine*. Am. J. Cardiol. 38:825, 1976.

19. SCHWARTZ, A. B., BANACH, S., SMITH, I. S., ET AL.: *Clinical efficacy of clonidine in hypertension*, in ONESTI, G., KIM, K. E., AND MOYER, J. H. (EDS.): *Hypertension: Mechanisms and Management*. Grune & Stratton, New York, 1973, p. 389.

20. ONESTI, G., KIM, K. F., SWARTZ, C., ET AL.: *Hemodynamic effects of antihypertensive agents*, in ONESTI, G., KIM, K. E., AND MOYER, J. H. (EDS.): *Hypertension: Mechanisms and Management*. Grune & Stratton, New York, 1973, p. 227.

21. HOOBLER, S. W., AND SAGASTUME, E.: *Clonidine hydrochloride in the treatment of hypertension*. Am. J. Cardiol. 28:67, 1971.

22. HÖKFELT, B., HEDELAND, H., AND DYMLING, J. F.: *Studies on catecholamines, renin and aldosterone following Catapresan (2-(2,6-dichlorphenylamin)-2-imidazoline hydrochloride) in hypertensive patients*. Eur. J. Pharmacol. 10:389, 1970.

23. HANSSON, L., HUNYOR, S. N., JULIUS, S., ET AL.: *Blood pressure crisis following withdrawal of clonidine (Catapres, Catapresan), with special reference to arterial and urinary catecholamine levels, and suggestions for acute management*. Am. Heart J. 85:605, 1975.

24. HUNYOR, S. N., HANSSON, L., HARRISON, T. S., ET AL.: *Effects of clonidine withdrawal: possible mechanisms and suggestions for management*. Br. Med. J. 2:209, 1973.

25. HANSSON, L., AND HUNYOR, S. N.: *Blood pressure over-shoot due to acute clonidine (Catapres) withdrawal: studies on arterial and urinary catecholamines and suggestions for management of the crisis*. Clin. Sci. Mol. Med. 45:181s, 1973.

26. CONOLLY, M. E., BRIANT, R. H., GEORGE, C. F., ET AL.: *A cross-over comparison of clonidine and methyldopa in hypertension*. Eur. J. Pharmacol. 4:222, 1972.

27. WEBSTER, J., JEFFERS, A., GALLOWAY, D. B., ET AL.: *Withdrawal of antihypertensive therapy*. Lancet 2:1381, 1974.

28. BAILEY, R. R.: *Clonidine (Catapres) overshoot, Letter*. N. Z. Med. J. 81:268, 1975.

29. WILKINSON, P., GOLDBERG, A. D., AND RAFTERY, F. B.: *The rebound phenomenon after clonidine therapy*. Circulation 51, 52 (Suppl. II):256, 1975.

30. STELZER, F. P., STUBENBORD, J. J., SREENIVASAN, V., ET AL.: *Late toxicity of clonidine withdrawal*. N. Engl. J. Med. 294:1182, 1976.

31. PETTINGER, W. A.: *Clonidine—a new antihypertensive drug*. N. Engl. J. Med. 293:1179, 1975.

32. PETTINGER, W. A.: *Letter to the editor*. N. Engl. J. Med. 294:845, 1976.

287

33. ONSTAD, A.: *Catapresan og anestesi, komplikasjon belyst ved et kasus.* Tidsskr. Nor. Laegeforen. 94: 1396, 1974.

34. WHITSETT, T. L., CHRYSANT, S. G., DILLARD, B., ET AL.: *Withdrawal of clonidine.* JAMA 235:2717, 1976.

35. DuCHARME, D. W. FREYBURGER, W. A., GRANAM, B. E., ET AL.: *Pharmacologic properties of minoxidil: a new hypotensive agent.* J. Pharmacol. Exp. Ther. 184:662, 1973.

36. CHIDSEY, C. A., GOTTLIEB, T. B., PLUSS, R. G., ET AL.: *The use of vasodilators and beta-adrenergic blockade in hypertension,* in ONESTI, G., KIM, K. E., AND MOYER, J. H. (EDS.): *Hypertension: Mechanisms and Management.* Grune & Stratton, New York, 1973, p. 357.

37. PLUSS, R. G., ORCUTT, J., AND CHIDSEY, C. A.: *Tissue distribution and hypotensive effects of a new vasodilator, minoxidil.* J. Lab. Clin. Med. 79:639, 1972.

38. KOCH-WESER, J.: *Correlation of pathophysiology and pharmacotherapy in primary hypertension.* Am. J. Cardiol. 32:449, 1973.

39. KOCH-WESER, J.: *Vasodilator drugs in the treatment of hypertension.* Arch. Intern. Med. 133:1017, 1974.

40. DORMOIS, J. C., YOUNG, J. L., AND NIES, A. S.: *Minoxidil in severe hypertension. Value when conventional drugs have failed.* Am. Heart J. 90:360, 1975.

41. WILBURN, R. L., BLAUFUSS, A., AND BENNETT, C. M.: *Long-term treatment of severe hypertension with minoxidil, propranolol and furosemide.* Circulation 52:706, 1975.

42. TARAZI, R. C., MAGRINI, F., DUSTAN, H. P., ET AL.: *Pulmonary hypertension with diazoxide and minoxidil.* Am. J. Cardiol. 35:172, 1975.

43. DUSTAN, H. P., TARAZI, R. C., AND BRAVO, E. L.: *Hemodynamic adjustments during long-tern drug therapy,* in MILLIEZ, P., AND SAFAR, M. (EDS.): *Recent Advances in Hypertension.* Laboratoires Boehringer Ingelheim, Reims, France, 1975, p. 247.

44. GILMORE, E., WEIL, J., AND CHIDSEY, C.: *Treatment of essential hypertension with a new vasodilator in combination with beta-adrenergic blockade.* N. Engl. J. Med. 282:521, 1970.

45. LIMAS, C. J., AND FREIS, F. D.: *Minoxidil in severe hypertension with renal failure. Effect of its addition to conventional antihypertensive drugs.* Am. J. Cardiol. 31:355, 1973.

46. PETTINGER, W. A., AND MITCHELL, H. C.: *Minoxidil—an alternative to nephrectomy for refractory hypertension.* N. Engl. J. Med. 289:167, 1973.

47. MARTIN, W. B., ZINS, G. R., AND FREYBURGER, W. A.: *The use of minoxidil, an experimental arteriolar dilator, in 510 patients with refractory hypertension.* Clin. Sci. Mol. Med. 48:189s, 1975.

48. MUTTERPERL, R. E., DIAMOND, F. B., AND LOWENTHAL, D. T.: *Long-term effects of minoxidil in the treatment of malignant hypertension in chronic renal failure.* J. Clin. Pharmacol. 16:498, 1976.

49. KLOTMAN, P. E., GRIM, C. E., WEINBERGER, M. H., ET AL.: *The effects of minoxidil on pulmonary and systemic hemodynamics in hypertensive man.* Circulation 55:394, 1977.

50. SCRIABINE, A., CONSTANTINE, J. W., HESS, H-J., ET AL.: *Pharmacological studies with some new antihypertensive aminoquinazolines.* Experientia 24:1150, 1968.

51. CONSTANTINE, J. W., McSHANE, W. K., SCRIABINE, A., ET AL.: *Analysis of the hypotensive action of prazosin,* in ONESTI, G., KIM, K. E., AND MOYER, J. H. (EDS.): *Hypertension: Mechanisms and Management.* Grune & Stratton, New York, 1973, p. 420.

52. FERNANDES, M., SMITH, I. S., WEDER, A., ET AL.: *Prazosin in the treatment of hypertension.* Clin. Sci. Mol. Med. 48:1815, 1973.

53. WOOD, A. J., PHELAN, F. L., AND SIMPSON, F. O.: *Cardiovascular effects of prazosin in normotensive and genetically hypertensive rats.* Clin. Exp. Pharmacol. Physiol. 2:297, 1975.

54. HESS, H-J.: *Biochemistry and structure-activity studies with prazosin,* in COTTON, D. W. K. (ED.): *Prazosin—Evaluation of a New Antihypertensive Agent.* Excerpta Medica, Amsterdam 1974, p. 3.

55. SAFAR, M. E., WEISS, Y. A., LONDON, G. L., ET AL.: *Short-term hemodynamic studies with prazosin,* in COTTON, D. W. K. (ED.): *Prazosin—Evaluation of a New Antihypertensive Agent.* Excerpta Medica, Amsterdam, 1974, p. 64.

56. MASSONI, A., TOMMASI, A. M., BAGGIONI, F., ET AL.: *Hemodynamic study in men of medium-term treatment with a new amino-quinazoline antihypertensive agent (prazosin),* in COTTON, D. W. K. (ED.): *Prazosin—Evaluation of a New Antihypertensive Agent,* Excerpta Medica, Amsterdam, 1974, p. 54.

57. LUND-JOHANSEN, P.: *Hemodynamic changes at rest and during exercise in long-term prazosin therapy of essential hypertension,* in COTTON, D. W. K. (ED.): *Prazosin—Evaluation of a New Antihypertensive Agent.* Excerpta Medica, Amsterdam, 1974, p. 43.

58. MAXWELL, M. H.: *Effects of prazosin on renal function and fluid-electrolyte metabolism,* in FREIS, E. D. (ED.): *Prazosin—Clinical Symposium Proceedings.* Postgraduate Medicine, Minneapolis, 1974, p. 36.

59. PITTS, N. E.: *The clinical evaluation of prazosin hydrochloride, a new antihypertensive agent*, in COTTON, D. W. K. (ED.): *Prazosin—Evaluation of a New Antihypertensive Agent*. Excerpta Medica, Amsterdam, 1974, p. 149.

60. STOKES, G. S., AND WEBER, M. A.: *Prazosin: preliminary report and comparative studies with other antihypertensive agents*. Br. Med. J. 1:298, 1974.

61. BOLLI, P., WOOD, A. J., AND SIMPSON, F. O.: *Effects of prazosin in patients with hypertension*. Clin. Pharmacol. Ther. 20:138, 1976.

62. GABRIEL, R., MEEK, D., AND GHOSH, B. C.: *Collapse after prazosin hydrochloride, Letters to the Editor*. Lancet 1:1095, 1975.

63. MROCZEK, W. J., AND FINNERTY, F. A.; JR.: *Prazosin—a double blind evaluation*, in COTTON, D. W. K. (ED.): *Prazosin—Evaluation of a New Antihypertensive Agent*. Excerpta Medica, 1974, p. 92.

64. THULIN, T., SAETRE, H., VIKESDAHL, O., ET AL.: *Multicenter study of the antihypertensive effect of prazosin hydrochloride (prazosin) on mild and moderate hypertension*, in COTTON, D. W. K. (ED.): *Prazosin—Evaluation of a New Antihypertensive Agent*. Excerpta Medica, Amsterdam, 1974, p. 126.

65. SCHNAPER, H. W., AND OBERMAN, A.: *Double-blind studies of the clinical effectiveness of prazosin*, in FREIS, F. D. (ED.): *Prazosin—Clinical Symposium Proceedings*, Postgraduate Medicine, Minneapolis, 1974, p. 83.

66. OKUN, R.: *Long-term efficacy and safety of prazosin in essential hypertension*, in FREIS, E. D. (ED.): *Prazosin—Clinical Symposium Proceedings*. Postgraduate Medicine, Minneapolis, 1974, p. 63.

67. TURNER, A. S., WATSON, O. F., AND PEEL, J. O.: *Clinical experience with prazosin hydrochloride*, in FREIS, E. D. (ED.): *Prazosin—Clinical Symposium Proceedings*. Postgraduate Medicine, Minneapolis 1974, p. 88.

68. HUA, A. S. P., MACDONALD, I. M., MYERS, J. B., ET AL.: *Studies with prazosin—a new effective hypotensive agent*. Med. J. Aust. 1:559, 1976.

69. HAYES, J. M., GRAHAM, R. M., O'CONNEL, B. P., ET AL.: *Experience with prazosin in the treatment of patients with severe hypertension*. Med. J. Aust. 1:562, 1976.

70. MARSHALL, A. J., BARRIT, D. W., POCOCK, J., ET AL.: *Evaluation of bendrofluoride beta-blockade, and prazosin in severe hypertension*. Lancet 1:271, 1977.

71. FERNANDES, M., AND FIORENINTI, R.: *Prazosin in the treatment of hypertension: Pharmacology and clinical use*, in ONESTI, G., AND LOWENTHAL, D. T. (EDS.): *The Spectrum of Antihypertensive Drug Therapy*. Biomedical Information Corp., New York, 1977, p. 41.

Hypertension in the Infant, Child, and Adolescent

Mary Allen Engle, M.D., Kathryn Hawes Ehlers, M.D., Arthur A. Klein, M.D., and Aaron R. Levin, M.D.

While the nationwide impact of hypertension in the adult is being recognized and measures are being taken to identify the often asymptomatic individuals as well as those with manifest problems and to offer them treatment with which they will comply, it is appropriate that the problem of hypertension in the pediatric population be addressed. Perhaps there are conditions associated with hypertension in the child which would respond to treatment at that young age before irreversible changes or complications of the hypertension, such as a stroke, had occurred in the adult. It seems reasonable to assume that essential hypertension in the adult begins in the childhood years. If so, how do we identify those at risk? If we are able to do that, how do we decide when to intervene and in what manner? Hypertension is such a common problem in later life, it must not be rare in children. It is not.

RECOGNITION

To diagnose hypertension, one must be alert to the possibility of its presence and have a routine way of looking for it. The foolproof way of screening on physical examination from the newborn infant on up is to palpate the peripheral pulses in arms and legs and to obtain the blood pressure (BP) in the arms. If there is a discrepancy in pulses between the two arms or between the arms and legs, or if the blood pressure in the arms is elevated, then the blood pressure should be measured in the legs as well (Fig. 1). This seems obvious and simple, but in babies and toddlers especially, it requires considerable patience to have the subject quiet for a valid reading. Furthermore, it requires a cuff of appropriate size.

Selection of Cuff

The size of the cuff is critical in babies and children of assorted sizes. If the cuff is too large, the blood pressure is artificially low; conversely, too small a cuff results in a spuriously high reading. The cuff should cover two thirds of the upper part of the extremity in which the measurement is being made, and the inflatable bladder should be long enough to more than encircle the upper arm or the thigh. Cuffs are commercially available in widths appropriate for premature infants (4 cm.), larger babies (5 and 7 cm.), and for children up to adult size (9, 13, and 15.5 cm.), and for the thigh of an adult (18 cm.).

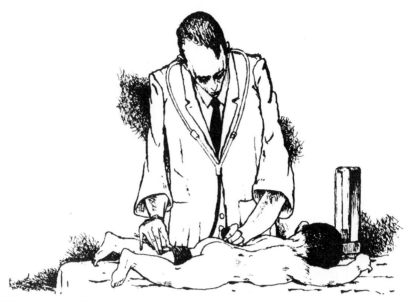

Figure 1. Measurement of blood pressure in leg of an infant, relaxed and quiet, with a cuff of appropriate size, utilizing a sphygmomanometer and listening in the popliteal space (from Jabloner, J., and Engle, M. A.: *High blood pressure in children*. Heart Bull. 13:84, 1964, with permission).

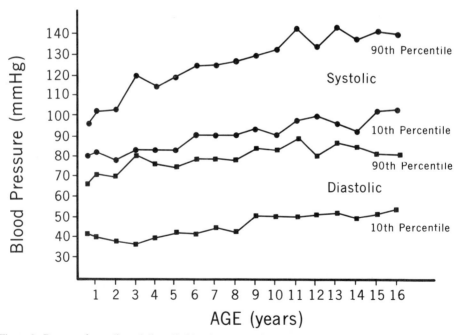

Figure 2. Ranges of systolic and diastolic blood pressures by years from birth through adolescence, based on composite data of Loggie and others (see text).

Measurement of Blood Pressure

The sphygmomanometer is the time honored method.[1] It is valid and it is applicable even to infants (Fig. 1). In young children, it is helpful first to inflate the balloon a reasonable amount and determine the pressure by palpation of the return of the radial pulses, before applying the stethoscope. That reading is usually 10 to 15 mm. Hg lower than the auscultatory reading. Diastolic pressure is recorded as the point of muffling (Korotkoff IV sound) and if the sounds continue beyond that, the point of cessation is also noted.[2, 3] The systolic pressure in the leg is normally slightly higher than in the arm, while the diastolic reading is approximately the same.

In an infant under two years of age, if a satisfactory reading is not obtained with the mercury manometer, a Doppler instrument can be used to record systolic and diastolic pressures. Less satisfactory are two other methods for use in babies that do not record the diastolic pressure. One is the observation of the bounce of the indicator needle or mercury column when the balloon is deflated and the systolic pressure is reached. The other is the "flush" technique,[6, 7] whereby a cuff of suitable size is wrapped around the wrist or ankle, the extremity is elevated, and mild local pressure is applied to produce blanching. The cuff pressure is quickly elevated to just greater than the anticipated systolic pressure and the extremity is placed flat again while the observer notes the point at which flushing appears as the cuff is slowly deflated. This pressure corresponds to a mean pressure, and often the reading in the leg is somewhat lower than that in the arm,[8] in contrast to the situation with auscultatory measurement.

For standardized conditions the BP should be determined with the subject resting quietly and supine and with the manometer at heart level. Leg pressures are recorded from the popliteal space with the subject prone (Fig. 1).

Normal Range of Blood Pressure

The systolic and diastolic pressures gradually rise from birth through adolescence, when they come to equal the adult values. This trend is shown diagrammatically in Figure 2, a synthesis of several studies, in particular those of Londe. The 10th and 90th percentiles are shown for boys and girls together.

Table 1 gives the percentile values for blood pressure by age for the 50th and 95th percentiles, an average of three studies.[9, 12, 13] This table was prepared by Mitchell and colleagues who served as a Committee on Arteriosclerosis and Hypertension in Childhood of the Council on Cardiovascular Disease of the Young of the American Heart Association.[14]

Though the foregoing guidelines were for both sexes, Lieberman advocated considering males and females separately after the age of 10 years. She used composite figures

Table 1. Percentile values for blood pressure by age

Age	Systolic pressure		Diastolic pressure	
	50%	95%	50%	95%
0 to 6 mo.	80	110	45	60
3 yr.	95	112	64	80
5 yr.	97	115	65	84
10 yr.	110	130	70	92
15 yr.	116	138	70	95

(From Mitchell, S. C., Blout, S. G., Jr., Blumenthal, S., et al.,[14] with permission.)

also from some of these same studies and put forward numbers that are easy to remember as upper limits of normal, with increments of increase of 10 mm. Hg in systolic and 5 mm. Hg in diastolic pressure for each age group from 0 to 3 up to 13 to 15 years (Table 2).[15]

The two tables and the graph provide similar information which seems to be close to the truth, even though the measurements in the different studies where data were combined were not always made under identical standardized conditions. Weiss and collaborators in Washington surveyed in a more uniform manner 7,119 children aged 6 to 11 years and reported on their blood pressure levels in relation to age, sex, race, and socioeconomic status.[16]

If the blood pressure reading obtained three times with a proper-sized cuff on a subject at rest and supine exceeds the 90th percentile of the normal range for the age, the person has hypertension. Measurement of blood pressure in the legs makes the diagnosis of generalized or of upper extremity hypertension. Serial determinations over the next hours, days, weeks, or longer permits a judgment that the hypertension is labile or is fixed and gives an idea of the range of elevation.

MANIFESTATIONS

The infant or child with hypertension may be asymptomatic, just as the adult. On the other hand, sudden onset of severe hypertension or longstanding severe elevation of pressure can lead to cardiac failure with pulmonary edema and peripheral edema or to cerebral complications with blurring of vision, coma, convulsions, or even, very rarely, a stroke. Headache is an infrequent complaint in normal children; so such a history should suggest the possibility of hypertension. Unexplained fatigue or anemia are also symptoms, particularly in the child with chronic renal disease and insufficiency.

The presence of cardiomegaly and of a gallop rhythm on physical examination as well as cardiomegaly with left ventricular enlargement on the roentgenogram (Fig. 3) give evidence of a cardiovascular burden of the hypertension. Left atrial enlargement on barium swallow occurs in the failing left ventricle or volume-overloaded heart. The electrocardiogram usually fulfills voltage criteria for left ventricular hypertrophy (Fig. 4) if the elevated pressure is not of recent onset. Rarely, because it is evidence of severe disease, ST segment depression and T wave inversion in leads V5 and V6 indicate left ventricular "strain." Funduscopic examination evaluates the severity of arteriolar disease.

MECHANISMS

Blood pressure is determined by several factors: the cardiac output and function of the left ventricle, the resistance of the peripheral vessels, the rebound of the elastic ar-

Table 2. Upper limits of normal blood pressure measurements in children

Sex	Age (yr.)	Pressure (mm. Hg)	
		Systolic	Diastolic
Male and Female	0 to 3	110	65
Male and Female	3 to 7	120	70
Male and Female	7 to 10	130	75
Male	10 to 15	140	80
Female	10 to 13	140	80
Female	13 to 15	140	85

(From Lieberman, E.,[15] with permission.)

294

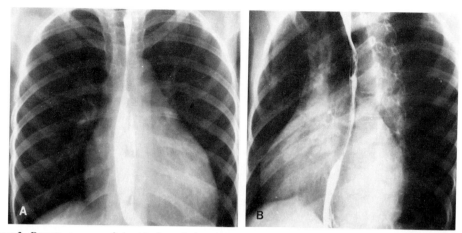

Figure 3. Roentgenogram of chest in frontal view (A) and in left anterior oblique projection (B) in child with hypertension and left ventricular enlargement causing increase in cardiothoracic ratio. There is no rib notching nor pulmonary edema. Case 1.

terial walls, the volume of blood within the vascular tree, and the viscosity of the blood. These are influenced by extravascular fluid volume, renin-angiotensin-aldosterone axis, and neural factors. Recent excellent reviews by Kirkendall and Overturk,[17] Skeggs,[18] Laragh,[19] and Peart[20] summarize the present state of understanding of these interrelationships. New and colleagues derived nomograms relating aldosterone excretion to urinary sodium and potassium in children.[21]

CAUSES

One may classify hypertension according to etiology as primary, if the cause is as yet unknown, or secondary. Table 3 lists the causes, beginning with those which have been identified, and ending with essential or primary hypertension. In early reviews of childhood hypertension from this institution[22] and elsewhere[23, 24] it was considered that most of the children with high blood pressure had it in association with a coexisting condition. Now, however, it is estimated that hypertension without apparent cause is about as frequent as is that with identifiable cause[25] and has a prevalence of about 1 percent, comparable to the incidence of congenital heart disease.

Renal

Acute and chronic glomerulonephritis continue to be the chief causes of recognized hypertension in the young. Acute nephritis spontaneously subsides in about 95 percent of instances, and so does the hypertension. Persistent hypertension is a common occurrence in any child with chronic renal disease of any of the forms listed in the table. It is considered to be renin- and/or volume-related. According to our colleague, Dr. John E. Lewy, Director of Pediatric Nephrology at this medical center, it is possible with hemodialysis to keep BP lower than in times prior to use of this modality.[26] In patients with renal transplant and one remaining kidney, BP is often elevated during the first few months after transplant, when steroid therapy and salt and water metabolism are being regulated, but once the proper balance is established, hypertension disappears.[26] In the patient with renal transplant and rejection, hypertension persists or returns.[26] In general, if the patient has not been hypertensive prior to transplant, he does not have hypertension afterward.[26]

Renovascular hypertension is illustrated in the following two children treated at our

295

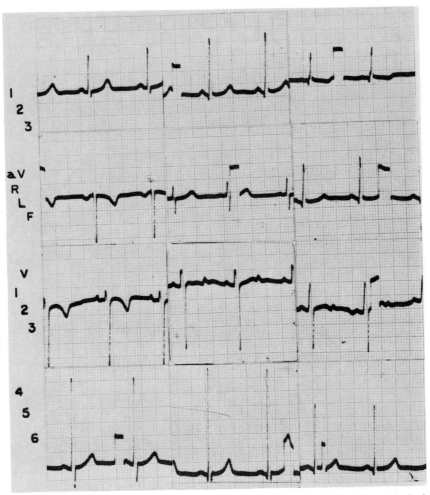

Figure 4. Electrocardiogram of a child with hypertension fulfills voltage criteria for left ventricular hypertrophy (R-V5 of 38 mm. and S-V1 of 25 mm.). The T waves and ST segments are normal; so there is no left ventricular "strain".

hospital, one with stenosis of a renal artery[27] and the other with a segmental renal lesion.[28]

Case 1: A 10-year-old girl was admitted because of a 4-month history of dyspnea, orthopnea, ankle swelling, and frequent emesis often associated with vague pain in the left flank. She was chronically ill with tachypnea, tachycardia, and hypertension of 150/110 mm. Hg in the arms and higher in the legs. She had an enlarged heart and was in heart failure. Chest x-ray films portrayed cardiac enlargement (Fig. 3). The electrocardiogram revealed left ventricular hypertrophy and "strain". Urinalyses showed a specific gravity of 1.010 to 1.015 and albuminuria. Urine cultures were negative. Urea clearance was normal, as were the results of tests for urinary catecholamines and 17 ketosteroids and hydroxysteroids.

She was immediately treated for heart failure with digitalis and salt restriction and was given reserpine and phenobarbital for the hypertension. Then the etiology of the hypertension was pursued further. Intravenous pyelogram showed de-

Table 3. Causes of hypertension in children

Renal: Unilateral or Bilateral Involvement	*Endocrine*
Glomerulonephritis, acute or chronic	Adrenal disorders
Primary	ACTH or cortisone administration
Secondary to:	Adrenogenital syndrome
Henoch-Schoenlein purpura	Cushing's syndrome
Lupus erythematosus	Adrenal tumors
Hypersensitivity reactions	Pheochromocytoma
Polyarteritis nodosa	Neuroblastoma
Pyelonephritis	Hyperaldosteronism, primary or secondary
Malformations	Enzymatic defect
Polycystic kidneys	Hyperthyroidism
Renal hypoplasia	
Hydronephrosis	*Central Nervous System*
Vascular anomalies	Infection
Renal artery obstruction	Encephalitis
Thrombosis	Poliomyelitis
Stenosis	Increased intracranial pressure
Aneurysm	Hemorrhage
Tumors	Trauma
Wilms' tumor	Tumor
Extrinsic tumor, as neuroblastoma	
or adrenal carcinoma	*Poisoning*
"Lower nephron nephrosis"	Plumbism
"Symmetrical cortical necrosis"	Acrodynia
Calculi	Ingestion excessive amounts of licorice
Trauma	
	Essential
Cardiovascular	
Coarctation of the aorta	
Lesions with wide pulse pressure, as:	
Patent ductus arteriosus	
Aorticopulmonary window	
Arteriovenous fistula	
Aortic insufficiency	

creased visualization of the left kidney. Cystourethrogram was normal. Test of differential renal function showed decreased flow of urine from the left kidney while that from the right was normal. Aortogram showed no opacification of the left renal artery (Fig. 5). Vessels of collateral circulation encircled the left ureter. The diagnosis was stenosis of the left renal artery with hypertension and heart failure.

Left nephrectomy was performed after splenorenal artery anastomosis could not be done. By the third postoperative day, her blood pressure dropped to 110/90 and by discharge, ranged from 90 to 120 over 60 to 80. Serum angiotensin levels, 35 to 50 percent above the mean preoperatively, dropped to normal. She remains asymptomatic and normotensive.[22]

Case 2: A six-year-old boy was known to be normotensive at 5 years of age but had been progressively and persistently hypertensive for the previous three months. Supine BP was 170/144 in the left arm and 184/134 in the leg. Physical examination was otherwise normal. Laboratory tests for evaluation of hypertension disclosed markedly elevated urinary aldosterone and peripheral plasma renin, both of

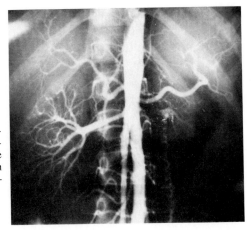

Figure 5 Aortogram in Case 1 shows normal opacification of right renal artery but absence of opacification of the left renal artery, due to stenosis of the left renal artery. Suprarenal artery is well seen on left. Note collateral vessel along course of left ureter.

which decreased with high sodium intake. Aortogram showed stenosis of the artery supplying the lower pole of the right kidney (Fig. 6). Plasma renin activity was normal and equal bilaterally in the right and left renal veins. However, at operation, renin activity was markedly elevated to 50 ng. per ml. per hr. from the vein draining the lower pole of the kidney while it was 19.6 ng. from the main renal vein. The lower pole of the right kidney was removed, and postoperatively the peripheral plasma renin activity and aldosterone decreased, and gradually the hypertension disappeared.[29]

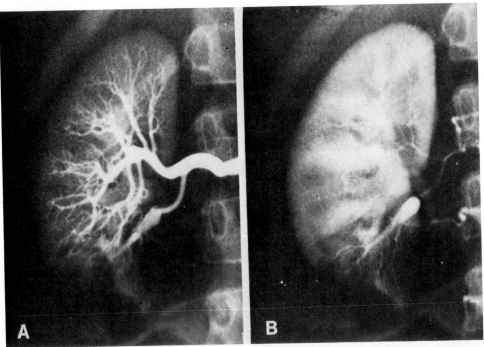

Figure 6. Arterial phase (A) and venous phase (B) of selective injection into right renal artery in Case 2 with segmental obstruction of right renal artery to lower pole of right kidney. Note the marked narrowing and poststenotic dilatation of this artery (A) and the evidence on venous phase of hypovascularity of the lower kidney (B).

Renal tumors are sometimes associated with hypertension but only uncommonly do patients present initially because of hypertension, as in the next case.

Case 3: A nine-month-old baby had a cough and failed to gain well. Examination revealed an enlarged heart and generalized hypertension of 170/100 mm. Hg. Electrocardiogram showed left ventricular hypertrophy with "strain" and left atrial abnormality, while cardiac series of chest roentgenograms with barium swallow showed marked left atrial as well as left ventricular enlargement. Urinalysis and tests of renal function were normal. Symptoms of her left-sided cardiac failure responded to digitalization, but hypertension persisted and increased. At one and one half years a mass become palpable in the left flank, and the suspicion of Wilms' tumor on the left was confirmed on pyelography and by removal of the left kidney and tumor. Hypertension lessened only slightly, her condition gradually deteriorated, a mass became palpable in the right flank, and she died of hypertensive cardiovascular disease from bilateral Wilms' tumors at the age of three years.

Cardiovascular

The next most common pediatric cause of hypertension is *coarctation of the aorta.* This anomaly has long been recognized as causing hypertension in the aorta and branches proximal to the coarctation, and a lower systolic pressure below. The hypertension of children with coarctation tends to have greater systolic than diastolic elevation. The narrowing is usually just distal to the left subclavian artery (Figs. 7 – 10) but it may rarely occur lower in the thoracic aorta or in the abdominal aorta.

Case 4: An eight-year-old girl referred to us for high BP was found to have severe hypertension in the arms, absent pulses in the legs, and a bruit over the lumbar area. At aortography, the coarctation was seen at the level of the renal arteries, both of which were quite small. Surgical attempt to resect the coarctation and to restore aortic continuity and renal arterial flow was unsuccessful. Her hypertension could be considered renovascular as well as that due to aortic blockage by coarctation.

Classically, coarctation of the aorta is considered to be a type of remediable hypertension, by surgical removal of the narrowing, but some children have higher pressures early in the postoperative period than they did preoperatively (paradoxical hypertension) and some individuals have persistent hypertension or late recurrence of hypertension following what was apparently satisfactory relief of the aortic narrowing. Infants who have required operation because of cardiac failure may, as they grow, develop a new hypertension in the arms and recurrence of coarctation due to failure of adequate growth of the anastomotic site (see Figs. 7 and 8).

Hyper-reactive hypertension seems to be more common in younger children, five years of age or less at the time of surgery, than in those around the age of 10 to 12 years. In 21 of 31 patients in Sealy's series at Duke University, this complication was noted.[30] All five of those reported by Ingomar to have reactive hypertension among the 33 children operated on were under age six.[31] In Toronto 43 percent of 65 young children had higher blood pressure in the first 48 hours postoperative than preoperatively.[32] Chronic postoperative generalized hypertension is less apt to be found in children operated on at age 10 to 12 years or younger than in adults in the older age group at surgery. For example, at Johns Hopkins University in long-term (11 to 25 years) postoperative followup of patients operated upon at a mean age of 20 years, 37 percent of the 59 studied had residual high blood pressure.[33] Yet in a younger population, Simon and Zloto of Michigan

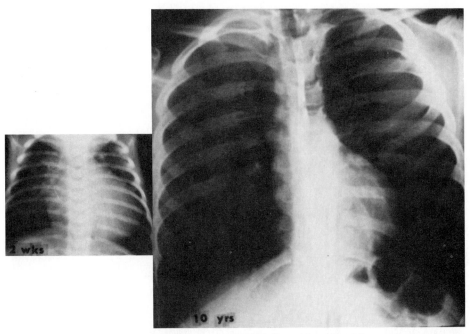

Figure 7. Chest roentgenogram on the left of a 1-month-old infant with cardiac failure and severe hypertension due to coarctation of aorta, showing marked cardiomegaly and pulmonary vascular congestion. Film was taken prior to surgery. On the left is film taken at age 10 years, showing average cardiothoracic ratio at time that hypertension in upper arm had returned (see Fig. 8).

found an incidence of 7 percent of persistent hypertension in their long-term followup (average 6.6 years) of 190 patients operated on beyond the age of 2 years. One hundred twenty-seven of these were 15 years of age or younger, and 45 were 16 to 30 years of age at the time of operation.[34]

Ever since successful surgical relief of the aortic block was first accomplished by Crafoord[35] and by Gross[36], investigators have attempted to define the cause(s) of arm hypertension in unoperated patients with coarctation and have noted and speculated on the cause(s) for pressures being higher than normal after repair.[37] Renal factors, though suggested,[38-40] might appear to have been refuted. Kirkendall and colleagues found normal renal hemodynamics and renin release rates in adult patients with uncomplicated coarctation of the aorta.[41, 42] Kioschos with Kirkendall[43] reaffirmed that renal blood flow and renal pressure were normal in such adults. In children with coarctation, Amsterdam and associates in Boston[44] and Strong and coworkers in Cleveland[45] also concluded that the renin-angiotensin system did not play a significant role in the hypertension preoperatively or postoperatively. However, of 15 subjects studied,[45] in only 3 of these was sodium restricted at preoperative study. They dismissed the finding of elevated peripheral plasma renin activity (PRA) in the first 4 postoperative days and they did not comment on the early hyper-reactive hypertension exhibited by three individuals. The patients were discharged on the fifth to seventh postoperative days with blood pressures still elevated; so the time when the elevated PRA and pressures returned to normal is not known. Blood pressure and PRA were in a normal range when studied about 3 months later. Markiewicz and coworkers in Poland reported in 1975 on a study of 11 patients from 5 to 20 years of age,[46] and they also concluded that the renin-angiotensin system was not involved directly in the maintenance of hypertension in patients with aortic coarctation. Plasma renin activity in the recumbent position was lower than

300

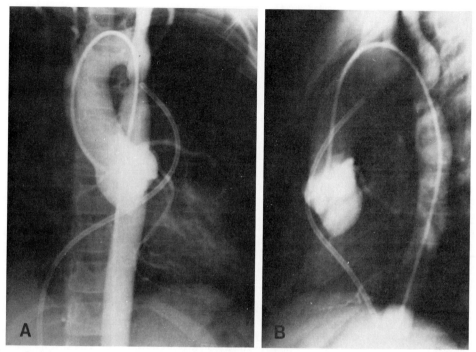

Figure 8. Aortogram in frontal (A) and lateral (B) projection of 10-year-old child whose chest x-rays are shown in figure 7. With growth of child but inadequate growth of anastomotic site, coarctation of the aorta had developed anew. Note constriction in descending aorta in usual place for coarctation and poststenotic dilatation of descending aorta.

in the upright position and was less preoperatively than in a control group. After surgery it rose to normal levels, but the time interval after operation when these values were determined was usually 4 to 6 months later. No information was provided on the blood pressure or renin levels in the early postoperative period. Rocchini and associates[47] have bridged some of this information gap in a study of 7 children, 5 of whom had paradoxical hypertension after coarctation resection. They found a rise in plasma renin activity by the third or fourth day that corresponded with the elevation in systolic and diastolic pressure and that coincided with abdominal pain.

Attention was paid to the characteristics of the arterial bed and pulsatile flow in the presence of coarctation prior to and following resection by Werko and associates,[48] and by O'Rourke and Cartmill[49] among others. They postulated that the problems of coarctation might be due not to increased resistance, but to decreased size of the arterial compression chamber. Counihan suggested that developmental narrowness in the small arteries might be responsible for residual postoperative hypertension.[37] Lorber and Lillehei,[50] Singleton,[51] and Sealy[30] were among the first to describe a true arteritis following resection of coarctation in the rare group of young children who developed abdominal complications with mesenteric arteritis. Some of these also manifested hyper-reactive hypertension postoperatively. This extreme situation may account for hypertension in a few, and perhaps lesser degrees of vascular reaction may be an explanation for some instances of acute or chronic hypertension postoperatively. Part of the reason for the greater likelihood of residual hypertension in adults than in children 10 to 12 years of age at surgery may lie in the changing characteristics of pressure wave transmission along the aorta with advancing age, as noted by O'Rourke and colleagues.[52] They found a decline in peripheral reflection coefficient resulting from decreased distensibility of peripheral arteries with increase in age. Whereas in children the amplitude of the pressure wave increased progressively along the aorta, in the elderly it did not.

Recently James and Kaplan of Cincinnati[53] and Kutayli with associates in Charleston[54] performed submaximal exercise testing on children several years after surgery utilizing the treadmill[53] or bicycle ergometer.[54] In both groups, systolic hypertension appeared in about half of those tested.

Reported series with long-term postoperative followup have often failed to differentiate residual pressure gradients between arms and legs, present from the moment of completion of repair, from "incomplete relief" or "recurrence" of coarctation. The last is usually a consequence of disproportionate growth of the anastomotic area in contrast to that of the rest of the aorta when operation has been undertaken in infancy or very early childhood (see Figs. 7 and 8). The first is due to the inability of the surgeon to construct a normal aorta because of hypoplasia of the transverse aortic arch in some patients (see Figs. 9 and 10). While coarctation of the aorta may be defined as a narrowing in the aorta sufficient to cause a systolic pressure gradient, and is classically a discrete, localized circumferential infolding of the aorta just distal to the left subclavian artery with normal aortic arch, there is sometimes hypoplasia of the whole transverse arch with progressive tapering from the innominate artery to the point of maximal narrowing at the coarctation diaphragm. There may be complete interruption of the isthmus of the aorta (Fig. 11). Even though the surgeon may resect the coarctation as completely as possible and restore aortic continuity to achieve as large a lumenal size as possible by end-to-end anastomosis or a circumferential or patch graft,[55, 56] he may not be able to abolish the pressure gradient completely.

It seems to us that neither preoperative nor postoperative hypertension in coarctation of the aorta is fully understood. While it is likely that the explanation of preopera-

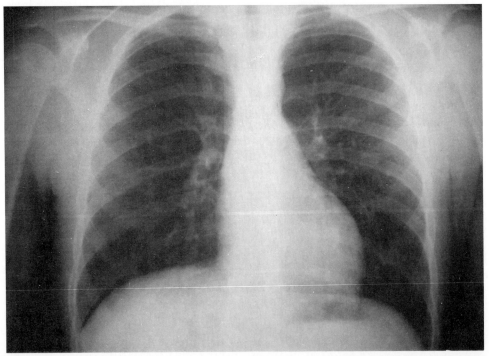

Figure 9. Roentgenogram of chest of a 10-year-old boy with BP in arms of 170/110 mm. Hg and with unobtainable BP in the legs shows an average-sized heart and slight notching of ribs. See Figures 10 and 11 for contrast visualization.

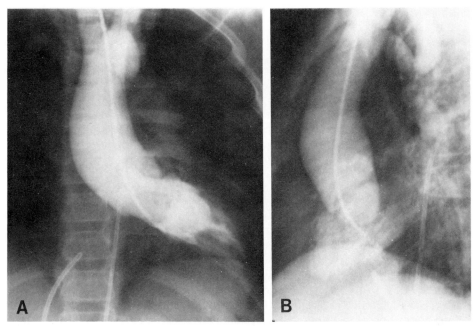

Figure 10. Left ventriculogram of 10-year-old boy (see Fig. 9) with complete interruption of isthmus of aorta. Frontal view on left with simultaneous lateral view on right shows normally contracting and normal-sized left ventricle with dilatation of the ascending aorta and innominate artery but hypoplastic transverse arch of aorta (seen in lateral view) and no opacification of descending aorta.

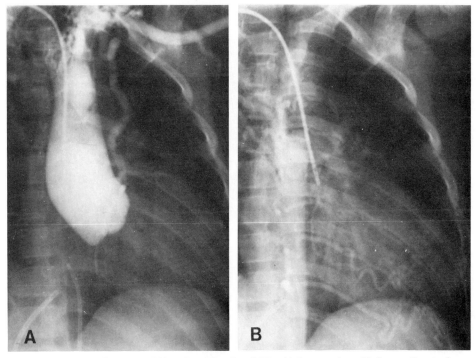

Figure 11. Aortogram of 10-year-old boy (see Figs. 9 and 10) with interruption of isthmus of aorta shows no opacification of descending aorta at time of filling of ascending aorta and collateral circulation (A) and late, faint filling of descending aorta (B) by means of the rich collateral blood supply.

303

tive hypertension lies in the resistance offered to aortic flow by the coarctation and by the collateral circulation (See Fig. 10), postoperative hypertension is more complex and may involve one or more factors whose roles remain to be elucidated.

Lesions with wide pulse pressure, such as an aorticopulmonary communication or aortic insufficiency, have systolic hypertension. In the first 12 to 24 hours after a moderately large patent ductus arteriosus has been surgically obliterated, generalized systolic and diastolic hypertension occurs. In instances with severe elevation of pressure, the electrocardiographic pattern of left ventricular "strain" is added to that of left ventricular hypertrophy. The condition spontaneously subsides as the systemic vascular bed dilates and systemic resistance falls, and as blood volume is readjusted. Only rarely is it necessary to use an antihypertensive agent during this period.

Endocrine

Several children have been referred to Dr. Maria New, Director of the Clinical Research Center, and have had cardiovascular evaluation by us for hypertension, which proved to be hormonally mediated.[57-70]

> **Case 4:** An infant was admitted in congestive heart failure and with generalized hypertension of 210/110 mm. Hg at the age of 2 months. She appeared Cushingoid. There was marked cardiomegaly by x-ray and left ventricular hypertrophy and "strain" on electrocardiogram. Prompt, full digitalization preceded intravenous pyelography, which showed poor visualization of the upper collecting system on the left and none on the right. At emergency laparotomy that day, with the diagnosis of adrenal tumor producing Cushing's syndrome and severe hypertension, the right adrenal gland with a tumor was removed. The left appeared normal. Postoperatively, cardiac failure and hypertension disappeared by the time of discharge eight weeks later. The tumor was an adrenal carcinoma.

> **Case 5:** A 17-month-old girl had been well until one month before admission when she began to grow excessively and to develop pubic hair. She was over the 84th percentile in height and weight and showed signs of precocious sexual development. Blood pressure was 170 to 190/90 mm. Hg in the arm and was higher in the legs. A firm, round mass was felt in the left side of the abdomen. Urinalysis and electrolytes were normal except for elevated 17-ketosteroid and 17-hydroxysteroid. Bone age was accelerated. Intravenous pyelogram showed slight displacement of the upper left kidney. The diagnosis was suprarenal tumor with hypertension and sexual precocity.
>
> At operation an encapsulated mass in the left adrenal gland 8 cm. in diameter was excised. No metastases were evident. The tumor was an adrenal carcinoma. Blood pressure and the 17-ketosteroid and hydroxycorticosteroid values became normal. Five years postoperatively, she was reported to be doing well.[22]

Central Nervous System

Hypertension is present in some children with increased intracranial pressure due to acute infection, intracranial hemorrhage, trauma, or tumor. Only rarely is it the presenting sign of the neurologic disorder.

Poisoning

Chronic ingestion of lead does occur in some toddlers who have pica and ingest paint containing lead. Their treatment consists of use of a chelating agent and elimination of the lead paint in the environment. An unusual kind of poisoning these days is illustrated by the following.

> **Case 6:** A 2-year-old girl was admitted because of progressive weakness and irritability. She and her siblings had been treated for chronic furunculosis with an ointment. She was pale, fretful and hypotonic. The blood pressure was 130/70 mm. Hg. Femoral pulses were stronger than the radials. A morbilliform rash was present, especially on the palms and soles. Urinalysis showed proteinuria. Twenty-four hour urine collection was positive for Hg. The lumbar tap was normal except for a protein of 81 mg. percent. Analysis of the ointment showed that it contained ammoniated mercury. Diagnosis was acrodynia caused by mercury poisoning.
>
> The treatment consisted of chelating agent (BAL) administered for 2 weeks. Physiotherapy was utilized and ointment was discontinued. Gradually she improved. After several months, there was no evidence of the rash or neurologic deficit, and the blood pressure was normal.[22]

Essential Hypertension

This form of hypertension, found only rarely in children in the past,[9-11, 15, 24, 25] is under intensive investigation now because of the assumption, which seems likely, that its onset is in childhood though its life threatening consequences may not appear until adulthood. In her clinic devoted to hypertensive children and adolescents, Loggie reported that the incidence of secondary hypertension has declined noticeably from 80 percent in 1972 to 58 percent in 1975 and that 55 percent of the teenagers referred have primary hypertension. Londe and Goldring[11] reported that 95 percent of 131 asymptomatic children with incidental hypertension were considered after investigation to have primary hypertension. Their experience resembled that in adults, approximately 90 percent of whom are designated as having essential or primary hypertension.[5]

It is possible now to predict which child might be at unusual risk of becoming hypertensive? The answer is not yet clear, but because of what is known from studies of adults one would anticipate that children with a family history of hypertension, black children, those who habitually add salt to food, and those who are obese would be in the group at risk.

Does labile hypertension portend later fixed hypertension? Again, longitudinal, prospective studies are needed for an answer.

Levine, Lewy, and New[62] screened students in a predominantly black high school and found 5.9 percent to be hypertensive. On re-examination, only 2.5 percent were still hypertensive. Twenty-eight students, or 1.5 percent of those initially screened, were admitted to the Clinical Research Center for further testing. Two had normal BP throughout hospitalization, while 26 demonstrated intermittent systolic and/or diastolic hypertension, the cause of which could not be identified. No followup data have yet been accumulated on those with labile or with persistent primary hypertension.

DIAGNOSTIC WORKUP

When a diagnosis of hypertension is made, how extensive should the diagnostic testing be? This depends on the degree of elevation of the blood pressure and on the likelihood of finding an underlying cause. The younger the child, under the age of 10 years, the more likely is the hypertension to be secondary.[15, 24] The more severe the pressure elevation, the more strenuous should be the search for a cause.

The advisory group on hypertension of the Intersociety Commission on Heart Disease Resources (ICHD)[63] advocated as the basic laboratory tests for adults the following: hematocrit, urinalysis, chest roentgenogram, electrocardiogram, BUN or creatinine, potassium, chloride, random blood sugar, and uric acid. Dustan[64] recommended adopting a simple and relatively inexpensive set of basic laboratory examinations, proposed by the Task Force of the High Blood Pressure Education Program.[65] The evaluation is directed toward determining the extent of vascular disease and identifying known causes. It is similar to the ICHD report and it includes a measure of renal excretory function (BUN or serum creatinine), urinalysis (to indicate renal parenchymal disease), serum potassium concentration (as an indicator of hyperaldosteronism), chest x-ray, and electrocardiogram. Special, detailed examinations are indicated in patients with hypokalemia, evidence of renal parenchymal disease or arterial stenosis, symptoms suggestive of pheochromocytoma, and in those in whom hypertension begins before the age of 30 or after 50 years. The latter recommendation was formulated by physicians caring for adults. We do not believe that extensive evaluation is needed in every infant, child, or adolescent with hypertension although the baseline studies recommended by these two expert groups are appropriate for the pediatric population. The cases reported illustrate some of the clues and tests for evaluation of suspected secondary hypertension.

TREATMENT

If the cause of the hypertension can be identified and eliminated, as in some of the foregoing case reports, the situation is ideal for treatment. If the cause can neither be identified nor corrected, what then for the baby, child or adolescent with hypertension?

A wide variety of antihypertensive drugs reflecting the multifactorial nature of hypertension is now available: diuretics, sympatholytics and vasodilators.[64] Dustan gave guidelines for rational therapy based on physiologic characteristics of various types of hypertension.[64] Laragh has proposed a classification based on the renin-sodium index for the two interacting components of vasoconstriction or volume excess and from this has proposed treatment for patients with essential hypertension.[66, 67] For those with the low renin profile, he advocated diuretics as treatment; and for those with high renin, he suggested the use of an antirenin drug such as propranolol. Frohlich discussed the therapy of the patient, based on certain hemodynamic concepts of hypertension.[68]

From the foregoing experiences of experts in adult hypertension, what can we extrapolate that is helpful in children? Londe and Goldring[11] as well as Loggie[25] and Sinaiko and Mirkin[69] point out that too little is known about the course of the child with labile or mild persistent hypertension to consider medication over what might be a lengthy period for the rest of their lives. The long-term effects on growing children of the drugs themselves are not known. Patient compliance in faithfully taking medication is a problem for most adolescents and for many others who are asymptomatic. These considerations point to the recommendation that only those with sustained, moderately severe hypertension that is considered primary be treated. For those children or adolescents with mild or labile hypertension, it might even be unwise to burden them with worry about their blood pressure, worry that might aggravate the condition as a response to this stress, and worry that might be unjustified to impose since we know so little of the natural history of this kind of hypertension.

If treatment is indicated which drug should be chosen, how should it be administered and for how long, and when should another agent be substituted or added? Loggie,[25] and Sinaiko and Mirkin[69] have published tables which give some of these answers as well as comments on time of onset, maximal effect, duration of action and side effects of the agents. The reader is referred to these excellent reviews for details, as well as to the article by Finnerty on critical considerations in the treatment of hypertension.[70] Table 4 is adapted from these sources.

In the acute hypertensive crisis, a potent and rapidly acting vasodilator such as di-

Table 4. Medical management of hypertension in children

Drug	Site of action	Acute				Chronic		Side effects
		Dose	Onset	Peak	If no response	Dose	Max.	
Diuretics								
Chlorothiazide (Diuril)	Arteriolar smooth muscle Sodium depletion	—	—	—	—	10–20 mg./kg./d.	2.0 gm./d.	Hyperglycemia, K depletion, hyperuricemia, dehydration
Furosemide (Lasix)	Volume depletion Increased renal blood flow	IV: 1–4 mg./kg./dose	15 min.	1 hr.	May increase to 100 mg./dose	—	—	Volume depletion, K depletion
Vasodilators*								
Hydralazine (Apresoline)	Arteriolar smooth muscle	IM: 0.25 mg./kg./dose	15–30 min.	1 hr.	Double dose 1–2 hr.	0.2–0.6 mg./kg. 4–6 hr.	300 mg./d.	Lupus, headache, palpitation
Diazoxide† (Hyperstat)	Arteriolar smooth muscle	Rapid IV: 5 mg./kg./dose	1–2 min.	Immediate	Repeat in 1 hr.	—	—	Does not produce hypotension
Sympathicolytics								
Reserpine (Serpasil)	Peripheral catecholamine depletion and central nervous system	IM: Test dose 0.2 mg.; 0.02 mg./kg./dose (not > 0.5 mg.)	1–3 hr.	Variable	Double dose 4–6 hr.	0.005–0.015 mg./kg./d.	2 mg.	Nasal congestion, sedation, bradycardia, depression
Methyldopa (Aldomet)	Unknown	—	—	—	—	10–60 mg./kg./d.	1.0–2.0 gm./d.	Hemolytic anemia, fever, leukopenia, abnormal liver function tests
Guanethidine (Ismelin)	Postganglionic sympathetic blockade	—	—	—	—	0.2–2.5 mg./kg./d.	100–150 mg./d.	Postural hypotension
Propranolol (Inderal)	Beta-receptors	PO: 1 mg./kg. in 4 doses/d. IV: q. 4–5 min. for 4 doses if necessary	15–30 min. 1–2 min.	2–3 hr.	Double dose 4–6 hr.	PO: 1–2 mg./kg./d. in 4 doses	4 mg./kg./d.	Slowing of pulse, fatigue, contraindicated in asthma, heart failure

*Nitroprusside (Nipride) has not yet been evaluated thoroughly in children, though it is promising in adults in treatment of hypertensive crisis as an intravenous infusion by microdrip, diluted in 5 percent dextrose in water to deliver 0.1 up to 8 micrograms/kg./min. If no response in 10 minutes, discontinue.
†Drug of choice for treatment of hypertensive crisis.

azoxide might be chosen. For the adolescent with moderately elevated BP, chronic use of an oral diuretic such as chlorothiazide, with potassium chloride supplementation as needed, is usually the initial choice for long range therapy.

CONCLUSION

Hypertension in the infant, child and adolescent is not uncommon. Often an identifiable cause can be found and removed by medical or surgical means. It is beginning to be increasingly appreciated that essential hypertension, so common in adults, has its origins if not its onset in the pediatric years. While advances have been made in drugs for relief of hypertension, much remains to be learned about the possible problems of their long-term use beginning in childhood. The goal in this field, as in other cardiovascular diseases, is immediate recognition and treatment of those who have the condition so as to prevent illness and premature death while ever seeking to understand the pathogenesis and to prevent the condition.

REFERENCES

1. KIRKENDALL, W. M., BURTON, A. C., EPSTEIN, F. A., ET AL.: *Recommendations for human blood pressure determination by sphygomomanometers.* Circulation 36:980, 1967.

2. BURTON, A. C.: *The criterion for diastolic pressure—revolution and counterrevolution.* Circulation 36: 805, 1967.

3. MOSS, A. J., AND ADAMS, F. H.: *Index of indirect estimation of diastolic blood pressure: muffling versus complete cessation of vascular sounds.* Am. J. Dis. Child. 106:364, 1963.

4. MCLAUGHLIN, G. W., KIRLEY, R. R., KEMMERER, W. T., ET AL.: *Indirect measurement of blood pressure in infants using Doppler ultrasound.* J. Pediatr. 79:300, 1971.

5. STEINFELD, L., ALEXANDER, H., AND COHEN, M. L.: *Editorial: Updating sphygomomanometry.* Am. J. Cardiol. 33:107, 1974.

6. GOLDRING, D., AND WOHLTMANN, H.: *Flush method for blood pressure determinations in newborn infants.* J. Pediatr. 40:285, 1952.

7. CAPPE, B. E., AND PALLIN, I. M.: *Systolic blood pressure determination in newborns and infants.* Anesthesiology 13:648, 1952.

8. MOSS, A. J., LIEBING, W., AUSTIN, W. O., ET AL.: *An evaluation of flush method for determining blood pressures in infants.* Pediatr. 20:53, 1957.

9. LONDE, S.: *Blood pressure in children as determined under office conditions.* Clin. Pediatrics 5:71, 1966.

10. FASOLA, A. F., MARTZ, B. L., AND ELMER, O. M.: *Plasma renin activity during supine exercise in offspring of hypertensive parents.* J. Appl. Physiol. 25:410, 1968.

11. LONDE, S., AND GOLDRING, D.: *High blood pressure in children: problems and guidelines for evaluation and treatment.* Am. J. Cardiol. 37:650, 1976.

12. ZINNER, S. H., LEVY, P. S., AND KASS, E. H.: *Familial aggregation of blood pressure in childhood.* N. Engl. J. Med. 284:401, 1971.

13. MOSS, A. J., AND ADAMS, F. H.: *Problems of Blood Pressure in Childhood.* Charles C Thomas, Springfield, Ill., 1962, p. 12.

14. MITCHELL, S. C., BLOUNT, S. G., JR., BLUMENTHAL, S., ET AL.: *The pediatrician and hypertension.* Pediatr. 56:3, 1975.

15. LIEBERMAN, E.: *Essential hypertension in children and youth: a pediatric perspective.* J. Pediatr. 85:1, 1974.

16. WEISS, N. S., HAMILL, P. V. V., AND DRIZD, T.: *Blood pressure levels of children 6-11 years. Relationship to age, sex, race, and socioeconomic status.* Vital Health Stat., 1973, series II, No. 135.

17. KIRKENDALL, W. M., AND OVERTURK, M.: *Plasma renin activity and systemic arterial hypertension.* Mod. Conc. Cardiovasc. Dis. 42:47, 1973.

18. SKEGGS, L. T.: *Biochemical relationships of the renin/angiotensin system.* Hosp. Prac. (March):145, 1974.

19. LARAGH, J. H.: *Vasoconstriction-volume analysis in treatment of hypertension.* Hosp. Prac. (June):55, 1974.

308

20. PEART, W. S.: *Renin-angiotensin system.* N. Engl. J. Med. 292:302, 1975.

21. NEW, M. I., BAUM, C. J., AND LEVINE, L. S.: *Nomograms relating aldosterone excretion to urinary sodium and potassium in the pediatric population: their application to the study of childhood hypertension.* Am. J. Cardiol. 37:658, 1976.

22. JABLONER, J., AND ENGLE, M. A.: *High blood pressure in children.* Heart Bull. 13:84, 1964.

23. SINGH, S. P., AND PAGE, I. B.: *Hypertension in early life.* Am. J. Med. Sci. 253:255, 1967.

24. LOGGIE, J. M. H.: *Systemic hypertension in children and adolescents.* Pediatr. Clin. North Am. 18:1273, 1971.

25. LOGGIE, J. M. H.: *Hypertension in children and adolescents.* Hosp. Prac. (June): 81, 1975.

26. LEWY, J. E.: Personal communication.

27. BROWN, J. J., FRASER, R., LEVER, A. F., ET AL.: *Renovascular and other renal hypertension.* Hosp. Prac. (February):107, 1975.

28. SCHAMBELAN, M., GLICKMAN, M., STOCKIGT, J. R., ET AL.: *Selective renal-vein renin sampling in hypertensive patients with segmental renal lesions.* N. Engl. J. Med. 290:1153, 1974.

29. BENNETT, S. P., LEVINE, L. S., SIEGAL, E. J., ET AL.: *Juvenile hypertension caused by overproduction of renin within a renal segment.* J. Pediatr. 84:689, 1974.

30. SEALY, W. C., HARRIS, J. S., YOUNG, W. G., ET AL.: *Paradoxical hypertension following resection of coarctation of aorta.* Surgery 42:135, 1957.

31. INGOMAR, C. J., AND TERSLEV, E.: *Hypertension after resection of coarctation of the aorta.* Br. Heart J. 23:370, 1961.

32. RATHI, L., AND KEITH, J. D.: *Post-operative blood pressures in coarctation of the aorta.* Br. Heart J. 26: 671, 1964.

33. MARON, B. J., HUMPHRIES, O., ROWE, R. D., ET AL.: *Prognosis of surgically corrected coarctation of the aorta: a 20-year postoperative appraisal.* Circulation 46:119, 1973.

34. SIMON, A. B., AND ZLOTO, A. E.: *Coarctation of the aorta. Longitudinal assessment of operated patients.* Circulation 50:456, 1974.

35. CRAFOORD, C., AND NYLIN, G.: *Congenital coarctation of aorta and its surgical therapy.* J. Thorac. Surg. 14:347, 1945.

36. GROSS, R. E., AND HUFNAGEL, C. A.: *Coarctation of the aorta. Experimental studies regarding its surgical correction.* N. Engl. J. Med. 233:287, 1945.

37. COUNIHAN, T. B.: *Changes in the blood pressure following resection of coarctation of the aorta.* Arch. Clin. Sci. 15:149, 1956.

38. SCOTT, H. W., AND BAHNSON, H. T.: *Evidence for a renal factor in the hypertension of experimental coarctation of the aorta.* Surgery 30:206, 1951.

39. TONELLI, L., BAISI, F., AND MALIZIA, E.: *Pre-and post-operative renal function in coarctation of the aorta and its relationship to the genesis of hypertension.* Acta Med. Scand. 148:35, 1954.

40. GENEST, J., NEWMAN, E. V., KATTUS, A. A., ET AL.: *Renal function before and after surgical resection of coarctation of aorta.* Bull. Johns Hopkins Hosp. 83:429, 1948.

41. KIRKENDALL, W. M., CULBERTSON, J. W., AND ECKSTEIN, J. W.: *Renal hemodynamics in patients with coarctation of the aorta.* J. Lab. Clin. Med. 53:6, 1959.

42. KROETZ, F. W., KIRKENDALL, W. M., AND KIOSCHOS, J. M.: *Renal blood flow (RBF) and renin release rates (RRR) in coarctation of the aorta.* Circulation 38:VI-120, 1968.

43. KIOSCHOS, J. M., KIRKENDALL, W. M., AND KROETZ, F. W.: *The effect of hydralazine on renin activity in patients with coarctation of the aorta.* Circulation 43, 44:11, 1971.

44. AMSTERDAM, E. A., ALBERS, W. H., CHRISTLIEB, A. R., ET AL.: *Plasma renin activity in children with coarctation of the aorta.* Am. J. Cardiol. 23:396, 1969.

45. STRONG, W. B., BOTTI, R. E., SILBERT, D. R., ET AL.: *Peripheral and renal vein plasma renin activity in coarctation of the aorta.* Pediatr. 45:254, 1970.

46. MARKIEWICZ, A., WOJCZUK, D., KOKOT, F., ET AL.: *Plasma renin activity in coarctation of the aorta before and after surgery.* Br. Heart J. 37:721, 1975.

47. ROCCHINI, A. P., ROSENTHAL, A., BARGER, A. C., ET AL.: *Pathogenesis of paradoxical hypertension after coarctation resection.* Circulation 54:382, 1976.

48. WERKO, L., EK, J., BUCHT, H., ET AL.: *Cardiac output, blood pressures and renal dynamics in coarctation of aorta.* Scand. J. Clin. Lab. Invest. 8:193, 1956.

49. O'ROURKE, M., AND CARTMILL, T.: *Influence of aortic coarctation on pulsatile hemodynamics in the proximal aorta.* Circulation 44:281, 1971.

50. LORBER, P. H., AND LILLEHEI, C. W.: *Necrotizing panarteritis following repair of coarctation of aorta: report of two cases.* Surgery 35:950, 1954.

51. SINGLETON, A. O., McGINNIS, L. M. S., AND EASON, H. R.: *Arteritis following correction of coarctation of the aorta.* Surgery 45:665, 1959.

52. O'ROURKE, M. F., BLAZEK, J. V., MORREELS, C. L., JR., ET AL.: *Pressure wave transmission along the human aorta. Changes with age and in arterial degenerative disease.* Circ. Res. 23:567, 1968.

53. JAMES, F. W., AND KAPLAN, S.: *Systolic hypertension during submaximal exercise after correction of coarctation of aorta.* Circulation 50:11, 1974.

54. KUTAYLI, F., TAYLOR, A., WEBB, H., ET AL.: *Submaximal standing exercise testing in coarctation of the aorta.* Presented at Proceedings, Scientific Sessions of Section on Cardiology, American Academy of Pediatrics, October 1975 (Washington, D.C.)

55. KING, H., KAISER, G., AND KING, R.: *Repair of coarctation of the aorta by patch grafting.* J. Thorac. Cardiovasc. Surg. 43:792, 1962.

56. REUL, G. J., JR., KABBANI, S. S., SANDIFORD, F. M., ET AL.: *Repair of coarctation of the thoracic aorta by patch graft aortoplasty.* J. Thorac. Cardiovasc. Surg. 68:696, 1974.

57. NEW, M. I., AND PETERSON, R. E.: *A new form of congenital adrenal hyperplasia.* J. Clin. Endocrinol. 27:300, 1967.

58. NEW, M. I., AND SEAMAN, M. P.: *Secretion rates of cortisol and aldosterone precursors in various forms of congenital adrenal hyperplasia.* J. Clin. Endocrinol. 30:361, 1970.

59. ZACHMAN, M., VOLLMIN, J. A., NEW, M. I., ET AL.: *Congenital adrenal hyperplasia due to deficiency of 11β-hydroxylation of 17-hydroxylated steroids.* J. Clin. Endocrinol. 33:501, 1971.

60. NEW, M. I., SIEGAL, E., AND PETERSON, R. E.: *Dexamethasone-suppressible hyperaldosteronism.* J. Clin. Endocrinol. 37:93, 1973.

61. BREST, A. N., AND BOWER, R.: *Renal arterial hypertension: incidence, diagnosis and treatment.* Am. J. Cardiol. 17:612, 1966.

62. LEVINE, L. S., LEWY, J. E., AND NEW, M. I.: *Hypertension in high school students. Evaluation in New York City.* N.Y. State J. Med. 76:40, 1976.

63. Hypertension Study Group: *Guidelines for the detection, diagnosis and management of hypertensive populations.* Circulation 44:A-263, 1971.

64. DUSTAN, H. P.: *Evaluation and therapy of hypertension—1976.* Mod. Concepts Cardiovasc. Dis. 45:97, 1976.

65. *Executive Summary of the Task Force Reports to the Hypertension Information and Education Advisory Committee,* National High Blood Pressure Education Program, National Institutes of Health, Bethesda, Md., Sept. 1, 1973, pp. 1–20.

66. LARAGH, J. H.: *Vasoconstriction-volume analysis for understanding and treating hypertension: the use of renin and aldosterone profiles.* Am. J. Med. 55:261, 1973.

67. LARAGH, J. H.: *The classification and treatment of essential hypertension using the renin-sodium index for vasoconstriction-volume analysis.* Johns Hopkins Med. J. 137:184, 1975.

68. FROHLICH, E. D.: *Hemodynamic concepts in hypertension.* Hosp. Prac. (November): 59, 1974.

69. SINAIKO, A. R., AND MIRKIN, B. L.: *Pediatric hypertension: current therapeutic considerations.* Pediatr. Ann. 5:98, 1976.

70. FINNERTY, F. A., JR.: *Critical considerations in the treatment of arterial hypertension.* Mod. Concepts Cardiovasc. Dis. 42:37, 1973.

Malignant Hypertension: Clinical Recognition and Management

James W. Woods, M.D.

The syndrome of malignant hypertension is characterized by an acute, and, if untreated, almost invariably fatal form of hypertensive disease. Essential clinical features include high diastolic blood pressure, usually over 130 mm. Hg, and papilledema. Many patients will also have proteinuria, microscopic hematuria, weight loss, progressive decline in renal function, and cardiac and central nervous system manifestations. Gross hematuria and microangiopathic hemolytic anemia may be present. Usually, but not invariably, this clinical syndrome is accompanied by a histologic lesion called malignant nephrosclerosis or necrotizing arteriolitis. A small percentage of patients may have a similar course with uremia and necrotizing arteriolitis without papilledema or with unilateral papilledema.[1] Severe hypertension with exudative retinopathy but without papilledema may be accompanied by necrotizing arteriolitis and has a similar prognosis to the malignant phase but is classified as accelerated hypertension. With the development and use of progressively more effective antihypertensive drugs over the past twenty years it has become possible to bring about resolution of the malignant phase with healing of necrotizing arteriolitis, and a significant increase in life expectancy for those patients who do not already have severe renal insufficiency at the time of diagnosis.

INCIDENCE

In view of the fact that these patients require specialized care, the case selection which enters into all published series makes the true incidence of malignant hypertension uncertain. Both Kincaid-Smith[1] and Bechgaard[2] estimated that the malignant phase develops in 1 percent of patients with the benign phase. There is also evidence that the malignant phase may develop de novo. In addition to essential or primary hypertension, malignancy may complicate a miscellaneous group of conditions all having elevated blood pressure in common and including chronic pyelonephritis, glomerulonephritis, renovascular disease, polyarteritis, radiation nephritis, Cushing's syndrome, primary aldosteronism, pheochromocytoma, and hypertension secondary to oral contraceptives.

If it were possible to promptly identify and adequately treat all individuals with sustained hypertension, the syndrome of malignant hypertension might disappear. It is unlikely that this will be achieved because of the ubiquity of hypertension and the frequent absence of symptoms in its uncomplicated phase.

311

PATHOLOGY AND PATHOGENESIS

It is apparent from the foregoing discussion that gross and microscopic pathologic examination of the kidneys may reveal, in addition to features of malignant nephrosclerosis, a variety of underlying renal diseases. In cases where malignant hypertension has developed de novo, the kidneys may be normal in size. The diagnostic feature on gross inspection is a "flea-bitten" appearance caused by petechial hemorrhages which are a result of arteriolar rupture. Microscopic features consist of proliferative endarteritis, necrotizing arteriolitis, and necrotizing glomerulitis. Proliferative endarteritis occurs in the afferent arterioles and small interlobular arteries, can develop rapidly, and produces extensive narrowing and obliteration of the vascular lumen. The increased tortuosity of segmental interlobular and arcuate arteries, cortical thinning, and tremendous diminution in the normal patterns of the cortical interlobular microvasculature resulting from malignant nephrosclerosis are illustrated in Figure 1B with normal renal vasculature shown for comparison in Figure 1A. Necrotizing arteriolitis also occurs in the afferent arterioles and is characterized by the deposition of polymorphonuclear leukocytes and fibrinoid material in the arteriolar wall. These vessels may contain thrombi and may rupture with resultant small hemorrhages giving the flea-bitten appearance seen on the surface of the kidney. The glomerulitis is similar to the necrotic lesion present in the afferent arterioles, and the two lesions are usually present in the same nephron. Necrotizing arteriolitis is found predominantly in the kidney and eye[3] but may also be found in other locations such as the pancreas, liver, gastrointestinal tract, adrenal, heart, and brain.

Effective antihypertensive drug therapy usually results in remission and healing of the acute arteriolar and glomerular lesions. The renal hilar arteries, however, which may reveal only slight subintimal changes in short-term survivors, may be almost occluded by subintimal hyperplastic fibrous tissue in long-term survivors.[4, 5] This change is illustrated in Figures 2 and 3. The latter lesion presumably reflects the damage inflicted upon the arteries during the pre-treatment period of uncontrolled hypertension and probably leads to the slowly progressive renal failure which eventually occurs in many treated patients.

The *pathogenesis* of malignant hypertension is not clear. Pickering[6] has assembled an impressive body of evidence which suggests that the severity of the hypertension or the height of the blood pressure itself is responsible for the clinical syndrome and pathological lesions. In support of his hypothesis are the following observations: 1) The blood pressure is higher in the malignant than in the benign phase. Cases which are exceptions to this observation have been reported but are uncommon. 2) The malignant phase may develop in patients with either primary hypertension or various types of secondary hypertension, all sharing a marked elevation of diastolic pressure. 3) Fibrinoid necrosis may occur in the pulmonary arteries of patients with severe pulmonary hypertension. 4) Postmortem studies revealed a high degree of correlation between the height of blood pressure during life and the presence of fibrinoid necrosis. 5) Hypertension produced in rats by partial constriction of a renal artery is followed by arteriolar necrosis, glomerulitis, and intimal proliferation in the contralateral kidney but not in the clamped one which was protected from high pressure. 6) Reduction of blood pressure for a period of time results in healing of the acute arterial lesion and disappearance of the syndrome of malignant hypertension.

There is also evidence suggesting that the renin-angiotensin-aldosterone system may play an important etiologic role in malignant hypertension since 1) high circulating plasma levels of these hormones are often present in this syndrome, 2) infusion of renin and angiotensin II in animals can produce arteriolar necrosis,[7] 3) angiotensin II blockade

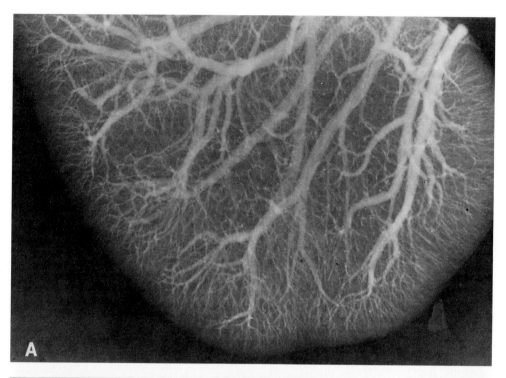

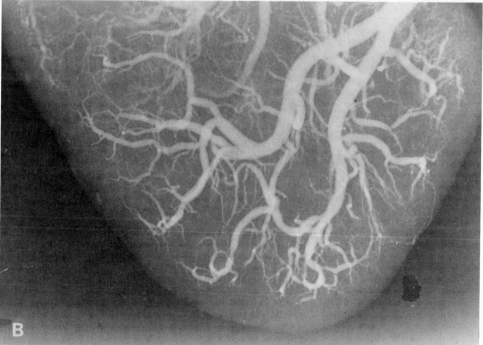

Figure 1. Radiographs of postmortem barium sulfate injected kidneys. (Courtesy of Dr. Richard Clark, Department of Radiology, University of North Carolina School of Medicine.)

313

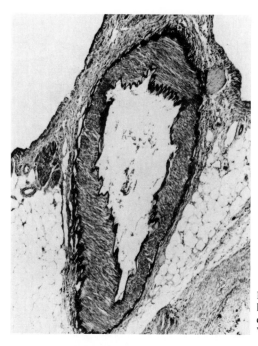

Figure 2. Minimal subintimal changes in a renal hilar artery of a patient dying one month after the diagnosis of malignant hypertension ($\times$ 40). (From Woods, Blythe, and Huffines,[5] with permission.)

with either the competitive inhibitor sar[1]-ala[8]-angiotensin II[8] or a converting-enzyme inhibitor[9] may lower blood pressure strikingly (but not to normal levels) in those patients with high renin levels, and 4) propranolol, which suppresses renin secretion, is said to be singularly effective in control of the hypertension in these patients.[10] Not all patients with malignant hypertension, however, have elevated levels of plasma renin activity (PRA). Of 22 malignant hypertensive patients studied by McAllister and associates,[11] when in balance on a 100 mEq. sodium diet, only 8 had elevated PRA (although 19 of 22 had elevated aldosterone secretion rates). These authors concluded that the reduction of renin, achieved by lowering blood pressure without sodium repletion, and the absence of elevated renin in many cases are consistent with the idea that high arterial pressure (rather than elevated renin) is the primary event in malignant hypertension producing the arteriolar damage which mediates the clinical syndrome. The possibility that even normal PRA levels may be inappropriately high in relation to body sodium has not been excluded. However, the weight of the evidence favors renal ischemia secondary to arteriolar disease as the most likely cause of elevated renin activity in this syndrome and the conclusion that hypersecretion of renin and/or aldosterone is not essential for the development of malignant hypertension, albeit as a secondary event this may intensify the disease.

An association between malignant hypertension and microangiopathic hemolytic anemia (MAHA) is now well recognized. The two main components of MAHA are excessive deposition of fibrin within the lumen and wall of small blood vessels and hemolytic anemia produced mainly by the fragmentation of erythrocytes as they pass through the fibrin mesh. Brain and his colleagues[12] believe that MAHA is secondary to the fibrinoid lesion, and that MAHA is a complication of the malignant phase. In the view of Gavras and coworkers,[13] intravascular coagulation is a necessary step in the development of the fibrinoid lesion and even if MAHA is not an essential element in the transition from benign to malignant hypertension, it is likely at least to aggravate the renal failure. These divergent concepts are unresolved. There is no convincing evidence that heparin or dipyridamole directed against intravascular coagulation re-

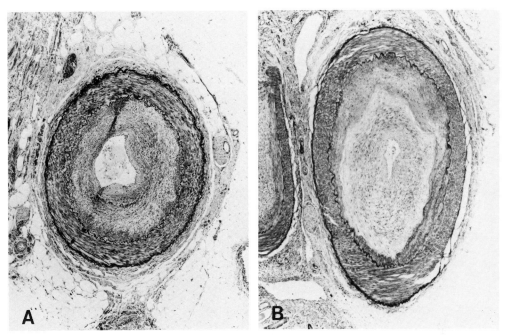

Figure 3. (A) Moderate subintimal hyperplasia in a renal hilar artery of a patient living for 15 months (reduced 15% from × 40), and (B) marked subintimal hyperplasia with severe reduction of the lumen in a patient living for 7.5 years (reduced 15% from × 40). (From Woods, Blythe, and Huffines,[5] with permission.)

sults in improvement of hypertension or renal function in malignant hypertension, whereas they do add to the increased risk of bleeding which accompanies this syndrome.

CLINICAL FEATURES

Several large studies are in agreement that malignant hypertension is more common in men than in women and that the peak incidence is in the fifth decade. Since it is more common in the Negro race and appears at an earlier age, medical centers serving a large number of black persons encounter malignant hypertension most frequently in black males in their 30's and 40's.

Severe headache of abrupt onset is one of the most characteristic symptoms. It is typically occipital in location and present on arising, but may occur in any part of the head and at any time of day or night. It is usually dull and aching in nature rather than throbbing. Blurring of vision, weight loss, anorexia, nausea, and vomiting commonly accompany the headache. Symptoms vary depending on the presence or absence of uremia and of congestive heart failure. A minority of patients present because of epistaxis, gross hematuria (10 to 20 percent), seizures, somnolence, or oliguria. Headache with papilledema may suggest brain tumor, and this diagnostic possibility may require exclusion, but the very high diastolic pressure usually points to the correct diagnosis.

In addition to the high blood pressure, physical examination typically reveals an ill patient and the presence of bilateral papilledema. Retinoscopic examination should be carried out either in a darkened room or best, after dilatation of the pupils with a short-acting mydriatic. Unequal pupils or the clinical suspicion of brain tumor contraindicates the latter, of course. The margins of the optic discs are blurred, the nerve head is elevated above the surrounding retina, pulsation of retinal veins is absent, the disc is hyperemic, and there are usually accompanying soft, fluffy, cotton-wool exudates and both linear and flame-shaped hemorrhages. Star figures are often present at the maculae. A scholarly review of the eye involvement in malignant hypertension has been published by Ashton.[3] Although it is often assumed that papilledema is a consequence of raised spinal fluid pressure, the association is not a constant one. If hypertension is relatively long-standing, retinal arterioles may show silver-wiring and there may be striking A-V crossing defects. On the other hand, in patients with the recent onset of severe hypertension, there may be segmental narrowing of retinal arterioles and no hemorrhages or exudates associated with papilledema. Although a few patients have reduced visual acuity, in most, vision is relatively good and is not changed by therapy. In addition to neuroretinopathy there may be a wide spectrum of neurologic abnormalities including encephalopathy and those associated with cerebral vascular disease.

Most patients will have cardiac enlargement, a sustained left ventricular thrust indicating hypertrophy, an audible atrial gallop or S_4 accompanied by a simultaneous visible and palpable "A" wave at the apex, and a short, functional systolic ejection murmur along the left sternal border. A ventricular gallop or an S_3 indicating left ventricular failure is present in some patients. Chest x-ray usually reveals left ventricular enlargement. The electrocardiogram can be expected to show left ventricular hypertrophy and, in addition, often reveals left atrial enlargement. The characteristic urinary finding is proteinuria which in our experience[14] has ranged between 0.4 and 4.0 grams excreted per 24 hours. Microscopic hematuria is frequently present, gross hematuria is not an uncommon finding as previously noted, and there may be hyalin and granular casts. Though occasional white cells may be present, pyuria is not a prominent feature unless pyelonephritis is present. Depending upon the degree of renal damage, a low, fixed specific gravity may or may not be present. A significant minority of patients will exhibit renal salt-wasting. The ability to conserve sodium is a critical determinant of the degree of sodium restriction which can be prescribed in treatment. The intravenous pyelogram may reveal underlying primary renal disease and normal size or bilaterally small kidneys, but often the kidneys are not visualized due to renal insufficiency so often present when the diagnosis is first made. In the presence of mild renal insufficiency, a double-dose of contrast medium with tomographic technique may successfully demonstrate the kidneys and ureters when the standard technique fails. Because of the gravity of this disease aortography should be carried out in those patients with good renal function in the hope that a remediable renal artery obstruction will be found. Most often, however, it reveals patent renal arteries with severe disease of the small arteries and arterioles, giving the so-called "pruned tree" appearance as has been illustrated in Figure 1.

Other laboratory abnormalities frequently include elevation of blood urea nitrogen, serum creatinine, PRA, and plasma aldosterone (secondary hyperaldosteronism). Very rarely primary aldosteronism may be complicated by the malignant phase and, in that case, plasma aldosterone is elevated but PRA is suppressed. In the presence of MAHA, schistocytes are seen in the blood smear and the reticulocyte count is elevated as is lactate dehydrogenase (LDH). Damage to the principal target organs, i.e., brain, heart and kidneys, may add other laboratory abnormalities. Uremia, of course, adds its own characteristic abnormalities in many organs.

It is thus apparent that the diagnosis of malignant hypertension may be made at a time when the patient has few symptoms and little evident organ damage but, all too often, only when he is critically ill with severe and irreversible damage to kidneys and heart. While spontaneous remissions may rarely occur in this disease, 85 to 90 percent of untreated patients are dead within 15 months—thus the term "malignant" hypertension. Uremia is the principal cause of death, followed by congestive heart failure and cerebral vascular accidents.

TREATMENT

The benefits of blood pressure reduction by means of antihypertensive drugs, in terms of survival and preservation of cardiac and renal function, have been clearly demonstrated in many studies. The most important factor determining prognosis is renal function at the time the treatment is initiated. Survival curves from two earlier, large series[15, 16] are shown in Figure 4 and illustrate the improvement in survival to be expected from effective therapy when it is begun before significant renal damage has occurred. The 38 percent survival in non-azotemic patients after 12 years found by Perry[16] and the 21 percent survival after 10 years found by Dollery[17] encourage the use of aggressive therapy for an otherwise rapidly fatal disease. We have shown that survival can be increased in malignant hypertension complicated by renal insufficiency.[14] Formerly, it was the general opinion that such patients rarely outlived their hospitalization and that reduction of blood pressure accelerated their demise by reducing renal blood flow. This has been shown not to be necessarily true, and even though renal function may not improve dramatically, further deterioration of renal function may be arrested, sometimes for many years. A survival curve for 20 patients with malignant hypertension and blood urea nitrogen levels (BUN) of 50 mg./100 ml. or higher at the time of diagnosis, treated aggressively, and followed closely to either death or the present time,[5] is shown in Figure 5.

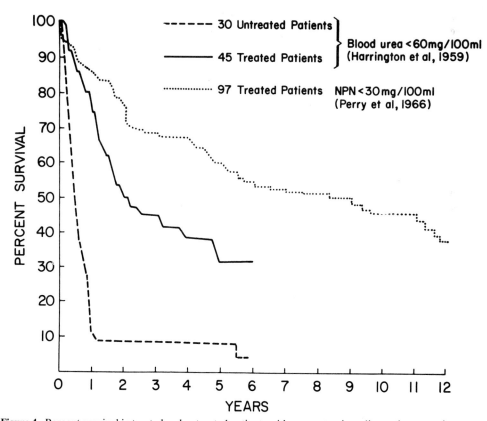

Figure 4. Percent survival in treated and untreated patients with nonazotemic malignant hypertension.

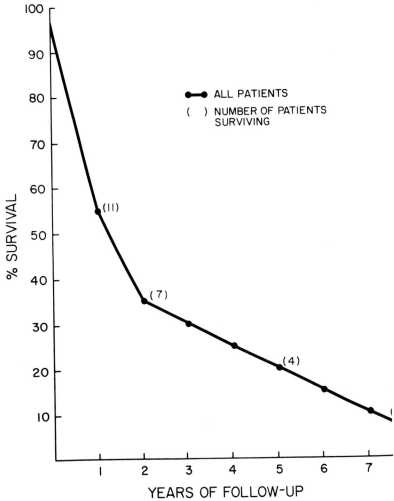

Figure 5. Survival curve for 20 patients with azotemic malignant hypertension. (From Woods, Blythe, and Huffines,[5] with permission.)

Successful therapy results in gradual resolution of retinal hemorrhages, exudates, papilledema and proteinuria within a few weeks time.

Antihypertensive Drugs Used Acutely

Because of the rapidity with which renal damage occurs and the risks of intracranial hemorrhage and pulmonary edema in this disease, patients with malignant hypertension should be promptly hospitalized, placed at bed rest, and should have their blood pressure lowered without delay. Consequently, administration of a rapidly acting parenteral drug is most often begun after the initial physical and laboratory examination and continued during more elaborate laboratory investigation. The four most useful drugs are listed in Table 1.

Diazoxide is inexpensive in terms of personnel time spent in its administration, and it

Table 1. Parenteral drugs used in initial management

Drug	Mode of Action	Onset	Peak	Duration	Dosage
Diazoxide	Decreased peripheral resistance by direct effect on arteriolar wall	1–2 min.	3–5 min.	4–12 hr.	300 mg. IV as a bolus; repeated as necessary
Sodium nitroprusside	Decreased peripheral resistance by direct effect on arteriolar wall; also dilates veins	0.5–1 min.	1–2 min.	3–5 min.	IV drip at 0.03–0.5 mg./min.
Hydralazine	Decreased peripheral resistance by direct effect on arteriolar wall	10–20 min.	20–40 min.	3–8 hr.	10–40 mg. IV or IM every 4–6 hr.
Reserpine	Decreased peripheral resistance by catecholamine depletion at nerve endings	2–3 hr.	3–4 hr.	6–24 hr.	0.5–5 mg. IM every 4–12 hr.

effectively lowers blood pressure in perhaps 80 percent of patients. Since high peak plasma levels are necessary for saturation of arteriolar receptors before inactivation by binding of the drug to albumin, it is given intravenously as a bolus. Close monitoring is required for 15 minutes and the dose may be repeated within 30 minutes if an inadequate response is obtained. Further doses are given as necessary in order to maintain diastolic blood pressure below 100 mm. Hg. Hypotension, hyperglycemia, and hyperuricemia are rarely problems. All vasodilators, and especially diazoxide, cause sodium retention and daily furosemide administration must accompany its repeated use.

Purely in terms of action *sodium nitroprusside*[18] is the best available drug since the onset is rapid, tachyphylaxis does not occur, toxicity is low, the blood pressure can be reduced to any desired level and maintained there, and the effect disappears within minutes of discontinuing the intravenous infusion. The dosage is not fixed and is determined by the desired response. Fifty milligrams is dissolved in a volume of glucose in water or normal saline appropriate to the fluid needs of the patient. Nitroprusside use requires constant monitoring in order to prevent hypotension, and, therefore, admission to an intensive care unit is usually necessary. Ideally, it is administered via an infusion pump with blood pressure measured frequently by means of an automatic blood pressure recorder such as the Arterisonde. The action of this drug is thought to be due to the nitroso (NO) group while toxicity is related to thiocyanate, a metabolic breakdown product. Thiocyanate blood levels are easily measured and should not exceed 10 mg. percent. If continued use of the drug is imperative in patients with complicating renal insufficiency and high thiocyanate blood levels, thiocyanate can be removed by dialysis.

Hydralazine is less potent, less predictably effective, and not infrequently results in reflex sympathetic stimulation with troublesome tachycardia and headache. Concomitant use of propranolol will counteract this stimulation and potentiate the antihypertensive effect. It does not result in hypotension, is easy to administer, and may adequately control blood pressure in some patients. It is most useful, however, in a continuing oral regimen after initial control has been established.

Reserpine has a delayed onset of action, is not predictably effective, and the therapeutic dose varies widely from one patient to another. Side effects include depression, somnolence, nasal stuffiness, increased gastric acid secretion, and occasionally a Parkinsonlike state. It is a last-choice drug which may be useful under certain circumstances.

Methyldopa can be given intravenously but is rarely effective, and *trimethaphan camsylate* is usually accompanied by the development of tachyphylaxis within 24 hours and, frequently, by urinary retention and constipation. In our institution both of these drugs have fallen into disuse.

Longer Term Management

After initial control of blood pressure has been achieved, thought must next be given to longer term therapy. Of prime importance is education of the patient about his disease and his regimen since understanding and compliance are absolutely critical to survival. Patients with malignant hypertension should obtain and be taught the use of equipment for home measurement of their blood pressure. General measures including achievement of ideal weight, discontinuance of smoking, and regular exercise tailored to physical capacity should not be omitted. Dietary sodium restriction is important, but sodium content of the diet must be reasonable in terms of the patient's ability to conserve sodium. Those with a degree of renal insufficiency may be renal salt wasters and may become severely sodium depleted if drastic sodium restriction is prescribed. Determination of 24 hour urine sodium excretion during ingestion of the prescribed sodium diet will verify this possibility.

Since the duration of parenteral therapy must be limited, an oral drug regimen is started simultaneously. Many drug combinations are possible including hydralazine-propranolol-diuretic, hydralazine-guanethidine-diuretic, methyldopa-diuretic, and clonidine-diuretic. If and when the potent vasodilator, minoxidil, receives FDA approval, it will no doubt have a place in therapy of this disease. Currently the first combination is our choice because of rapid onset of therapeutic effect, and absence of troublesome side effects including orthostatic hypotension, impairment of sexual function, drowsiness, dry mouth, etc. Propranolol prevents reflex sympathetic stimulation associated with hydralazine. It is necessary that hydralazine (50 mg.) and propranolol (40 to 80 mg.) be given every 6 or 8 hours, but the frequency of dosage is more acceptable to the patient than are major side effects. If this regimen fails, we would next initiate hydralazine and guanethidine (with a daily dose of diuretic). We find that the guanethidine loading plan recently described is useful.[19]

Significant cardiac and/or renal decompensation require additions to the regimen directed to their stabilization or improvement. Since some patients present with oliguric renal failure or uremia, peritoneal dialysis may be needed to sustain the patient over the short-term until renal function improves. Since excess extracellular fluid volume (which can be contributed to by many of the antihypertensive drugs) is a principal reason for resistance of blood pressure to antihypertensive therapy, excess fluid must be removed by means of diuretics or dialysis. When control of fluid volume and heavy drug therapy fail to control blood pressure in malignant hypertensives with severe renal insufficiency, bilateral nephrectomy and chronic hemodialysis may have to be considered. Fortunately, this is rarely necessary. There is evidence that such patients may represent a subgroup with the highest levels of PRA.[20]

CONCLUSION

The past two decades have seen advances in our understanding of this severe disease and a steadily expanding armamentarium of potent drugs which has significantly improved survival. This is encouraging. Even more encouraging is the current national

320

interest and effort toward detection and control of high blood pressure in the general population. Success in this effort could lead to a marked reduction in the frequency of the malignant phase.

REFERENCES

1. KINCAID-SMITH, P., McMICHAEL, J., AND MURPHY, E. A.: *The clinical course and pathology of hypertension and papilloedema (malignant hypertension).* Q. J. Med. 27:117, 1958.

2. BECHGAARD, P.: *The natural history of benign hypertension,* in BOCK, K. D., AND COTTIER, P. T. (EDS.): *Essential Hypertension: An International Symposium.* Springer-Verlag, Berlin, 1960, p. 198.

3. ASHTON, N.: *The eye in malignant hypertension.* Trans. Am. Acad. Ophthalmol. Otolaryngol. 76:17, 1972.

4. McCORMACK, L. J., BELAND, J. E., SCHNECKLOTH, R. E., ET AL.: *Effects of antihypertensive treatment on the evolution of the renal lesions in malignant nephrosclerosis.* Am. J. Pathol. 34:1011, 1958.

5. WOODS, J. W., BLYTHE, W. B., AND HUFFINES, W. D.: *Management of malignant hypertension complicated by renal insufficiency. A follow-up study.* N. Engl. J. Med. 291:10, 1974.

6. PICKERING, G. W. *High Blood Pressure,* ED 2. Churchill, London, 1968.

7. GIESE, J.: *Renin, angiotensin and hypertensive vascular damage: a review.* Am. J. Med. 55:315, 1973.

8. BRUNNER, H. R., GAVRAS, H., LARAGH, J. H., ET AL.: *Angiotensin II blockade in man by sar^1-ala^8-angiotensin II for understanding and treatment of high blood pressure.* Lancet 2:1045, 1973.

9. GAVRAS, H., BRUNNER, H. R., LARAGH, J. H., ET AL.: *An angiotensin converting-enzyme inhibitor to identify and treat vasoconstrictor and volume factors in hypertensive patients.* N. Engl. J. Med. 291:817, 1974.

10. BUHLER, F. R., LARAGH, J. H., BAER, L., ET AL.: *Propranolol inhibition of renin secretion: A specific approach to diagnosis and treatment of renin-dependent hypertensive disease.* N. Engl. J. Med. 287:1209, 1972.

11. McALLISTER, R. G., VAN WAY, C. W., III, DAYANI, K., ET AL.: *Malignant hypertension: Effect of therapy on renin and aldosterone.* Circ. Res. 28 and 29 (Suppl. II): 160, 1971.

12. BRAIN, M. C., DACIE, J. V., AND HOURIHANE, D. O.: *Microangiopathic hemolytic anemia: Possible role of vascular lesions in pathogenesis.* Br. J. Haematol. 8:358, 1962.

13. GAVRAS, H., BROWN, W. C. B., BROWN, J. J., ET AL.: *Microangiopathic hemolytic anemia and the development of the malignant phase of hypertension.* Circ. Res. 28 and 29 (Suppl. II):127, 1971.

14. WOODS, J. W., AND BLYTHE, W. B.: *Management of malignant hypertension complicated by renal insufficiency.* N. Engl. J. Med. 277:57, 1967.

15. HARINGTON, M., KINCAID-SMITH, P., AND McMICHAEL, J.: *Results of treatment in malignant hypertension. A seven-year experience in 94 cases.* Br. Med. J. 2:969, 1959.

16. PERRY, H. M., SCHROEDER, H. A., CATANZARO, F. J., ET AL.: *Studies on the control of hypertension. VIII. Mortality, morbidity, and remissions during twelve years of intensive therapy.* Circulation 33:958, 1966.

17. DOLLERY, C. T.: *Treatment of malignant hypertension.* Mod. Treatm. 3:39, 1966.

18. PAGE, I. H., CORCORAN, A. C., DUSTAN, H. T., ET AL.: *Cardiovascular actions of sodium nitroprusside in animals and hypertensive patients.* Circulation 11:188, 1955.

19. SHAND, D. G., NIES, A. S., McALLISTER, R. G., ET AL.: *A loading-maintenance regimen for more rapid initiation of the effect of guanethidine.* Clin. Pharmacol. Ther. 18:139, 1975.

20. VERTES, V., CANGIANO, J. L., BERMAN, L. B., ET AL.: *Hypertension in end-stage renal disease.* N. Engl. J. Med. 280:978, 1969.

Hypertension in Blacks*

Herbert G. Langford, M.D.

The purpose of this chapter is to note resemblances and differences in blood pressure problems of blacks and whites in the United States, and to evaluate the practical and theoretical significance of any observed differences. Genetic and socioeconomic factors, which are correlated and perhaps causal of the differences in hypertension, will also be discussed. We shall end by observing that the major differences between blacks and whites in terms of amount of hypertension and amount of hypertensive cardiovascular disease is probably environmental rather than genetic, though a genetic contribution cannot be excluded. Also, the risk associated with equivalent amounts of hypertension is no greater for the individual black than for the white patient.

BLOOD PRESSURE AND THE FREQUENCY OF HYPERTENSION IN BLACKS AND WHITES

Every population study of blood pressure in the United States has shown that from an early age blacks have higher pressures than whites. This finding holds whether expressed as mean blood pressure or as percent of the population that is hypertensive. In a population-based study, Comstock conclusively demonstrated the increased blood pressure and frequency of hypertension in blacks.[1] We among others have confirmed Comstock's finding which showed that by the age of 14 years, blacks have higher pressures than whites.[2]

The latest National Health and Nutrition Survey reported that the mean diastolic pressure in white males aged 18 to 24 was 76.4 mm. Hg, and in black males 74.2 mm. Hg. At 25 to 34 years the figures were 80.8 (white) and 84.3 (black). By 35 to 44 years, the mean for whites had risen to 84.2, and the mean for blacks to 91.2.

The prevalence rate for definite hypertension ($\geq$160 mm. Hg systolic or 95 mm. Hg diastolic) follows the same trends. At 25 to 34 years 8.2 percent of the white men and 17.7 percent of the black men were hypertensive by the foregoing definition; and at 35 to 44 years, 17.3 percent of the white men and 38.2 percent of the black men reached or surpassed 160 mm. Hg systolic and/or 95 mm. Hg diastolic.[3] Why the latest National Health and Nutrition Survey failed to demonstrate higher blood pressures in blacks than whites before the age of 24 is not clear. Perhaps it is related to the planned oversampling of the poor. As will be outlined later, the poorer the individual, the higher the

*Supported in part by Grant HE 10726, Grant 1MOIRR 00626, Grant 1ROLHL 18891-01 and a grant from the Hartford Foundation

blood pressure. Therefore, if an excess of poor young white men were sampled, the black/white difference would be decreased or eliminated.

In various surveys the differences in mean blood pressure vary depending, among other factors, on the age, social class, and geographical site of the groups being studied. The difference in mean blood pressure may often be quite small. As the standard deviation of a group's blood pressure increases as the mean blood pressure increases and as the blood pressure distribution in all populations is skewed to the right, a small difference in mean pressure will produce a large difference in percentage of hypertensives in the population. The blood pressure difference in blacks and whites decreases by the age of 50 years and is comparatively small by 70 years. The most likely explanation for this finding is differential mortality, the blacks having been removed from the population due to death from hypertension, whereas the whites have been removed at a slower rate and with less attrition due to their blood pressure.

Because of the aforementioned considerations and because of a variety of criteria used to define hypertension, a wide range of values may be ascribed for the relative frequency of hypertension in the two races.

BLACK/WHITE DIFFERENCES IN MORTALITY RELATED TO HYPERTENSION

The blood pressure differences previously outlined are accompanied by a marked difference in mortality from hypertension. To choose an extreme example, death from stroke is six times more frequent in the 30-year-old black male than in the white male.[4] Howard and Holman analyzed black/white hypertension mortality ratios by occupation and socioeconomic class.[5] They found the mean black/white ratio runs as high as 12.49 to 1 for the young lower class socioeconomic group. Hypertension mortality increases in the white with decreasing social class but not as drastically as in the black. For the highest socioeconomic class, the black/white ratio of hypertensive mortality is approximately 3.

IS HYPERTENSION WORSE IN BLACKS?

Regardless of how black/white ratios of hypertension-related mortality are examined, blacks have a much higher hypertension-related death rate. In epidemiologic terms, the population ascribable mortality related to hypertension is markedly increased. From this dramatic and unequivocal fact there has grown the assumption that the risk for a black person with hypertension is greater than that for a white person with the same blood pressure, i.e., the individual ascribable hypertensive risk is greater for blacks. In the only study that I have found which directly addressed the question, *the opposite turned out to be the case.* The individual ascribable risk for hypertension was *less* for black men than for white men in Evans County, Georgia.[6] The authors did not attempt to explain this finding. However, studies done by Stamler and his colleagues in Chicago more than a decade ago suggest an explanation. Black men at that time had significantly lower blood cholesterols and they smoked less.[7] Evans County, Georgia, and Chicago, Illinois, are far removed. It is likely that the black laborer of Evans County of a decade and a half ago (when the subjects were originally entered in the study), had even lower levels than Chicago blacks of such risk factors as cholesterol and smoking. In addition, the blacks of Evans County probably did more physical work than the whites of that area. As physical exertion probably prevents death from cardiovascular causes, the blacks of Evans County were receiving considerable prophylaxis against heart attacks at that time.

Therefore, it seems fair to conclude that individual ascribable risk is that of the known risk factors which *do not include skin color*. As there is a significant but low order correlation between skin color and blood pressure which will be discussed in the next section, skin color could be considered a surrogate for blood pressure in a multi-variate risk function. But the sphygmomanometer is a much better way to determine blood pressure.

POSSIBLE CAUSES OF EXCESS HYPERTENSION IN BLACKS

Factors Related to Social Class and Environment

A significant increase of mean blood pressure correlates with the downward trending social class in blacks and whites. In addition, there is an urban/rural blood pressure gradient with blood pressure usually being higher in individuals in rural areas than in persons from the cities.[2] There is also a north/south gradient with southern blacks and whites having a higher hypertensive death rate than their northern counterparts.[8] In general, the poorer, the more rural, and the more southern the individual, the higher the blood pressure. As the American black is on the average poorer and more likely to live in the south, the overall higher blood pressures of blacks can be viewed as a logical consequence of sociologic phenomenon.

For the following reasons, the foregoing argument is less than a rigorous explanation of the black/white difference. The explanation suggests that if we equate whites and blacks on education, income, occupation, or other indicators of social class, the black/white blood pressure difference would be abolished. This does not occur. Even with such stratification the blacks will have higher pressures or higher hypertension-related death rates than whites.

Therefore there may be a residual genetic contribution to the hypertension of blacks. On the other hand, it is at least equally tenable that the sociological forces identified as social class are still acting more strongly in the black than in the white, even if the black has attained the same income or education.

A sociologic explanation of black/white differences in blood pressure will require an elucidation of the physiological route by which the sociological forces operate. There are at least three suggestions available in the literature.

Diet

We,[9] Grim,[10] and Cullen[11] have noted a higher urinary sodium/potassium ratio in blacks than in whites, accompanying the higher blood pressures of the blacks. Meneely and Dahl showed that potassium protected rats against salt hypertension.[12, 13] Part of the route by which socioeconomic forces may affect blood pressure may be a dietary path; fruits cost more than other sources of calories, and "southern cooking" with its prolonged simmering of vegetables may further leech out potassium from its natural sources.

Obesity

At least part of the socioeconomic blood pressure gradient may be related to the gradient of obesity. Part of the black/white difference may be explained on the same grounds. How obesity affects blood pressure is not known. It is quite unlikely that all the socioeconomic and racial blood pressure differences can be explained on this basis.

Factors Operating Through the Mind

If it is postulated that psychic stresses increase progressively with lowered socio-economic status and rural southern living, the urban/rural, north/south and black/white blood pressure differences can be explained. Unfortunately our ability to define and measure these stresses is rudimentary. Harburg and coworkers are making a valiant effort to quantitate indices of stress and blood pressure in Detroit.[14]

Genetic Factors and Blood Pressure in Blacks

Boyle, working in Charleston, has shown a direct linear correlation between blackness of skin and blood pressure.[15] Long has shown a significant positive correlation between blood group constellations indicating African ancestry in blacks and blood pressure.[16] These two studies could be interpreted as proving that a genetic factor predisposing to hypertension is highly correlated with Negro ancestry.

It would be unwise to arrive at such a conclusion at this time. Socioeconomic status is still correlated with skin color in blacks, with the lighter blacks being of higher socioeconomic status. Skin color and blood groups may be merely elaborate ways to determine education and income in United States blacks.

PHYSIOLOGIC MECHANISMS AND PATHOLOGIC PROCESSES WHICH MIGHT BE RESPONSIBLE FOR BLACK/WHITE BLOOD PRESSURE DIFFERENCES

Russell, Masi, and Richter[17] demonstrated a significant association between hypertension and the presence of adrenal adenomas. This association was stronger in blacks than in whites. If a hormone secreted by adenomas is the proximate cause of hypertension, a mechanism for some of the excess hypertension found in blacks would be demonstrated.

Also, low-renin hypertension is commoner in blacks than in whites. This fact could be related to a mild excess of mineralocorticoid secretion and could represent hormones produced by the aforementioned adenomas. Grim has shown that blacks excrete a sodium load slower than whites.[10]

If we make the following assumptions: (1) that the regional and socioeconomic pressure gradients, which have been described already, have an environmental origin which is probably related to either too much sodium or too little potassium in the diet, (2) that blacks often have a diet with relatively more sodium and less potassium, and (3) that they apparently have more difficulty excreting sodium, then it seems possible that the black/white difference could be due to a special racial susceptibility as well as to a greater exposure to an unfavorable, hypertension-producing electrolyte intake.

TREATMENT OF THE BLACK HYPERTENSIVE PATIENT

Since hypertension is significantly more frequent in blacks than whites, we can anticipate that any complete survey of a black population will show more individuals on antihypertensive therapy than a comparable white population. However, as there is a slight but not overwhelming correlation of lower socioeconomic status or education with poorer compliance, we can anticipate that a somewhat smaller proportion of the hypertensives will be receiving continual care in a black community.

There are some theoretical grounds to suggest that the identified blacks should be easier to treat, physiologically speaking, than white hypertensives. More blacks have low-renin hypertension than do white hypertensive patients. As the low-renin state seems to predict good control with diuretics, it is reasonable to postulate that, from the pharmacologic standpoint, the black hypertensive should have a better chance of blood pressure control with simple diuretic therapy than a white patient with the same initial blood pressure.

IMPLICATIONS FOR THE FUTURE

As blacks are incorporated into the mainstream of American life, they should benefit from one likely effect on their cardiovascular risk status, and suffer from an opposing one.

Hypertension should be a lesser problem for blacks in the future; for as the blacks ascend the socioeconomic ladder and leave the rural south, blood pressure should be lower.

There is evidence that accompanying the beneficial effect of decreasing poverty there will be increased blood cholesterol, increased smoking and probably decreased physical activity. The possible cardiovascular consequences are frightening; if elevated cholesterol, smoking, and inactivity exact their toll before an improved socioeconomic status lowers the blood pressure of blacks, they may be faced with an epidemic of myocardial infarction.

IMPLICATIONS FOR RESEARCH

Neither the underlying defect leading to the development of essential hypertension, nor the nature of the environmental factors responsible for differences in the prevalence of hypertension are known. The black/white and socioeconomic differences discussed in this chapter are admirably suited for the testing of hypotheses about the underlying and contributing causes of hypertension.

REFERENCES

1. COMSTOCK, G. W.: *An epidemiologic study of blood pressure levels in a biracial community in the southern United States.* Am. J. Hyg. 65:271, 1957.
2. LANGFORD, H. G., WATSON, R. L., AND DOUGLAS, B. H.: *Factors affecting blood pressure in population groups.* Trans. Assoc. Am. Phys. 81:135, 1968.
3. Advance data from vital and health statistics of the national center for health statistics. No. 1, 1976, pp. 1–7.
4. BORHANI, N. O.: *Epidemiology of Stroke in Medical Basin of Comprehensive Community Stroke Program,* National Institutes of Health, 1968, pp. 25–35.
5. HOWARD, J., AND HOLMAN, B. L.: *The effects of race and occupation on hypertension and mortality.* Milbank Mem. Fund Q. 48:263, 1970.
6. DEUBNER, D. C., TYROLER, H. A., CASSEL, J. C., ET AL.: *Attributable risk, population attributable risk, and population attributable fraction of death associated with hypertension in a biracial population.* Circulation 52:901, 1975.
7. BERKSON, D. M., STAMLER, J., LINDBERG, H. A., ET AL.: *Socioeconomic correlates of atherosclerotic and hypertensive heart diseases.* Ann. N.Y. Acad. Sci. 84:835, 1960.
8. ACHESON, R. M.: In: *Cerebrovascular Disease Epidemiology. A Workshop.* Public Health Monograph 1966, pp. 24–40.
9. LANGFORD, H. G., AND WATSON, R. L.: *Electrolytes and hypertension,* in PAUL, O. (ED.): *Epidemiology and Control of Hypertension.* Stratton Intercontinental Medical Book Corp., New York and London, 1974, pp. 119–128.
10. GRIM, C. E., McDONOUGH, J. R., AND DAHL, L. K.: *Dietary sodium, potassium and blood pressure. Racial differences in Evans Co., Ga.* Circ. Res. 61, 62 (Suppl. 3):85, 1970.
11. CULLEN, L.: Personal communication to R. L. Watson.

12. MENEELY, G. R., BALL, C. O. T., AND YOUMANN, J. B.: *Chronic sodium chloride toxicity: Protective effect of added potassium chloride.* Ann. Int. Med. 47:263, 1957.

13. DAHL, L. K. LEITL, G., AND HEINE, M.: *Influence of dietary potassium and sodium/potassium molar ratios on the development of salt hypertension.* J. Exp. Med. 136:318, 1972.

14. HARBURG, E., ERFORT, J. O., CHAPE, O., ET AL.: *Socioecological stressor areas and black-white blood pressure.* J. Chronic Dis. 26:595, 1973.

15. BOYLE, E., JR.: *Biological patterns in hypertension by race, sex, body weight and skin color.* JAMA 213:1637, 1970.

16. LONG, W. K.: *African genes and hypertension.* N. Engl. J. Med. 283:708, 1970.

17. RUSSELL, R. P., MASI, A. T., AND RICHTER, E. D.: *Adrenal cortical adenomas and hypertension.* Medicine 51:211, 1972.

Index

330